HEALTH PROMOTION:
New Discipline or Multi-Discipline?

T0206861

HEALTH PROMOTION
New Discipline or
Multi-Discipline?

Edited by

RICCA EDMONDSON

and

CECILY KELLEHER

IRISH ACADEMIC PRESS
DUBLIN • PORTLAND, OR

First published in 2000 by
IRISH ACADEMIC PRESS
44, Northumberland Road, Dublin 4, Ireland

and in the United States of America by
IRISH ACADEMIC PRESS
c/o ISBS, 5804 NE Hassalo Street,
Portland, OR 97213 3644

Website: www.iap.ie

British Library Cataloguing in Publication Data
Health promotion: new discipline or multi-discipline? –
   (Social sciences research centre series)
   1. Health promotion
   I. Edmondson, Ricca. II. Kelleher, Cecily.
   613

   ISBN 0–7165–2657–3 hbk
       0–7165–2711–1 pbk

Library of Congress Cataloging-in-Publication Data
Health promotion: new discipline or multi-discipline?/edited by Ricca Edmondson and
Cecily Kelleher.
        p.   cm. — (Social Sciences Research Centre Series)
     Includes index.
     ISBN 0–7165–2657–3 (hb) — ISBN 0–7165–2711–1 (pb)
        1. Health promotion. 2. Health promotion—Social aspects.   3. Health planning—
Social aspects. I. Kelleher, Cecily. II. Edmondson, Ricca. III. Series.
RA427.8.H524 2000
613—dc21   00–035044

Typeset in 11 pt on 12.5 pt Ehrhardt
by Carrigboy Typesetting Services, County Cork
Printed by Creative Print and Design (Wales), Ebbw Vale

Contents

PART ONE. THE INTERFACE BETWEEN HEALTH PROMOTION AND PUBLIC HEALTH: THEORIES AND METHODOLOGIES

List of Contributors

DR TIM ALLEN teaches at the Development Studies Institute of the London School of Economics and is also Visiting Senior Lecturer at the Open University. In addition to television programmes his recent publications include *In Search of Cool Ground: War, Fight and Homecoming in Northeast Africa* (1996), *The Media of Conflict* (edited with Jean Seaton, 1999), and *Divided Europeans: Understanding Ethnicities in Conflict* (edited with John Eade, 1999). He is currently working on a new edition of *Poverty and Development*, the best-selling textbook he edited with Alan Thomas, first published in 1992.

PROF. JOHN ASHTON is Regional Director of Public Health and Regional Medical Officer for the North-West of England. He holds chairs in public health at both John Moore's University, Liverpool and the University of Liverpool, and is a visiting professorial fellow at the Liverpool School of Tropical Medicine. One of the founders of the WHO Healthy City Initiative, among other works he was co-author of the best-selling book, *The New Public Health*.

PROF. GEORGE DAVEY SMITH is Professor of Clinical Epidemiology at the Department of Social Medicine in the University of Bristol. His initial work in epidemiology concerned the influence of health promotion programmes, and he has worked on coronary heart disease, sexually transmitted disease and HIV/AIDS prevention initiatives. His main current research interests concern the influences of exposures acting across the lifecourse on the development of disease in adulthood.

DR KATHRYN DEAN, M.S.W., R.N., is a research and training consultant for population studies on health and behaviour, and Adjunct Professor in the School of Nursing, University of Minnesota, and the Gerontology Research Center, Simon Fraser University, Vancouver, B.C. She served for many years as the Leader of the WHO Collaborating Center for Health Promotion Research at the Institute of Social Medicine, University of Copenhagen, working extensively in the areas of health promotion, lifestyle and life situation influences on health. She writes and consults on methodological issues affecting the quality and validity of survey research on health and health-related behaviour.

PROF. SHAH EBRAHIM is Professor in the Epidemiology of Ageing at the University of Bristol and is co-ordinating editor of the Cochrane Heart Group, as well as principal investigator of the British Women's Heart and Health Study.

DR RICCA EDMONDSON lectures in the Department of Political Science and Sociology at the National University of Ireland, Galway. After a D.Phil. in the theory of the social sciences she published *Rhetoric in Sociology* (1984), then carried out research at the Max Planck Institute for Human Development in Berlin (*Rules and Norms in the Sociology of Organisations*, 1987). She is editor of *The Political Context of Collective Action: Power, Argumentation and Democracy* (1997), author of *Ireland: Culture and Society* (written for the German Open University in 1998) and a former co-editor of *The Irish Journal of Sociology*. Her interests include ageing, health and cultural theory, on which she is currently writing a new book.

DR MATTHIAS EGGER is Senior Lecturer in Epidemiology and Public Health Medicine at University of Bristol. His research interests include methods in clinical epidemiology and the epidemiology and prevention of HIV infection and other sexually transmitted diseases.

DR JOAN FEATHER is the Coordinator of the Prairie Region Health Promotion Research Centre, and a Research Scientist in the Department of Community Health and Epidemiology at the University of Saskatchewan in Canada. Her career has embraced research in health services and health status; currently she focuses on processes of building capacity for health promotion at individual and organisational levels, with an emphasis on new decentralised health authorities.

DR FRANK FUREDI is Chairperson of Development Studies and Senior Lecturer in Sociology at the University of Kent. In recent years he has written widely around the theme of the construction of social problems. His *Population and Development* (1997) examined the construction of the population problem. *The Culture of Fear* (1997) explored the construction of panics about risk and his *The Silent War* (1998) investigated the sociological construction of the race issue. At present he is writing a text focusing on the theme of the medicalisation of social problems, and he comments widely on related problems in the international press.

DR MARCIA HILLS is the Director of the Community Health Promotion Centre and an Associate Professor at the School of Nursing, the University of Victoria, Canada. Her career has focused on creating participatory approaches to research, education and practice in health promotion. Her current interests include transforming mainstream health professionals' practices, developing alternative health-care models and creating frameworks for emancipatory education.

PROF. CECILY KELLEHER holds the Foundation Chair of Health Promotion at The National University of Ireland, Galway, and is Director of the multi-disciplinary Centre for Health Promotion Studies at Galway. Research interests include nutrition and general lifestyle risk-factor surveillance and settings evaluations, particularly in the workplace and primary care. She has worked on a range of innovative programmes on the education of adults across the health sector.

DR RONALD LABONTE has worked in health promotion, community development, healthy public policy development, and health research/evaluation for 25 years in a variety of government and NGO settings. He currently divides his time between teaching health promotion/community development in universities in Canada and elsewhere, consulting to health authorities in Canada, the United States, the UK, Australia, New Zealand and Latin America, and undertaking independent research.

DR ANNE MACFARLANE is a research officer at the Centre for Health Promotion Studies, the National University of Ireland, Galway. As a research fellow, from 1992 to 1998, she completed an M.A. and Ph.D. in Health Promotion under the supervision of Professor Cecily Kelleher. She has been a contributor to the health promotion and Social Care teaching programmes within the department, and her main research interests are health-seeking behaviour and health services research.

PROF. KLIM MCPHERSON works at the London School of Hygiene and Tropical Medicine. He has been Professor of Public Health Epidemiology in the Department of Public Health and Policy, where he set up an M.Sc. and a new Unit of Health Promotion. Now he is currently Acting Head of another new unit – the Unit of Cancer and Public Health in the Department of Epidemiology and Population Health.

DR SAOIRSE NIC GABHAINN is Research Fellow at the Centre for Health Promotion Studies, the National University of Ireland, Galway, with degrees in psychology and health promotion from Galway and Nottingham. Her research has been concerned, among other topics, with the evaluation of school health education and the interaction between formal and informal social support during recovery from alcohol problems. She acts as Assistant

Academic Director in the Centre for Health Promotion Studies, working on a range of evaluation and basic research projects in the area of young people and schools' health promotion.

DR DESMOND O'BYRNE is Chief of Health Education and Health Promotion in the WHO, Geneva. Prior to joining the WHO in Copenhagen in 1984 he was head of research and information in the Health Education Bureau in Dublin. He is a graduate of the National University of Ireland, Galway, where he took his B.A. and M.A. degrees, and of Oxford University, where he wrote his D.Phil.

DR RANDY PAGE is Professor and Coordinator of Health Education at the University of Idaho, Moscow. His research and writing focuses in particular on adolescent health risk behaviour.

JANE SIXSMITH is currently Director of Adult and Outreach Education in the Department of Health Promotion, the National University of Ireland, Galway. She qualified as a registered general nurse and has worked in a variety of applied areas related to health before undertaking further study in community nursing and health promotion.

PROF. KEITH TONES is Professor of Health Education at the University of Leeds. After beginning his career in teaching, he has been involved since 1972 in research and training in health education and health promotion. He has published widely, including a popular book on evaluation, *Health Education: Effectiveness, Efficiency*. He is editor of the international journal, *Health Education Research: Theory and Practice*.

PROF. MARKUS WÖRNER is head of the Department of Philosophy at the National University of Ireland, Galway; he is currently also Mercator Professor in Philosophy at the Free University, Berlin. His major works include *Performative und Sprachliches Handeln* (1978), *Das Ethische in der Rhetorik des Aristoteles* (1990), and *Thomas von Aquin: Summa Contra Gentiles IV* (1996). He is at present preparing books on human lifetime and on hermeneutics and argument.

List of Figures

Chapter Seven

Chapter Twelve

Chapter Fifteen

Chapter Sixteen

Introduction

RICCA EDMONDSON AND
CECILY KELLEHER

To promote health is difficult. That is true whether we think of health promotion as a general term describing efforts to attain a widely held human goal or as a recognised activity in professional or academic practice, one informed by a theoretical rationale. It is difficult in large part because it involves reflection and change on so many levels, many of which have conventionally been regarded as disparate or even incompatible. But this is just what makes health promotion so exciting and potentially so creative. Even though principles and practices in the arts and the sciences have often been mutually opposed, and even though principles and practices in public organisations can be hard to make compatible with those of everyday life, in health promotion these tensions must somehow be reconciled. Thus, if health is to be promoted effectively, its promotion will be based on advances in understanding action and thought in all these areas. The results of these advances will be tangible, not only in enhanced health-related features of people's daily living, but also in terms of our understanding of health itself – a fundamental aspect of what it is to be a human being.

Health promotion as it is currently understood and practised worldwide has its origins in two distinct sources – sources whose combination in the contemporary field furnish it with its characteristic breadth and diversity. First, it emerges from a tradition of health education that fostered individuals' knowledge and skills in matters of personal lifestyle, developed and delivered in the main through primary health care, schools and the mass media. However, it is also heir to the public health movement, which had its origins in the nineteenth century. This began as a means of improving living conditions, particularly in urban areas, and it emphasised issues such as sanitation and infectious disease control, and the regulation of environmental and housing conditions. A century ago in Europe and the 'developed' world generally, the greatest threats to human health came from transmissible and infectious diseases, affecting the very young in particular. Throughout the twentieth century, new threats to human health emerged, mainly in adulthood,

1

exemplified by the epidemic pattern of coronary heart disease and the increasing incidence of cancers, principally of the digestive system, the lung, prostate and breast, or new life-threatening diseases like Acquired Immunodeficiency Syndrome. In the period since the Second World War an increasing interest has developed in the components of these major threats to human health which are seen as preventable, in principle, with a focus on adult lifestyle practices such as smoking, eating and drinking habits, patterns of exercise and sexual activity.

The growth of preventive medicine to combat chronic diseases was in essence an attempt to replicate the successful strategy of infectious disease control by so-called risk-factor identification and treatment. Intervention could not have been contemplated had the science of epidemiology not contributed to our knowledge of what caused ill health but also had we not learned so much from the systematic study of individuals and societies in social and behavioural sciences such as sociology, psychology and anthropology. At this stage the health education and public health strategies began to identify common ground, both focusing on the personal behaviour of the individual. But it was increasingly argued throughout the 1970s that this strategy had its limitations. First, critics questioned the appropriateness of placing responsibility for health at the level of the individual without due recognition of the circumstances that influenced that person's lifestyle; after all, population health is strongly influenced by sociopolitical circumstances. Secondly, there was criticism of the idea that our understanding of human health and well-being could be reduced to a purely biological level. Finally, there was a sense that it was unproductive to focus on illness prevention rather than its converse, health maintenance. An approach was required that would embrace human health as a complex but positive characteristic and that would somehow reconcile these sometimes conflicting perspectives and dimensions. Not alone that, to be effective, this approach would also have to be practical, operational and amenable to evaluation.

The World Health Organisation was responsible for the much-discussed holistic and aspirational definition of health as a state of complete physical, mental and social well-being and not merely the absence of disease. Its approach to health promotion was strongly influenced by public policy developed in Canada, and it was in this spirit that the first World Conference on Health Promotion in Ottawa in 1986 sought to redefine health promotion as a process that enables people to increase control over their own health. From the beginning it was recognised that health promotion required a number of elements in concert. Overall public policy should be conducive to the health of the populations it was designed to serve, the development of personal capacities would remain a crucial element at all life stages, health services needed to be reoriented to focus much more on primary care and proactive health maintenance programmes, and immediate social environments should be supportive to those wishing to promote their own health and well-being. Finally it was believed that processes of community empowerment and development might also facilitate positive health. It can hardly be sufficiently stressed that, just as health promotion has abandoned a chiefly biomedical model of health change, it so has abandoned a chiefly individualistic one. In exploring areas which include healthy public policy, sociopolitical and economic change, and participative community action, health promotion now emphasises the bonds between people and groups and the relations these may have to health.

This ambitious framework self-evidently requires cross-sectoral action and also the participation of a range of disciplines. Traditional public health requires the input of many health professionals, particularly epidemiologists, but also engineers and environmental scientists, while health education requires the skills of teachers, psychologists and other social scientists. The new concept of health promotion embraces an even wider range of participants across public life and it derives its theories and models of practice from a wide spectrum of social science and biomedical specialities.

Thus, the health promotion movement is now a global one, and this collection tries to reflect the scope of the debate it involves. One of the main thrusts of the text's enquiry derives from the question of whether an applied area such as health promotion can emerge in its own right as a discipline, given its diversity of source disciplines and the diversity of practices it currently embraces. Are its theories grounded only in those disciplines from which it emerged or are there new or modified theories informing practice, based on growths in knowledge? This question gains in pertinence from the fact that, both in the natural sciences and in the humanities, models, practices and theories – however commonplace they may seem to those who are familiar with them – inevitably imply specific views of what human beings are, how they are influenced and influence each other, what knowledge consists of and how explanations are to be framed. One of the main concerns of a work such as this must therefore be methodological: what are the main types of approach involved in the field? Can they be united to form a coherent approach to health-related change?

Secondly, there are of course many ethical and political aspects to these issues, by no means all of which can be covered here, but our contributors reflect the experience of four continents, a spectrum of disciplines ranging from the humanities and social sciences to the biomedical sciences and a variety of contexts and issues across the human lifespan. It is sometimes assumed that health promotion is a defensive field and it is certainly true that it attracts much debate about theories and practice, both within the field itself and from commentators in related fields looking on; this is hardly surprising given the range of knowledge sources which health promotion requires to operate. To change anything in society requires ensuring that the change is as likely as can be established to be beneficial, that adequate resources exist to undertake the change and that appropriate processes of choice on the course of action in question have been engaged in. Finally, therefore, at an operational level, how are we to know if and how health promotion works? How is it to be practised in different countries and settings on a day-to-day basis?

Currently, settings-based approaches are prominent among both theories and practices in health promotion. Many of these are predicated on the idea that some form of socio-economic and political change is the most ethical and effective way to promote health; to this extent they incorporate aims and criteria from almost all of the above-mentioned areas at once. Health promotion has moved a long way from exclusively biomedical and individualistic interventions, but these multi-faceted, multi-disciplinary new developments illustrate the fact that special forms of communication and decision will be needed if we are to mediate between the diverse aspirations and standards involved, and to reconcile them with expectations about argument held in the natural sciences. The examples of different disciplinary approaches collected in this volume are intended, therefore, both to provide the reader with insight into a fast-developing area and to explore sources of creative tension as new ideas on promoting health emerge.

Taken as a whole the contributions in this collection, wide-ranging and diverse in background and content as they are, share central themes which are currently crucial in health promotion circles. What emerges from reading this volume is a common curiosity to understand what constitutes health and well-being, a lively discourse on appropriate methodologies and research questions, and recurring political and ethical questions about the nature, purpose and justification of health promotion interventions.

The book is comprised of two sections; the first underscores the blend in health promotion between orientation to practical policy and reflection on methods and their implications. It combines a number of accounts of the health promotion movement itself with competing or complementary views on how research in health promotion should be carried out. John Ashton asserts in his opening contribution that modern health promotion is a movement to which practitioners across the entire spectrum of education and public health can contribute. He believes that the Ottawa Charter initiative in 1986 was not intended to establish an independent or new discipline, but to redefine what health promotion actions might be undertaken by a diversity of practitioners.

The next two chapters counterpoise contributions to a hotly contested debate in the practice of health promotion. George Davey Smith and his colleagues provide an epidemiological perspective. They contend that randomised controlled trials, or RCTs, are a robust design for removing the bias of self-selection in whatever context they are employed. If the outcome of a health promotion intervention appears not to be proven, then researchers should reappraise the intervention's content rather than criticise RCTs as a methodology of evaluation. Davey Smith et al. provide a variety of examples to illustrate this argument; they also underline the obligations to the public which ensue from the use of public money. Keith Tones takes a somewhat different position. He points out that health promotion is a complex and often very long-term process, particularly where educational objectives are concerned; RCTs are unrealistic, he argues, for routine use in everyday real-life situations. An intervention's link to morbidity or mortality should not have to be intrinsic to each evaluation, he believes, as the point, if proven once, does not need to be proven again. Such a constraint would divert effort, focus and resources from the process of the intervention. In any case, out-come expectations in a health-promotion setting may possess their own scale of magnitude, modest for pharmacological research but realistic in social circumstances. Though both these articles argue for appropriate interventions and the application of suitable outcome measures, the challenge is to decide what is appropriate or suitable, and when. Tones wishes to introduce a 'judicial review' based on standards of acceptability taken from diverse intellectual and practical areas – substantially dissenting from the claim that RCTs should be used in social and educational as well as epidemiological settings. Davey Smith and colleagues conclude by arguing for wider-scale social change interventions, but this has considerable ethical and political implications, touched upon in further contributions to the text.

The next two contributions concern current World Health Organisation policy on health promotion. The fourth international conference in Jakarta was a stage along a process developed by the WHO over two decades, according to Des O'Byrne, and the cultural challenges in the modern world are immense. O'Byrne outlines likely future developments and plans for the next meeting in the series in Mexico in 2000; his contribution has the special function of expressing a point of view direct from the WHO itself. The Jakarta conference, according to Cecily Kelleher's personal account of the meeting, provided a focus in microcosm for many current health promotion debates, both in focusing on relevant ethical and political questions and in seeing a shift in evaluation strategies. There is evidence in health promotion rhetoric and in supporting research that more holistic, community-development approaches are now being adopted. However, we should not assume automatically that any given methodological approach is absolutely para-mount over others. There also continue to be problems in the definition of health itself and hence in concepts of health promotion, brought into sharper relief because this is an active, highly politicised process.

Ricca Edmondson then examines basic issues in understanding the importance of culture and context as influences on how we act or interpret situations at the level of meaning, of motivation and of the philosophical aspects of action. She illustrates her argument with examples from her own research on this issue, particularly in Germany and Ireland. We underestimate the complexity of these levels, so is it any wonder when simplistic approaches fail to have the desired effect, either in understanding how people behave or in terms of how they respond to health promotion interventions? Edmondson concludes that we need to make appropriate responses to the different types of knowledge which are relevant to health, distinguishing between using knowledge for technical and for participative decisions, and the next authors continue this theme. Ron Labonte and his colleagues, long advocates of a constructionist approach to health promotion and of the use of appropriate qualitative methodologies, document the usefulness of a particular story-telling technique they have developed for reflecting on and transmitting experiential knowledge. This is a narrative process that, in a health research setting, formalises techniques used in human discourse for centuries. The authors of these two articles, therefore, emphasise the need to reappraise the value we place on different means of uncovering truth and reality.

Parallel questions are examined in a quantitative fashion by Kathryn Dean, who uses a number of examples to outline the danger of oversimplification by using measures that do not adequately discriminate between constituent components or allow for the likely impact of their application in different types of situation. She criticises the untimely use of crude interventions whose relative impact in specific situations or population subgroups have not been estimated, and argues for the need to develop more subtle observational methods for measuring constructs before undertaking intervention work.

Klim McPherson discusses how a preference for or against any type of intervention on the part of participants in unblinded intervention studies may not only influence outcome, but could and should be considered and, if possible, quantified. Such a preference effect might itself form the explanation for an apparent benefit attached to one intervention over another, all other things being biologically equal. McPherson shows algebraically that even in a simple situation of an additive effect with just one comparison the impact may be considerable. Given that the reality of such interaction is likely to be much more complex in any real-life situation, this is an important potential confounder for any main effect in a study. The implications for health promotion intervention are relevant, both when there is an apparent benefit to an intervention and also, presumably, when there is an advantage to the reference area. Whether a qualitative or a quantitative approach is taken, the lessons from these four contributions again coincide to the extent that all argue that more subtlety and more consideration of context and interaction are required in health promotion research.

The second section examines health promotion in different settings and situations. Tim Allen explores the issue of context in how we understand health, illness and disease. Biomedicine as a dominant paradigm in the Western world often functions as a closed system based on a microbiological understanding of disease. What drives health-care systems in many cultures (exemplified here from his own African experience) is very different. Allen explores the clash of cultures which occurs when medical aid workers try to establish Western-based health-care systems without an adequate under-standing of the setting in which they are working. Such workers need a more sensitive understanding of what is going on around them if their objective really is to improve other people's health; this is especially important in areas where biomedicine's input is strongly related to advice about behavioural change, for instance in areas where HIV rates are high. In the course of this argument Allen examines the nature of systems of thought as such; are cultural systems as hermetically sealed as some contemporary theorists argue? How easy will it be to communicate about health between cultures – in Africa and elsewhere?

Two central tenets of health promotion have been personal skills develop-ment and healthy public policy. Furedi examines these issues as they are embodied in current approaches to the question of increasing global population numbers. Is the problem really that we have too many people on the planet or do the problems lie in the distribution of material and political resources? Furedi charts a succession of approaches, from traditional straightforward population reduction strategies through to neo-Malthusian and feminist perspectives on the issue. While the personal development of women has become part of health-related policies worldwide, can this sometimes be used to repackage neo-Malthusian concerns about fertility rates? Is the right of the individual to decide his or her own numbers of children being subordinated to a form of cultural imperialism in the name of population control? Furedi's chapter illustrates some pitfalls in applying sociopolitical principles on a global level – particularly when some of these principles can so easily masquerade as others.

Turning to another area of major current interest, Anne MacFarlane discusses the attitudes of older people to their health and goes on to describe qualitative interviews undertaken with a group of older Irish people. Among three dimensions to their definition of health, she finds that a functional definition predominates – though not for functional reasons. Interestingly, this is true not just of feeling healthy at present but of maintaining health in general. MacFarlane argues for public policy choices which will much more tangibly support older people in their aspirations to make active contributions to their own and others' lives. Markus Wörner continues this theme of ageing with a discussion on the necessary conditions for a good life; his contribution exemplifies an approach to the way in which philosophy can contribute to the study and practice of health promotion. Wörner explores how we explain to ourselves and are motivated by a sense of the purpose of life. If we are to incorporate well-being into our concept of health then a respect for this sense of purpose, or, as he styles it, the cultivation of sensibility and of friendship, is of the utmost importance for the individual and for society as a whole. In this context Wörner outlines some of the conditions of the good life advocated in ancient 'arts of living', which include – only apparently paradoxically – learning how to die.

In a collection reflecting the global health promotion movement, it is pertinent to include an input from the North American school of health promotion research, which combines epidemiological surveillance with a concern for individual change and for enhancing 'social capital' in contemporary societies. Randy Page summarises the US experience that adolescents' biggest health risks result from their lifestyle. Shyness and loneliness, his research suggests, are associated with higher risk behaviours, and skills programmes to tackle these are being developed. He concludes that gender differences have emerged in both the smoking habit and motivation to smoke, and that low self-esteem may not be an issue connected with smoking for girls in the way it is for boys. He suggests that in fashioning interventions we should take account of young people's own perception of risk behaviour prevalence, and of the effects of their pastimes.

Saoirse Nic Gabhainn continues a related theme, particularly in relation to drug and alcohol misuse, and argues that these two issues should not be confused, as both motivation for them and influences on them may be quite different. Alcohol is quantitatively a bigger problem than drug misuse and is also qualitatively different, in that it is a legal drug which forms part of the mystique of adult culture. She suggests that we now have good evidence on what might be effective strategies but the implementation of these strategies is complex. Cross-sectoral collaboration, regularly advocated in health promotion circles, requires more thought on operational issues and the true assimilation of guidelines into routine practice. Research techniques and methodologies vary and, besides good data, we need to be aware of problems in interpreting data for its many users.

The smoking habit is probably the most discussed lifestyle risk-factor of the last thirty years and it remains, like the ancient riddle of the sphinx, a complex and seemingly insoluble problem. The review of this issue by Kelleher and Sixsmith is in two parts. The first, based on a review of Irish studies on smoking, suggests that the problem in Ireland is similar to that elsewhere in that it has special salience for young people and the economically disadvantaged. The second part of the article reviews likely strategies for intervention and urges more regard for the different motivations to smoke according to gender and age, and an appreciation that the smoking habit is a subtle proxy for health promotion practice generally, requiring multi-sectoral interventions to make an effective impact.

Since the Centre for Health Promotion Studies was established in 1991 as a constituent of the Social Sciences Research Centre in Galway, there have been rapid developments in the field of health promotion. The centre's own approach to research has been multi-disciplinary from the outset. It has developed research activity in a diversity of settings, requiring only that such work should be characterised by the aim of facilitating individuals' and groups' capacities to maintain or develop their health potential.

The contributors to this volume are members of the National University of Ireland, Galway (Cecily Kelleher, Ricca Edmondson, Markus Wörner, Saoirse Nic Gabhainn, Anne MacFarlane and Jane Sixsmith), or were invited visitors with recognised international expertise who participated either in our annual summer school conferences (John Ashton, Des O'Byrne, George Davey Smith, Keith Tones, Klim McPherson and Randy Page), in other academic meetings (Ron Labonte and Kathryn Dean) or in the annual Social Science Research Centre lecture series (Frank Furedi and Tim Allen). Together, these authors bring personal but complementary approaches to many of the issues which are most central to health promotion today.

All editors hope that people will read their book; we hope you will not only read this one but do so in sequence and as a whole, because it provides for a stimulating and witty journey from beginning to end. While we like to be hospitable to our guests and welcomed each with pleasure to Galway, there is a certain paradox in the fact that several are encountering each other's contribution for the first time through these pages. Whether it is a multi-disciplinary activity or a new discipline in itself, health promotion as an endeavour has a social contribution to make!

For their invaluable support we thank Ms Mary Silke in the SSRC and Ms Linda Longmore at Irish Academic Press. We wish to thank each of the contributors to this volume, as well as those whose funding made it possible: the Western, North-Western and Mid-Western Health Boards, who support the NUI,G annual summer school in health promotion, and the Social Sciences Research Centre, NUI,G, in whose series this book appears.

RICCA EDMONDSON
& CECILY KELLEHER
Galway, June, 2000

PART ONE

The Interface between Health Promotion and Public Health:
Theories and Methodologies

ONE

Policy Perspectives

JOHN ASHTON

The views expressed in this paper come with a health warning, because they seem to upset people. I confess to finding this intriguing, because the essence of public health is the struggle to improve the health of the population in general and that of the most disadvantaged in particular. I suspect that the raw nerve which I am touching connects to the anti–public–health tendency towards professionalisation which has characterised the field since the earliest days and which remains rampant, despite rhetoric to the contrary.

To start with some definitions; that originally enunciated by Winslow in 1920 has enjoyed renewed currency in recent years, as a result of its having been re-packaged in the Acheson Report on 'Public health in England', which was published in 1988 (Acheson Report 1988, Winslow 1920). Winslow wrote:

> Public Health is the science and art of preventing disease, prolonging life and promoting physical health and efficiency through organised community efforts for the sanitation of the environment, the education of the individual in principles of personal hygiene, the organisation of medical and nursing services for the early diagnosis and preventive treatment of disease, and the development of the social machinery which will ensure to every individual in the community a standard of living adequate for the maintenance of health.

What is remarkable about this definition (apart from its omission of any clear reference to mental and social health) is, on the one hand, its comprehensive embrace of the environmental, personal prevention and therapeutic components of public health strategy, and on the other hand the very modern-sounding recognition of the social nature of the enterprise and the blend of art and science which is needed. I have described elsewhere the chronologically unfolding layers of dominant themes of public health in developed countries before the New Public Health appeared on the scene

(Ashton and Seymour 1988): the environmental (1840–1880), personal prevention (1880–1920) and therapeutic (1930–1970) approaches. Suffice it to comment here on the irony that Winslow's balanced understanding was about to be submerged under a deluge of pharmaceuticals and scientific reductionism which would take the best part of fifty years to play itself out, when Donald Acheson would be in a position to restate Winslow's wisdom with any confidence that it would be understood.

One final comment on this piece of the jigsaw is to note the tussle for control of the field of public health in the United Kingdom between the physicians, the engineers and others; this was decided decisively in favour of the former, perhaps surprisingly in view of his hostility towards them, by Edwin Chadwick in 1842. He proposed the establishment of the post of Medical Officer of Health in his 'Report on the Sanitary Conditions of the Labouring Population', arguing that:

> for the general means necessary to prevent disease, it would be good economy to appoint a district medical officer, independent of private practice, with the securities of special qualifications and responsibilities, to initiate sanitary measures and reclaim execution of the law (Acheson 1990; Chave 1984).

The fact that doctors were given the leadership role was arguably to be a source of both strength and weakness in the battles for health which were to follow over the next hundred years: a strength when they used their public credibility and moral authority to champion the poor, a weakness when they became identified as a tribal craft-group pursuing their own self-interest and failing to accord proper recognition to the contribution of others. It was this latter failing which in due course led to seething and uncontainable resentment from environmental health officers, social workers and others, and in the English case to the break-up of the once powerful Local Authority Public Health departments in 1970, with the creation of separate directorates for Environmental Health and Social Services. This was followed by the dissolution of the Public Health Department altogether in 1974 and the removal of the public health doctors, now recast as community physicians, to the health authorities. These latter were shorn of their direct power and influence over the policy areas that impact on public health and left to dabble with the clinical agenda whilst notionally maintaining the public health flame. Is it really any wonder that things became fragmented and ineffectual?

Onto the stage at this juncture strode health promotion! 'Strode' may perhaps be overstating the case, but the concepts of health promotion had been emerging in the early 1970s with a strong Canadian background, born of the Lalonde report of 1974 and the subsequent disillusionment at the victim–blaming emphasis in much of the renewed interest in public health, which emphasised health education focusing on individual lifestyle (Labonte and Penfold 1981; Lalonde 1974). A great deal of the background thinking which lay behind the notion of health promotion can be attributed to the work of the World Health Organisation, beginning with the Alma Ata declaration on Primary Health Care in 1977, continuing with the development of the strategy of Health for All which was adopted in 1981, and culminating in the production of the Ottawa Charter for Health Promotion in 1986 (WHO 1978, 1981, 1984). Writing in 1984, I described health promotion as 'Any combination of health education and political, economic and organisational activity designed to improve or protect health through its effect on the human environment and on behaviour' (Ashton 1984). There are clear resonances here with Winslow, but looking back I can see now how my thinking was influenced by those such as Draper and Milio who were so certain of the need to connect the technical and managerial to the political (St George and Draper 1981, Milio 1986). The Ottawa Charter itself, when it appeared, very much influenced by Ilona Kickbusch of the European office of the World Health Organisation, stressed the role of 'Healthy Public Policy' as the foundation of health promotion and the New Public Health – with its emphasis on creating supportive environments, developing personal skills and reorientating health services. The role of professionals of whatever hue was seen as being to enable, to mediate and to be advocates for public health. It is my contention that the creation of another cadre of health worker, 'the health promotion officer', was not top of the agenda for the delegates at Ottawa.

Despite the clear framework presented in the WHO pamphlet on the subject of health promotion in 1984 and its subsequent elaboration in the Ottawa Charter two years later, it is a sad reality that too often the term has been used to market old wine in new bottles (individually-orientated health education or the repositioning of one professional group or another, each using the rhetoric of the concepts in an attempt to raise status). It is still not uncommon to hear people speak of 'Health Education Health Promotion' in one breath, rather like a very long German word, as if there were no difference in meaning between the two terms.

The 1980s are still too close for us to have a completely clear perspective on what happened then; however, I think some aspects are beginning to come into focus. This was in many ways a period of transition from old ways of seeing and doing things to new ways, and of a search for a new paradigm that could accommodate a generation born after the war and accustomed to challenging orthodoxy – whilst bringing its own orthodoxy in the form of the ephemera of consumerist values. At first these values became focused on lifestyles and the narcissistic pursuit of eternal life through jogging and brown bread, but with the '90s this began to give way to a concern with the environment and the reconciliation of the way we live with this habitat called 'Earth'. The challenge of this is well described in the recent report of the Environmental Health Commission, *Agendas for Change*. Central to the synthesis of the three agendas – biomedical, environmental and social – which make up public health as we approach the millennium is the reorientation of our value-systems towards sustainability and equity, and the reorientation of 'the organised efforts of society' in such a way that our organisational forms are fit for their purpose. Here structure should follow a clear understanding of function. Part of our structure is the way in which professional workers are trained and operate, their value-systems and orientation. If professionals in the field of public health are not to be a conspiracy against the public, we must be clear about their roles as partners. I would suggest that it is time to resolve some of the core issues in favour of genuine multi-disciplinary partnership of professional public health workers united under one description, that of 'public health', and to resist the calls for the creation of new professional tribes with specialist labels that are usually the precursors of guild preciousness and restrictive practice.

This seems to apply particularly when the term 'Health Promotion' is used as a proper noun or a job description rather than an adverb. If the task is to produce public health organisations that are heath promoting, wherein everybody has a part to play, we must end the confusion that comes from having people called Health Promotion Officers though nobody can tell you what they do; we should unpack the task of public health to make explicit the contributions of each individual, whether lay, professional or public servant, and of each organisation, whether private household, voluntary group, private firm or public body. In this mission different people will lead with different tasks and hopefully we can escape the diversion that comes from tribal ambition. Within this clear view of public health, I am certain that there is an important role for health education! It is a logical next step to conclude that Directors of Public Health should not need to be physicians.

REFERENCES

Acheson, R., 1990. 'The Medicalisation of Public Health in England: The United Kingdom and the United States contrasted', *Journal of Public Health Medicine*, 12, 1: pp. 31–8.

Acheson Report, 1988. *Public Health in England: The Report of the Committee of Enquiry into the Future Development of the Public Health Function in England.* London: HMSO (Cmnd 289).

Ashton, J., and Seymour, H., 1988. *The New Public Health*. Open University Press.

Ashton, J., 1984. *Health in Mersey: A Review*. Liverpool: University of Liverpool Department of Public Health.

Ashton, J., 1992. ed. *Healthy Cities*. Open University Press.

Chartered Institution of Environmental Health Officers, 1997. *Agendas for Change: The Report of the Environmental Health Commission*. London: Chadwick House.

Chave, S., 1984. 'The First Medical Officer of Health', *Community Medicine*, 6: pp. 61–71.

Lalonde, M., 1974. *A New Perspective on the Health of Canadians*. Minister of Supply and Services Canada.

Labonte, R., and Penfold, S., 1981. 'Canadian Perspectives in Health Promotion: A critique', *Health Education*, April: pp. 4–9.

Milio, N., 1986. *Promoting Health through Public Policy*. Ottawa Canada: Canadian Public Health Association.

St George, D., and Draper, P., 1981. A Health Policy for Europe', *Lancet*, ii: pp. 463–5.

Winslow, C.E., 1920. 'The Untilled Fields of Public Health', *Science*, 51: p. 23.

World Health Organisation, 1978. *Alma Ata 1977. Primary Health Care*. Geneva: WHO/UNICEF.

World Health Organisation, 1981. *Global Strategy for Health for All by the Year 2000*. Geneva: WHO.

World Health Organisation, 1984. *Health Promotion: A Discussion Document on the Concepts and Principles*. Copenhagen: WHO.

World Health Organisation, 1986. *Ottawa Charter for Health Promotion*. Ottawa: Canadian Public Health Association.

TWO

Should Health Promotion be Exempt from Rigorous Evaluation?

GEORGE DAVEY SMITH, SHAH EBRAHIM AND MATTHIAS EGGER

The concept of health promotion covers a wide range of activities, but an important concern of health promotion in general, and health education in particular, is to influence the behaviours and lifestyles of populations. In the United Kingdom considerable resources have been allocated to this enterprise. However, the changes produced by, and the methods used in evaluations of, health promotion and health education are a matter of ongoing debate (Speller *et al.* 1997).

It has been suggested that health promotion interventions require a different basis for evaluation than is considered appropriate for other medical interventions; for example, evaluations of the effectiveness of drug treatments (Nutbeam 1996; Speller *et al.* 1997). The proponents of an alternative approach to the evaluation of health promotion activities claim that more emphasis should be given to the process of the intervention, rather than to effectiveness, and that observational designs and qualitative research should be used, rather than randomised controlled trials (Speller *et al.* 1997). The proposals for alternative evaluation techniques have sometimes directly followed on from findings using established methods which suggested that the health promotion programmes were ineffective. For example, the finding that a community-based demonstration programme to prevent cardiovascular disease in Wales produced no net changes in risk factors over and above those observed in a matched control area in north-east England led the investigators to suggest that the quasi-experimental design they had employed was inappropriate (Tudor Smith *et al.* 1998). On the other hand, the implementers of poorly-designed evaluations of health promotion activities have made extravagant claims about the effectiveness and cost-effectiveness of such programmes. For example, based on an uncontrolled before–after comparison it was claimed that training doctors and midwives in a 'baby friendly' health education intervention in India greatly improved the feeding practices of mothers (Prasad and de L. Costello 1995). However, a randomised controlled trial testing the effectiveness of essentially the same intervention in Nepal showed no improvement of feeding practices (Bolam *et al.* 1998).

In this chapter we shall argue for rigorous evaluations of health promotion activities aimed at behavioural and lifestyle change, and for wider acceptance of the results of such evaluations by the health promotion and health education community. Few will dispute that patients should only be treated with interventions proven to have favourable ratios of benefit to risk, and cost to benefit. Health promotion seeks to influence the lives of large numbers of people, most of whom feel healthy. Before imposing lifestyles on healthy people we should demonstrate that such activities will in fact lead to an objective improvement of health and quality of life, and at a reasonable cost.

THE PERILS OF OBSERVATION: THE (UN)PROTECTIVE INFLUENCE OF BETA-CAROTENE

It is important to remember the degree to which even well-designed observational or quasi-experimental studies can produce misleading findings. The protective effect (that wasn't) of ß-carotene provides an excellent example of this. Fruit and vegetables have been viewed as essential constituents of a healthy diet for centuries. Their health-maintaining properties and contribution to longevity have been promoted in self-help manuals since these were first produced. In earlier times the promotion of fruit and vegetable consumption was often combined with promoting physical exercise, frequent bathing and religious observance, combined with advice to avoid alcohol, tobacco and sexual indulgence (Shryock 1947). The moral nature of such advice is clear, but with the discovery of vitamins and the recognition that fruit and vegetables were a prime source for several of these, a scientific rationale for nutritional advice was developed (Peto *et al.* 1981).

A considerable research effort has gone into both observational and randomised controlled trials testing the hypothesis that low consumption of antioxidant vitamins increases the risk of cardiovascular disease and cancer (Jha *et al.* 1995; Peto *et al.* 1981). The results of these studies are worth detailed evaluation, since a considerable body of evidence exists to show that people who consume a diet low in antioxidant-rich vitamins are also those whose behaviours with respect to smoking, alcohol consumption and exercise, and whose socio-economic characteristics, place them at high risk of cardiovascular and cancer mortality. Such confounding could produce apparent protective effects of antioxidant vitamin consumption which are not indicative of any causal relationship, but reflect the similar nature and

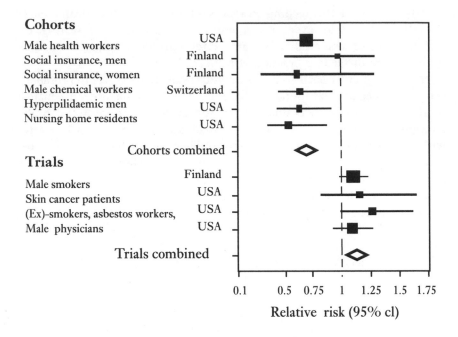

Figure 1. Meta-analysis of the association between beta-carotene intake and cardiovascular mortality. Results from observational studies indicate considerable benefit, whereas the findings from randomised controlled trials show an increase in the risk of death.

direction of confounding in the various observational studies which have been carried out. A homogeneous set of observational results could be produced in this way.

Several antioxidant vitamins have been studied in relation to disease. Beta-carotene has been most extensively discussed and was the subject of a seminal *Nature* article (Peto *et al.* 1981). We have therefore focused on this antioxidant and have conducted meta-analyses (Egger *et al.* 1998) of the observational studies that were recently reviewed by Jha *et al.* (1995) as well as of the published randomised controlled trials (The Alpha-Tocopherol Beta Carotene Trial Research Group 1994; Hennekens *et al.* 1996; Omenn *et al.* 1996). Figure 1 displays the associations found with cardiovascular disease mortality. For observational studies, results relate to a comparison between groups with high and low beta-carotene intake, whereas in trials participants randomised to beta-carotene supplements were compared with participants randomised to a placebo.

Using a fixed-effects model, the meta-analysis of the cohort studies suggested a highly significant reduction in the risk of cardiovascular death among those consuming greater amounts of beta-carotene (relative risk reduction 31%, 95% CI 41 – 20%, p<0.0001). Combining the results from the randomised trials indicates a moderate adverse effect of beta-carotene supplementation (relative increase in the risk of cardiovascular death 12%, 95% CI 3–22%, p=0.005). Similar discrepant results are observed for cancer incidence and mortality. The results of the observational studies, together with the ease with which plausible mechanisms could be advanced, left some investigators unable to believe the negative results of the first trial, from Finland. The disappointing findings were at that time dismissed as 'demonstrating the extreme play of chance' (Hennekens *et al.* 1994), but further trials (Hennekens *et al.* 1994; Omenn *et al.* 1996) demonstrated that they were valid.

In the individual observational studies, considerable efforts had been made to control for confounding. These generally led to very small changes in the estimates of reduction in risk in relation to antioxidant vitamin intake. This may well be another example of the difficulty of adequate adjustment for confounding factors in observational studies (Davey Smith and Phillips 1992). The findings of the observational and experimental studies of antioxidants should remain as a demonstration of how cautious we need to be with respect to trusting observational data.

Non-experimental and quasi-experimental evaluations of health promotion activities suffer from all of the potential biases and distortions to which observational epidemiological studies – such as those relating beta-carotene to cardiovascular disease – are prone. It has been suggested that it is not useful pointing out that non-randomised evaluations of health promotion programmes can produce highly misleading findings (Baxter *et al.* 1998), a response which simply fails to realise the very different basis which randomised evidence gives to assertions that health promotion programmes have either produced some benefits (and therefore are not simply a waste of resources) or have not had detrimental effects.

PROMOTING HEALTHY HEARTS: THE MULTIPLE RISK
FACTOR INTERVENTION TRIAL

A similar comparison of observational or quasi-experimental findings and the results of rigorous randomised controlled trials can be seen with respect to interventions aimed at reducing coronary heart disease risk through modifying risk factors. Several community-based intervention programmes for example, the celebrated North Karelia project (Puska *et al.* 1976) were claimed to have produced dramatic reductions in coronary heart disease

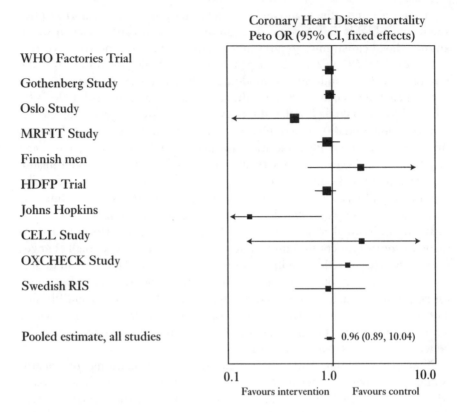

Figure 2. Meta-analysis of the effects of multiple risk factor interventions and cardiovascular mortality. Pooled effects of intervention are not significant. Trials among hypertensive patients show evidence of benefit, whereas those conducted among primary care and workplace participants do not.

mortality in the communities involved. There have also been a series of randomised controlled trials of multiple risk factor interventions aimed at reducing cardiovascular disease (Ebrahim and Davey Smith 1997).

In these trials, the study populations differed: some targeted the whole population, whereas others identified 'high risk' subjects, and others conducted a combined approach in the workplace. Trials also differed in the types of intervention used, although most included dietary modification, giving up smoking and increasing exercise. Some studies included pharmacological treatment of high blood pressure and raised blood cholesterol, whereas others did not. Common to all the trials was an aim to intervene on more than one risk factor in the belief that multiple risk factor intervention would be more effective than focusing on a single risk factor.

The effect of multiple risk factor intervention on both total and CHD mortality was insignificant (Figure 2). Reductions in mortality were observed in studies involving hypertensive participants and in which pharmacological treatment was also used. The pooled effects of intervention were statistically insignificant but a small benefit of intervention (an 11% reduction in CHD mortality) may have been missed. This evidence does not prove the null hypothesis (i.e. it is not possible to say that there is no benefit from multiple risk factor intervention) but, rather, the evidence does not refute the null hypothesis and does not give support to the alternative hypothesis of attributing benefit to intervention.

Community interventions can be (but usually are not) evaluated rigorously. Probably one of the best planned randomised controlled trials at the community level in health promotion was the COMMIT study. This involved eleven community pairs, one community within each pair being randomised to receive smoking cessation activities through public education, through health-care provider programmes, through work-site interventions and through improving smoking cessation resources in the community (COMMIT Research Group 1995). Ten million dollars were spent on these activities, with the intention that there would be multiplier effects through matched funding. The process evaluation indicated that the intervention went ahead as planned; the primary aim was to reduce the prevalence of heavy smoking. The outcome was a non-significant net reduction of 0.7% (95% confidence intervals to -3% + 2%). The cost-effectiveness was around $50,000 per heavy smoker who quit (although the confidence intervals included a negative value, i.e. the resources put into the programme could have actually increased the numbers of heavy smokers). It is clear that the additional resources implemented during such programmes are not yielding the expected benefits.

Most of the quasi-experimental community-based cardiovascular disease prevention projects have produced rather disappointing findings, in line with the more rigorously evaluated COMMIT study (Carleton *et al.* 1995; Luepker *et al.* 1994, 1996). The exceptions, like North Karelia, appear to be cases where secular trends have been misinterpreted as the effects of the health promotion programmes. Figure 3 presents the declines in ischaemic heart disease mortality in North Karelia compared to elsewhere in Finland, and demonstrates that they were not different (Valkonen, 1992). The North Karelia project serves as an example of the King Canute principle in health promotion (Davey Smith *et al.* 1994). In popular imagination – if not in mythology or fact (Larson 1912) – King Canute sat on the beach and, in order to demonstrate the enormous extent of his power, instructed the tide to stop coming in. His supposed failure in this enterprise is his lasting contribution to British folklore. Health promotion, on the other hand, has learnt from Canute's experiences, choosing instead to sit on the beach while the tide is going out and applauding. In this situation, it is then possible to claim that the ebbing tide is a direct outcome of the applause.

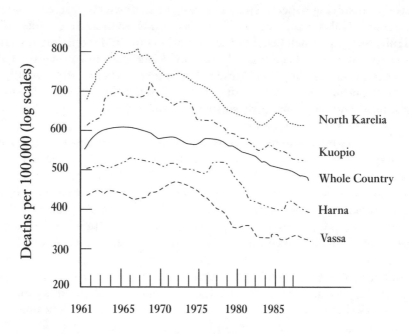

Age standardised mortality from ischaemic heart disease selected countries in Finland 1961–87, three year moving averages, males aged 35–64. From Valkonen 1992, *Int J Health Services.*

Figure 3. Declining trends in mortality occurred throughout the provinces of Finland and the whole country. Major investments were made in health promotion during the 1970s in North Karelia. The similar trends in other provinces raises the question, would these mortality declines have occurred without the programme?

Similar considerations apply to other projects which claim dramatic success, for example the Rotherham Heart Health Promotion Project (Baxter *et al.* 1997). In this project a greater reduction in cigarette smoking and some other apparent improvements in two intervention communities compared to a control community were claimed to demonstrate the dramatic success of the health promotion activity, with the authors being confident enough to claim that 'the estimated cost per life year gained was £31'. If this were true it would be a stunning finding and the rapid redirection of a considerable bulk of health services resources should follow. Unfortunately, the evidence for these claims is thin. The evaluation was based on a before–after comparison in two intervention communities and

| Social class | Current prevalence of smoking (%) | | | | Decline in current smoking (%) | |
| | 1991 | | 1995 | | 1991–5 | |
	Men	Women	Men	Women	Men	Women
I & II	22	22	20	18	10	18
III Non-manual	27	29	27	26	0	10
III Manual	35	35	33	30	6	17
IV & V	38	35	38	35	0	0

Figure 4. Changes in prevalence of current smoking and percentage decline by social class in 1991 and 1995.

one control community. These communities were not well matched, with the control community being more deprived and having a higher unemployment rate and higher mortality from coronary heart disease at baseline. The clear evidence of widening socioeconomic differentials in smoking would, therefore, be expected to produce an apparent beneficial effect of the project on smoking. Indeed, social class differences in smoking from the 1991 and 1995 health surveys for England show that the prevalence of current smoking did not fall in social classes IV and V, whereas, in social classes I and II combined, relative percentage declines in the prevalence of current smoking of 10% and 18% occurred among men and women respectively (Figure 4). The differential trends in smoking habits found between the intervention and control communities may thus be explained in terms of confounding by social circumstances.

CONCLUSIONS

The call for alternative evaluation techniques for health promotion following the disappointing results of community intervention trials aiming at reducing the risk of cardiovascular disease is misguided. It is not the evaluation technique that did not work, but the interventions. There are many examples of interventions which have been shown to be effective in community intervention trials; for example, a carefully designed randomised trials in eight US cities showed that the training of popular opinion leaders who then endorsed safe sex practices reduced the rate of sexual risk behaviours among homosexual men visiting gay bars (Kelly *et al.* 1997). A randomised community study in urban Bangladesh showed that an educational intervention which included the training of volunteers, group discussions, community-wide meetings, stories and games led to an improvement of water-sanitation behaviours and to a reduction of the incidence of childhood diarrhoea (Stanton and Clemens 1987).

Rather than searching for new evaluation techniques we should scrutinise the interventions, and the assumptions which have led to their development. An important lesson to learn is that the importance of counselling the individual has been overestimated, and more emphasis must be given to the social context (Mant 1996). Fiscal and legislative changes that aim to reduce smoking, improve diet and increase the facilities and opportunities for exercise should be given higher priorities (Ebrahim and Davey Smith 1997). Social policies that reduce socio-economic inequalities may provide the most cost-effective measures to promote the public health.

REFERENCES

Alpha-Tocopherol Beta Carotene Trial Research Group, 1994. 'The Effect of Vitamin E and Beta Carotene on the Incidence of Lung Cancer and other Cancers in Male Smokers', *New England Journal of Medicine*, 330: pp. 1029–35.

Baxter, T., Milner, P., Nicholl, J., and Wilson, K., 1998. Authors' reply. *British Medical Journal*, 316: p. 705.

Baxter, T., Milner, P., Wilson, K., Leaf, M., Nicholl, J., Freeman, J., 1997. 'A Cost Effective, Community Based Heart Health Promotion Project in England: Prospective Comparative Study', *British Medical Journal*, 315: pp. 582–5.

Bolam, A., Manandhar, D.S., Shrestha, P., Ellis, M., and de L. Costello, A.M., 1998. 'The Effects of Postnatal Health Education for Mothers on Infant Care and Family Planning Practices in Nepal: A Randomised Controlled Trial', *British Medical Journal*, 316: pp. 805–11.

Carleton, R.A., Lasater, T.M., Assaf, A.R., Feldman, H.A., McKinlay, S., and the Pawtucket Heart Health Program Writing Group, 1995. 'The Pawtucket Heart Health Program: Community Changes in Cardiovascular Risk Factors and Projected Disease Risk', *The Americal Journal of Public Health*, 85: pp. 777–85.

COMMIT Research Group, 1995. 'Community Intervention Trial for Smoking Cessation (COMMIT), II: Changes in Adult Cigarette Smoking Prevalence', *American Journal of Public Health*, 85: pp. 193–200.

Davey Smith, G., and Phillips, A.N., 1992. 'Confounding in Epidemiological Studies: Why "Independent" Effects May Not Be All They Seem', *British Medical Journal*, 305: pp. 757–9.

Davey Smith, G., Ströbele, S.A., and Egger, M., 1994. 'Smoking and Health Promotion in Nazi Germany', *Journal of Epidemiological Community Health*, 48: pp. 220–3.

Ebrahim, S., and Davey Smith, G., 1997. 'Systematic Review of Randomised Controlled Trials of Multiple Risk Factor Interventions for Preventing Coronary Heart Disease', *British Medical Journal*, 314: pp. 1666–74.

Egger, M., Schneider, M., and Davey Smith, G., 1998. 'Spurious Precision? Meta-Analysis of Observational Studies', *British Medical Journal*, 316: pp. 140–4.

Hennekens, C.H., Buring, J.E., and Peto, R., 1994. 'Antioxidant Vitamins: Benefits Not Yet Proved', *New England Journal of Medicine*, 330: pp. 1080–1.

Hennekens, C.H., Buring, J.E., Manson, J.C., Stampfer, M., Rosner, B., Cook, N.R., *et al.* 1996. 'Lack of Effect of Long-Term Supplementation with Beta Carotene on the Incidence of Malignant Neoplasms and Cardiovascular Disease', *New England Journal of Medicine*, 334: pp. 1145–49.

Jha, P., Flather, M., Lonn, E., Farkouh, M., and Yusuf, S., 1995. 'The Antioxidant Vitamins and Cardiovascular Disease', *Annals of Internal Medicine*, 123: pp. 860–72.

Kelly, J.A., Murphy, D.A., Sikkema, K.J., McAuliffe, T.L., Roffman, R.A., and Solomon, L.J., 1997. 'Randomised, Controlled Community-Level HIV-Prevention Intervention for Sexual-Risk Behaviour among Homosexual Men in US Cities', *Lancet*, 350: pp. 1500–5.

Larson, L.M., 1912. *Canute the Great*. New York: G.P. Putnam & Sons.

Luepker, R.V., Murray, D., Jacobs, D., Mittlemark, M., Bracht, N., and Carlaw, R. 1994. 'Community Education for Cardiovascular Disease Prevention: Risk Factor Changes in the Minnesota Heart Health Program', *American Journal of Public Health*, 84: pp. 1383–93.

Luepker, R.V., Rastam, L., Hanham, P.J., Murray, D.M., and Gray, C., 1996. 'Community Education for Cardiovascular Disease Prevention: Morbidity and Mortality Results from the Minnesota Heart Health Programme', *American Journal of Epidemiology*, 144: pp. 351–62.

Mant, D., 1996. 'Health Promotion and Disease Prevention: The Evaluation of Health Services Intervention', in M. Peckam and R. Smith, eds., *The Scientific Basis of Health Services*. London: British Medical Journal Publishing Group.

Nutbeam, D., 1996. 'Health Outcomes and Health Promotion: Defining Success in Health Promotion', *Health Promotion Journal of Australia*, 5: pp. 58–60.

Omenn, G.S., Goodman, G.E., Thornquist, M.D., Balmes, J., Cullen, M.R., and Glass, A., 1996. 'Effects of a Combination of Beta Carotene and Vitamin A on Lung Cancer and Cardiovascular Disease', *New England Journal of Medicine*, 334: pp. 1150–5.

Peto, R., Doll, R., Buckley, J.D., and Sporn, M.B., 1981. 'Can Dietary Beta-Carotene Materially Reduce Human Cancer Rates?', *Nature*, 290: pp. 201–8.

Prasad, B., and de L. Costello, A.M., 1995. 'Impact and Sustainability of a "Baby Friendly" Health Education Intervention at a District Hospital in Bihar, India', *British Medical Journal*, 310: pp. 621–3.

Puska, P., Koskela, K., Pakarinen, H., Puumalainen, P., Soininen, V., and Tuomiletho, J., 1976. 'The North Karelia Project: A Programme for Community Control of Cardiovascular Diseases', *Scandinavian Journal of Social Medicine*, 4: pp. 57–60.

Shryock, R.H., 1947. *The Development of Modern Medicine: An Interpretation of the Social and Scientific Factors Involved.* Wisconsin: University of Wisconsin Press.

Speller, V., Learmonth, A., and Harrison, D., 1997. 'The Search for Evidence of Effective Health Promotion', *British Medical Journal*, 315: pp. 361–3.

Stanton, B.F., and Clemens, J.D., 1987. 'An Educational Intervention for Altering Water–Sanitation Behaviours Related to Reduce Childhood Diarrhoea in Urban Bangladesh. II: A Randomized Trial to Assess the Impact of the Intervention on Hygienic Behaviours and Rates of Diarrhoea', *Americal Journal of Epidemiology*, 125: pp. 292–301.

Tudor-Smith, C., Nutbeam, D., Moore, L., and Catford, J., 1998. 'Effects of the Heartbeat Wales Programme over Five Years on Behavioural Risks for Cardiovascular Disease: Quasi-Experimental Comparison of Results from Wales and a Matched Reference Area', *British Medical Journal*, 316: pp. 18–22.

Valkonen, T., 1992. 'Trends in Regional and Socio-Economic Mortality Differentials in Finland', *International Journal of Health Services*, 3/4: pp. 157–66.

THREE

Evaluating Health Promotion: Judicial Review as a New Gold Standard

KEITH TONES

Evaluation is the process of determining the extent to which certain valued goals have been achieved. There have been many sporadic demands over the years for health promotion or, perhaps more accurately, health education, to justify its existence. More recently, however, with the advent of evidence-based medicine, these demands have become rather more persistent. Clearly, it is important that the effectiveness of health promotion should be subjected to critical scrutiny along with all other health services. Unfortunately there has been a tendency to utilise inappropriate criteria for assessing health promotion's worth and, at the same time, to specify which research methods should be employed to evaluate programmes and interventions. These methods are quite often largely irrelevant since they fail to acknowledge the peculiar characteristics and complexities of health promotion. This chapter will, therefore, seek to challenge the traditional 'gold standard' for evaluating health-related research, i.e. the randomised controlled trial (RCT). It will, in its stead, propose the adoption of a new gold standard – based on a process of 'judicial review'.

Here we shall, first of all, consider the importance of acknowledging the variety of stakeholders involved in any research enterprise, together with the typical power imbalance intrinsic to the stakeholder community and associated political imperatives. The primacy of the RCT will be challenged and special emphasis placed on (1) the fact that health promotion programmes are inherently more sophisticated and complex than the interventions typically associated with clinical trials, (2) the centrality of empowerment and participation in health promotion and the associated importance of action research and (3) the quest for illumination which is central to the development of effective programmes. The question of validity must be seriously addressed by those who design and operate health promotion programmes and its importance will be briefly explored in the context of a discussion of what are termed Types I, II and III errors. Type III error is of particular importance for health promotion programmes and the efficacy paradox associated with this will be considered. Given the limitations of RCTs and other forms of experimental design, the use of qualitative methods together with the principles and practice of triangulation will be advocated as a basis for *judicial review* – a new and more appropriate paradigm. By way of an epilogue, the chapter will conclude with a few thoughts on post-modernism.

EVALUATION AND THE STAKEHOLDER COMMUNITY

Quite simply, evaluation is concerned with the extent to which any given enterprise or endeavour achieves certain valued outcomes. It is, however, essential to recognise that those involved in the health promotion enterprise will almost certainly have different values – and, what is worse, may not know it. It is salutary to compile a list of the various individuals having a stake in the success (or failure!) of any given programme. Figure 1 provides a simplified map of this stakeholder community.

Most of the stakeholders will have different hopes and ambitions relating to the outcomes of, say, a drop-in sexual health service for young people. Funders will hope to see value for money and evidence that the centre has achieved whatever goals underpin the funding organisation. Managers may have a similar concern but will also be concerned to show that the service is efficiently run – and may also have an eye on the renewal of their contracts or promotion prospects. Politicians, on the other hand, may have particular sensitivities about public opinion, in addition to their own personal views, preferences or inhibitions about sex. They might well be pleased to have evidence of failure so that an embarrassing service can be closed down. If, however, the community at large is shown to welcome the service, the political imperative of re-election may well override politicians' personal views. The community itself is manifestly a key stakeholder and may have different requirements for the service. On the reasonable assumption that practitioners will be committed to the programme, they will doubtless be desperate to demonstrate success – probably because they consider sexual health promotion is of great importance and because they also wish to keep their jobs!

It might be thought, at first glance, that researchers and theoreticians would adopt a rather detached, distinctly scientific and neutral stance. This is, of course, myth. Theoreticians will often be interested not only to build theory but also to demonstrate the superiority of the particular theory or theories to which they subscribe. Researchers may well adopt a somewhat detached, even Olympian, stance (unless they are also theoreticians), since

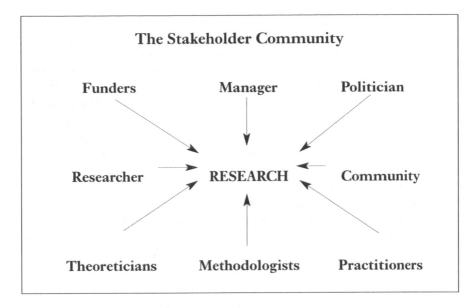

Figure 1. The Stakeholder Community.

their goal may be to produce high-quality research (whether the outcome of the study be disappointing or satisfactory from the point of view of the other stakeholders). On the other hand, if the researchers subscribe to the ideological principles of health promotion, they may seek to actively involve the community and identify with it. They may then play an active part in guaranteeing a successful outcome – at least from the community's perspective.

Researchers and theoreticians are also likely to possess particular methodological partialities – a point of particular relevance to this chapter. For example, researchers who espouse a participatory approach in their work may well have a sociological background and be strong advocates of a qualitative, ethnographic approach. Researchers from an epidemiological or psychological discipline are more likely to feel comfortable with a quantitative approach and subscribe to the ideology of positivism.

Readers will, of course, recognise that power is not necessarily equally shared within this peculiar community. At the risk of caricature, we might say that managers and funders within the health service will quite probably be influenced by a preventive medicine agenda which defines success in terms of epidemiological or behavioural outcomes. They are thus more likely to fund research which adopts a quantitative approach – preferably the RCT/true experimental design. For a number of historical and economic reasons, the advocates of such an approach are likely to have greater power and influence than those adopting a more salutogenic, ethnographic paradigm.

INDICATORS OF SUCCESS

Before commenting further on the appropriate use of indicators for assessing effectiveness and efficiency, it is worth noting that health promotion involves a synergistic interaction between health education and what the World Health Organisation has called healthy public policy. Accordingly, we might expect to judge the success of any genuine health promotion programme in relation to two complementary measures: the effective development and implementation of policy and sound educational interventions.

A second assertion will be made at this point. Epidemiological indicators (such as mortality or morbidity) should never be used to judge the success of health promotion programmes. Instead, a judicious mixture of indirect, intermediate and outcome indicators should be used. The reason for this somewhat dogmatic statement will be more evident if we consider the steps involved in two typical health promotion programmes. Figure 2 below provides a simplified summary of the first of these.

This first programme consists of a fairly typical mass media campaign. The figure shows not only the psychological stages in the process of influencing individual behaviours, but also what might be expected by way of success at each of the stages shown. For instance a properly constructed media programme would be expected to attract attention in 65% of the target group. However, only 20% of that group who have received the message

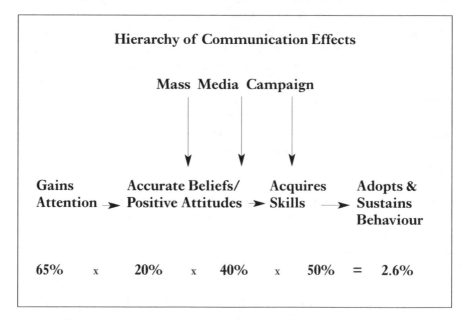

Figure 2. Hierarchy of communication effects in a mass media campaign.

would be likely to believe all aspects of the persuasive communication and/or have a positive attitude to the recommended behaviour. Nor would it be surprising if only 40% of that group had the necessary skills to adopt the recommended behaviour and if some 50% of those then proceeded to adopt and sustain the healthy action in question. The net success rate in this hypothetical example would then be 2.6% of the target group. Apart from anything else, this example should serve to remind us that mass media programmes are unlikely to achieve substantial behaviour change – and, accordingly, appropriate standards should be built into the programme objectives.

The programme would, then, be evaluated in relation to the extent to which it had attracted attention, influenced beliefs and attitudes and provided skills. Each of these psychological measures can be described as intermediate indicators representing milestones along the road to achieving a successful outcome. The adoption and maintenance of behaviours – such as healthy eating habits – would, on the other hand, be considered as outcome indicators.

Ideally, mass media should provide one particular educational element within a broader community-wide programme that includes not only education but also supportive health policy. The campaign analysed in Figure 2 might thus be part of a more extensive and comprehensive programme designed to promote healthy eating. It would, ideally, be supported by nutrition policies at both national and local level. For instance the national nutrition policy might be reflected at the organisational level – in the workplace or school. A health-promoting school would, in turn, be expected to have a taught curriculum accompanied by appropriate policy. Such a policy would, by definition, ensure that the nutrition education curriculum was consonant with the food served in its canteens and tuck shops.

The reality would, of course, be more complex, since most sophisticated programmes will build on what has gone before and the likelihood of achieving healthy outcomes might well depend on the effectiveness of a number of previous interventions. Figure 3 seeks to demonstrate this point by outlining the kinds of intervention that might be needed to increase the likelihood of women aged 50 and over responding to invitations to attend for cervical screening. It also illustrates the three major kinds of indicator of success.

The assumption is made that the ultimate goal of the programme is that of reducing the incidence and prevalence of cervical cancer. Before this can happen, any abnormality must be detected and the target group of women must visit their general practitioners for a smear test. Clearly there must also be an efficient laboratory service and an effective call and recall service if maximum uptake of the service is to take place. A mass media campaign

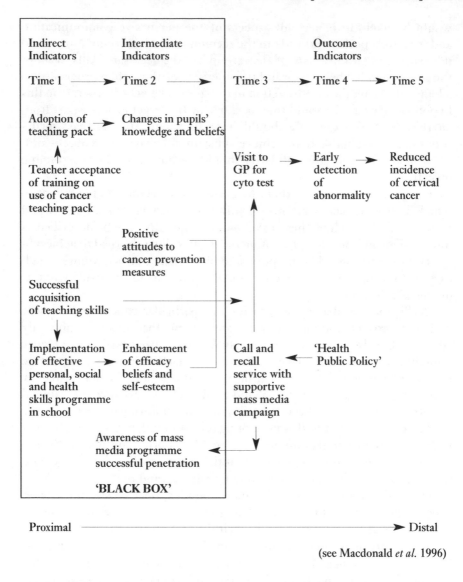

Figure 3. The kinds of intervention that might increase the likelihood of women aged 50 and over attending for cervical screening.

might be required to publicise the service and encourage women to attend. Moreover, it is reasonably clear that, even where such a service exists, many women will fail to respond to invitations to attend due to that cluster of beliefs and attitudes which are subsumed under the term 'cancerophobia'. The reduction of this unrealistic fear of cancer will, clearly, require a number of interlocking educational activities. These should not be delivered in a one-off fashion but should involve a judicious mix of biology together with personal and social education. The total package should create a sound understanding of cellular function, leading not only to an understanding of cancer but to a belief that there are a number of cancers having different characteristics and differential cure rates. It should also contribute to more general capabilities such as self-efficacy, beliefs in manageability, meaningfulness and a general commitment to living. The ensuing sense of coherence will, of course, be enhanced by the supportive ethos of a health-promoting school. Needless to say, these manifold influences will occur over rather a long period of time. Ignoring the important effects of primary socialisation and the family, some forty years might elapse between the first biology lessons and the decision to attend for screening!

INTERMEDIATE INDICATORS

There are, then, a large number of intermediate indicators which might be used to chart progress during this forty-year period:

- Children's biological understanding
- Children's knowledge and beliefs about cancer
- Children's self-efficacy beliefs in relation to adopting preventive activities
- Children's level of self-esteem
- Children's assertiveness skills
- Adults' general level of cancerophobia
- Adults' sense of coherence

And, as a result of the mass media campaign:

- Adults' awareness of the campaign
- Adults' beliefs and attitudes in relation to the service
- Adults' self-efficacy beliefs in relation to using the service

INDIRECT INDICATORS

It will be seen from Figure 3 that there are a number of indirect indicators which should be used to assess the effectiveness and efficiency of the whole programme. These are viewed as indirect, since they assess interventions which contribute to the success or failure of the programme as a whole. For instance, cancer education in secondary schools might be enhanced if teachers were to use an appropriate teaching resource; it would certainly be enhanced if teachers were to be trained! It is, moreover, self-evident that the effectiveness of both teaching packs and training courses should be evaluated. The indicators used for this are described here as indirect indicators.

Indirect indicators would also be required for evaluating any other supportive activity or programme – including any policy initiative which would enhance the effectiveness of the main programme under consideration. Of course both intermediate and outcome indicators might well be required to evaluate many such programmes in their own right.

OUTCOME INDICATORS

Figure 3 includes four indicators of programme outcome: visit to a GP or screening service; efficient detection of abnormality; reduced incidence of cervical cancer; efficient call and recall service. While it is important to assess each of these, only one is truly a health promotion indicator – the behavioural outcome of visiting the GP. Although essential to an effective health promotion programme, a proper call and recall service is the concern of health service managers and clinicians, and efficient detection of abnormalities by GPs is manifestly a matter of medical competence! More problematical perhaps is the assertion made earlier in this chapter that epidemiological outcomes should never be used to indicate the effectiveness of health promotion. The major reasons for this assertion are simple enough.

It should be patently obvious that using fluctuations in the incidence of cervical cancer to evaluate the effectiveness of school health education (and associated teacher training) some forty years earlier would require a longitudinal research design of bewildering complexity. In any case the link between behavioural outcomes such as use of a service and outcomes such as incidence or prevalence of a disease is essentially an epidemiological matter. Clearly it would be pointless mounting a health promotion programme of this kind unless it had been proven beyond reasonable doubt to have an impact on medical status. If that were not the case, the programme should not be running! If the link has been established, it is superfluous to use epidemiological data to assess the effectiveness of health promotion. In other words, morbidity and mortality data provide justification for developing health promotion programmes but not the means for evaluating their effect. Consequently the most 'distal' measures of success will be individual behaviours or some cluster of behaviours involved in a composite risk score.

Some of the components of the programme can be justified in their own right. The enhancement of self-esteem or the provision of interaction skills may well contribute to medically desirable outcomes but they are also intrinsically worthy. Indeed, in many cases an intermediate indicator of a successful preventive programme may, at the same time, be an outcome indicator for a successful educational programme or a programme which has as its major goal the enhancement of well-being.

CHALLENGING THE GOLD STANDARD

We turn now to a consideration of evaluation methodology. Just as we have argued that epidemiological indicators are not appropriate for assessing health promotion, so we argue that the research techniques considered to be essential in the pursuit of evidence-based medicine are rarely relevant for evaluating health promotion. In short the randomised controlled trial (RCT) or its educational/behavioural science equivalent, the True Experimental Design, is viewed as a gold standard to which all evaluations should aspire. A full discussion of this question is beyond the scope of this chapter (see Tones 1997, 1998, for further consideration of this and related issues). However, the most important limitations of the RCT in health promotion are listed here:

- Randomisation is difficult or impossible in real-life situations.
- The health promotion enterprise is intrinsically more complex and qualitatively different from a typical clinical trial.
- The RCT is ideologically unsound, since maximal client participation is desirable in health promotion.
- The results of health promotion evaluations should provide illumination, not merely a response to the simple question, 'Has this programme worked?'

Some of these points will receive further clarification below.

EFFECTIVENESS, EFFICIENCY AND EFFICACY: A TALE OF THREE ERRORS

The terms 'effectiveness' and 'efficiency' are in quite common use; the term 'efficacy' is less commonly used as a distinct concept. Before considering this important notion, we shall recall the meaning of the two former criteria for health promotion success.

In brief, effectiveness refers to the extent to which a given programme has achieved its goals. Efficiency, on the other hand, is a measure of relative effectiveness in that it compares the results of a given intervention with alternative and competing measures (e.g. health promotion for prevention of a disease versus treatment of that disease; the relative effectiveness of education for smoking cessation compared with increased taxation in reducing prevalence). Cost effectiveness is in fact an efficiency measure which assesses the superiority of one or other measures in relation to financial criteria.

We might note, incidentally, that certain health education/health promotion interventions are demonstrably efficient according to the stringent requirements of cost benefit analysis. For instance, the cost of a hip replacement (itself considered to be a very effective surgical procedure) has been calculated as £750 per quality adjusted year of life gained (QUALY). The cost of simple smoking-related advice provided by a GP, on the other hand, would appear to be a bargain at a mere £167 per QUALY! However, since effective health promotion can result in the prolongation of life and, arguably, a proportionate increase in medical costs, cost-effectiveness measures of efficiency should be used with great caution!

As noted above, efficacy has no universally accepted meaning. However, the definition adopted by Brook and Lohr (1985) is most useful for our present discussion. In short, according to the authors, efficacy refers to the probability of benefit under ideal conditions. 'Effectiveness has all the attributes of efficacy except one: it reflects performance under ordinary conditions by the average practitioner.' To ignore these precepts will typically lead to the practitioner or researcher being guilty of a Type III error.

EFFICACY AND TYPE III ERROR

The RCT is designed primarily to combat what may be termed Type I error. In other words, it seeks to avoid the situation where practitioners or researchers wrongly claim that a programme has been successful because they have failed to take account of a competing explanation. Randomisation to experimental and control groups protects against this kind of inappropriate interpretation.

Type II error, on the other hand, involves wrongly claiming that a programme has failed – perhaps because the devices used to measure outcomes have been insufficiently sensitive. For instance an inappropriately standardised and validated self-esteem scale may fail to demonstrate that a mental health programme has had any effect on clients' sense of self-worth. If the same programme had been assessed by semi-structured interviews the real effect of the programme might have been revealed. But Type III error is committed much more frequently in evaluating health promotion programmes. In short, an evaluation might demonstrate a programme has not been effective when it would be quite clear to the professional that there was no chance of it ever succeeding due to an inappropriate design or inadequate input. In other words, the ideal conditions that could have produced success, i.e. led to efficacy, had not been supplied. For example, it is clear that many so-called health education interventions, involving, say, only the provision of a booklet exhorting people to increase their consumption of fruit and vegetables, are doomed to failure. A more sophisticated programme would be needed before success could be achieved. A further enlightening instance is provided by Kirby (1995), who argued that a successful sex education programme should have the following characteristics:

- Should be based on Social Learning Theory
- Should have a narrow focus on sexual risk-taking
- Requires a minimum of 14 hours' teaching in small groups
- Should use active learning methods
- Must provide basic information
- Should address the issue of social pressure
- Should provide clear messages and reinforce them
- Should include modelling
- Teachers must be properly trained to deliver the programme

Assuming that these assertions are soundly based, evaluating a sex education programme that does not meet these requirements would be to commit a Type III error.

THE EFFICACY PARADOX

The paradoxical implications of seeking to avoid Type III errors in the pursuit of efficacy will doubtless not have escaped the reader. On the one hand, it is pointless providing an inadequate health promotion programme; on the other hand, it is rarely, if ever, possible to provide an ideal programme which meets all health education requirements together with supportive healthy public policy. Fortunately, the reality is not quite so problematic. Programme planners should strive to meet ideal programme requirements and, if they fail, should then ask whether a more limited but pragmatic programme might achieve sufficiently worthwhile results. For instance, the provision of smoking advice by GPs (to which reference was made earlier) could doubtless have been more effective if the consultation time had been longer, the GP had proven counselling skills and the clients had enlisted in a self-help group. However, the results of the brief intervention were 'good enough'.

ILLUMINATION AND PARTICIPATION

Summative evaluation refers to the evaluation of a completed programme. It typically involves a comparison of the results of pre-tests with the results of post-tests. (Of course if the RCT model had been adopted, the differences between the pre- and post-test results of the experimental group which received the programme would be compared with a control group to which subjects had been randomly allocated.) Apart from any other objections levelled against the RCT, summative evaluation can have little practical value in that it will merely show how well a programme has performed and, perhaps, whether objectives have been achieved. It rarely, however, yields data which provide insight into why particular parts of a programme have been successful or unsuccessful. In other words, rather in the fashion of the lamp-post and the drunk, it supplies support rather than illumination.

The addition of process evaluation – i.e. a record of what actually happened during the programme – can help shed light on the proceedings. However, even assuming that relevant documentary evidence has been accumulated, the RCT fails to meet the full requirements of those health promotion initiatives which not only seek to maximise client participation but also endeavour to use research to achieve meaningful and rapid social change.

PARTICIPATION AND ACTION RESEARCH

We noted earlier that an integral part of the philosophy of health promotion – and therefore of health promotion research – was the importance of enabling people and communities to increase control over their lives and their health. Vanderplaat (1995), writing about research for empowerment, approvingly cites Raeburn (1987) as follows:

> Community people decide what their own needs are, set their own goals, and take action themselves; these projects are owned, controlled and determined by the people whom they are intended to benefit; at the heart of the system is a fundamental principle – that of people deciding what they want for themselves.

The importance of formative evaluation has long been acknowledged in relation to training and education. It refers to the use of various assessment measures throughout a given programme. These measures are then used to modify the programme in response to participants' responses. Typically this would involve various remedial inputs to maximise the chance of the whole target group achieving the programme objectives – a kind of guarantee of success. Formative evaluation clearly involves more than mere process evaluation: it utilises process to initiate change during the programme rather than to provide a degree of illumination after it has been completed. It has some features in common with two important philosophies of evaluation: the notion of the reflexive practitioner and action research.

The philosophy underlying the concept of the reflexive practitioner urges practitioners to improve their practice by constant pragmatic research and evaluation. Action research involves a continuous cycle of researching a problem, applying the results of the research to the solution of the problem and then assessing the impact of the actions which emerge. Action research is especially relevant for health promotion, since health promotion is or should be a radical movement seeking to create active participating communities which will challenge the status quo in order to remedy health -damaging social and environmental circumstances.

AN ALTERNATIVE EVALUATION PARADIGM: THE CASE FOR JUDICIAL REVIEW

For the various reasons outlined above, we have questioned the relevance of the RCT and related paradigms for evaluating health promotion programmes. However, this must not mean abandoning the search for validity. Validity refers to the extent to which any given evaluation succeeds in measuring what it sets out to measure. For example, in order to be valid, a claim that a sex education programme has been effective must be based on convincing evidence that programme objectives have been met, e.g. that the client group in question has now acquired knowledge, beliefs, attitudes and skills which were lacking prior to the programme. We observed earlier how a pro- gramme's internal validity could be damaged by Type I error and how the RCT provided a powerful means of avoiding such an error. It may also have been apparent that both the use of the RCT and an unswerving demand for efficacy in order to avoid Type III error could reduce the likelihood of external validity – i.e. the transferability of successful programmes to other 'real life' situations. For all of these reasons, it is argued here that we need to adopt a new paradigm which utilises a principle of 'judicial review'.

Now although this term is used in legal parlance to refer to attempts to reassess previous judicial decisions and alleged miscarriage of justice, the general approach and the use of evidence would seem particularly appropriate to making decisions about the effectiveness of health promotion programmes. In the real world of education and health, managers and practitioners are faced continually with making resource allocation decisions. They will be fortunate indeed if they can access valid and unequivocal evidence from research to support their decisions. The current vogue for Cochrane-type reviews that purport to provide an evidence base for medicine are not especially helpful in guiding action in the field of health promotion. What managers and practitioners need is rapidly generated evidence – preferably incorporating assessment of community perceptions and needs in addition to the usual normative information provided by traditional epidemiology (a fact which explains the increasing popularity of rapid participatory appraisal). The judicial principle adopted here would adopt the kinds of standard that would offer at least two criteria for action: the more risky option associated with the notion of a balance of probabilities and the tougher standard of 'beyond reasonable doubt'.

Interestingly, it is possible to adapt the well-known criteria for establishing cause-and-effect relationships in clinical medicine 'beyond reasonable doubt' to the requirements of health promotion. A valid basis for ascribing outcome to a given programme would therefore meet the following requirements:

- There should be a strong, consistent and specific association
- There should be a temporally convincing 'dose–response' relationship (see comments on avoiding Type III error)
- The presumed cause–effect relationship should be theoretically plausible (the theory in question being primarily social science and educational theory).

In the context of action and decision-making, two additional criteria (body text) might be applied:

- Transferability – the potential for applying the present programme to other similar settings and contexts
- 'Catalytic validity': a term coined by Janesick (1998) to indicate the extent to which there is evidence that a programme would generate significant change

THE CASE FOR TRIANGULATION

Perhaps the most useful tool for assessing the validity of health promotion interventions is that of triangulation. Denzin (1978) provided an almost definitive list of different kinds of triangulation as follows:

- Data triangulation
- Investigator triangulation
- Theory triangulation
- Methodological triangulation

In the formulation adopted here, it is assumed that consistency between the different perspectives provided by these techniques will increase the conviction that a given result is valid. Clearly, overall validity will depend on the reliability and validity of the individual techniques.

Janesick (1994, 1998) added a fifth dimension to this list that she called interdisciplinary triangulation. Perhaps modifying her meaning slightly, we might assert that evidence from the judicious use of the creative arts could add to the collection of evidence on which decisions are to be made.

ONE CHEER FOR POST-MODERNISM

By way of a final observation, it should not be assumed that the rejection of research methods dear to the hearts of those addicted to the view that truth is only knowable through positivism necessarily implies the adoption of a cynical post-modernist stance. Although the post-modern tendency has had salutary effects in emphasising the social construction of reality, the author of this chapter is sympathetic to the point of view recently expressed by the venerable sociological researcher William Foote Whyte (1997). In response to an assertion that there is 'no longer any such thing as fiction or non-fiction, there is only narrative', he confidently claimed that 'There are such things as physical and social facts.' He went on to satirise some of the more labyrinthine and esoteric expressions of post-modern writings by drawing attention to a physicist colleague's submission to an academic journal. The article was entitled, 'Transgressing the Boundaries: Toward a Transformative Hermeneutics of Quantum Gravity'. Despite the fact that the paper was a spoof and had been deliberately written as gobbledegook, it was in fact published. For those interested, it may apparently be found in the journal *Social Text* (1996)!

We should perhaps add that at least some aspects of the so-called post-modern predicament are not new. It has been apparent to sociologists for many a year that social norms, their associated practices and the values and beliefs underpinning them differ to greater or lesser extents from culture to culture. Variations exist between subcultures and are frequently challenged by the prevailing social constructions of counter-cultures. There may be cultural commonalities but there is no universal culture. This variability is created by the process of socialisation.

For instance, the socialisation principle is apparent if we consider the various attempts of health education to gain access to the 'secret garden' of the school curriculum. Even before the relatively recent explosion of knowledge, it was evident that the content of the curriculum was partial in its representation of reality. Schools did not merely inculcate an agreed and finite body of knowledge and a universally accepted set of values. Rather, they sought to manipulate and shape their pupils in accordance with what the particular society considered to be most worthwhile – or, to be more precise, in accordance with the ideology of the most powerful in that society. As we have seen in recent years, the very teaching methods used are not so much subject to the technical requirements of learning but rather to ideological dictates. In other words, the school is an excellent example of a socialisation agency.

This lack of certainties and the relativism inherent in the situations described above does not mean that we should respond by merely giving a bemused shrug of the shoulders. Rather, we acknowledge cultural vari- ability, analyse its implications and, in the school example cited above, we seek to challenge and influence the ideologies which are incompatible with the values of health promotion (or more precisely those consistent with the Ottawa Charter); where successful, we should take practical steps such as the construction of a health career to help counter 'unhealthy' influences and structure efficient inputs consistent with our values.

At the level of the individual rather than the social, it has been quite clear for decades that there is no one-to-one relationship between external sensory inputs and internal constructions of reality. Individual beliefs (i.e. *subjective* probabilities) about common phenomena and experiences may differ quite substantially. The study of illusions have – at least since the 19th century – shown unequivocally that people may differ in their very *perception* of sensory information. They frequently 'see' or 'hear' what they expect to be the case rather than actually reproducing 'reality'. And of course, in accordance with the dictates of wish fulfilment, humans have an annoying tendency to interpret incoming information to match their prevailing motivation – their values and prejudices and even their bodily drives.

We have, then, known for some time that uncertainty exists (even at sub- atomic level!). This is no excuse for not seeking to impose meaning on multiple realities – or for not taking action. After all, health promotion is, or should be, the militant wing of public health. What is more, theory is an essential part of this process of understanding and acting. No one theory is perfect; some theories are more useful than others in certain circumstances. We do, however, have a quite substantial theoretical grasp of, for example, the psychological, social and environmental determinants of health-related actions – and indeed about the educational processes involved in fostering efficient learning (Tones and Tilford 1994).

With reference to the evaluation of effectiveness and efficiency of health promotion, we should, of course, avoid simplistic conclusions drawn from naïve quantification. Indeed, this chapter has emphasised the folly of doing so. We must, however, use an eclectic mix of approaches to gain a reasonably sound handle on reality in defining community needs and in evaluating the quality of our health promotion endeavours. As I have argued vehemently in this chapter, this may be achieved by a principle of judicial review, using multiple methods based on sound theory – and, of course, to be consistent with the ideology underlying our interventions, these endeavours should be carried out *in collaboration with* rather than *on* individuals and communities.

REFERENCES

Brook, R., and Lohr, K., 1985. 'Efficiency, Effectiveness, Variations and Quality', *Medical Care*, 23: pp. 710–22.

Denzin, N.K., 1978. *The Research Act: A Theoretical Introduction to Sociological Methods* (2nd ed). New York: McGraw-Hill.

Janesick, V.J., 1994. 'The Dance of Qualitative Research Design: Metaphor, Methodolatry and Meaning', in N.K. Denzin and Y.S. Lincoln, eds., *Handbook of Qualitative Research*. London: Sage.

Janesick, V.J., 1998. *Stretching Exercises for Qualitative Researchers*. Thousand Oaks, CA: Sage.

Kirby, D., 1995. *A Review of Educational Programme Designed to Reduce Sexual Risk-Taking Behaviours among School-Aged Youth in the United States*. Washington, DC: US Congress Office of Technology Assessment and the National Technical Assessment and the National Technical Information Service.

Macdonald, G., Veen, C., and Tones, K., 1996. 'Evidence for Success in Health Promotion: Suggestions for Improvement', *Health Education Research*, 11, 3: pp. 367–76.

Raeburn, J., 1987. 'People Projects: Planning and Evaluation in a New Era', *Health Promotion*, Winter: pp. 2–13.

Tones, B.K., and Tilford, S., 1994. *Health Education: Effectiveness, Efficiency and Equity*. London: Chapman and Hall.

Tones, B.K., 1997. 'Beyond the Randomized controlled Trial: A Case for "Judicial Review"' *Health Education Research*, 12, 2: i–iv.

Tones, B.K., 1998. 'Effectiveness of Health Promotion', in D. Scott and R. Weston, eds., *Evaluating Health Promotion*. London: Stanley.

Whyte, W.F., 1997. *Creative Problem Solving in the Field: Reflections on a Career*. Walnut Creek: Altamira Press.

Vanderplaat, M., 1995. 'Beyond Technique: Issues in Evaluating for Empowerment', *Evaluation*, 1, 1: pp. 81–96.

FOUR

The Future of Health Promotion: Jakarta Conference

DESMOND O'BYRNE

INTRODUCTION

The first formal commitment at an international conference to health promotion was made at the First International Conference on Health Promotion, Ottawa, Canada, 1986. However, the beginning of modern health promotion goes back to the Lalonde Report (1974), which really set up Canada to take a lead role in the initial development of health promotion. The first World Health Assembly Resolution on Health Promotion (WHA5l.12) was formulated in May 1998. The WHA resolution recognised that the Ottawa Charter for health promotion has been a world-wide source of guidance and inspiration for health promotion development through its five essential strategies – to build healthy public policy, create supportive environments, strengthen community action, develop personal skills and reorient health services. Between these two time-periods – Ottawa, 1986, to WHA, May 1998 – health promotion has grown and developed. This chapter will briefly examine some of those developments and then look forward to the new millennium with its many challenges and opportunities.

To give some background on the health promotion perspective, I shall briefly refer to some key definitions and principles.

HEALTH DEFINITIONS

Health is defined by the WHO Constitution as a state of complete physical, social and mental well-being, and not merely the absence of disease or infirmity. Within the context of health promotion, health has been considered less as an abstract state and more as a means to an end which can be expressed in functional terms, as a resource for everyday life, which permits people to live an individually, socially and economically productive life (*cf.* WHO, Health Promotion Glossary, 98.1).

46

Today, the spiritual dimension of health is increasingly often recognised. The Constitution of WHO states that: 'The enjoyment of the highest attainable standard of health is one of the fundamental rights of every human being without distinction of race, religion, political belief, economic or social conditions.' Correspondingly, all people should have access to basic resources for health. The Constitution goes on to state 'that informed opinion and active cooperation on the part of the public are of utmost importance in the improvement of the health of the people. Health promotion is the process of enabling people to increase control over, and to improve their health' (Ottawa Charter). This is further developed in the Health Promotion Glossary, to 'stress that Health Promotion is the process of enabling people to increase control over the determinants of health and thereby improve their Health'.

MILESTONES ON THE ROAD INTO THE TWENTY-FIRST CENTURY

The *Ottawa Conference and Charter* (1986) ushered in modern-day health promotion with its three strategic areas of advocacy, enabling and mediating, and its five interrelated action areas of policy, environment, community action, personal skills and reoriented health services.

The *Adelaide Conference* (1988) started from the premise that health is both a fundamental human right and a sound social investment. The conference urged governments to promote health through linked economic, social and health policies. The conference identified four priority areas for health public policy:

- improving the health of women
- food and nutrition
- tobacco and alcohol
- creating supportive environments

Since 1988, many international organisations, countries and regional/local governments have adopted public health policies which embody the spirit of Adelaide.

The *Sundsvall Conference* (1991) highlighted the link between health and physical environments. A supportive environment is of paramount importance for health; the two are interdependent and inseparable. The Sundsvall Statement urged that the achievement of both be made central objectives in setting priorities for development, and that this should be given precedence in reconciling competing interests in the everyday management of government policies.

- widespread absolute and relative poverty
- demographic changes: ageing and the growth of cities
- epidemiological developments: continuing high incidence of non-communicable diseases, injuries and violence
- global environmental threats to human survival
- new technologies: information and telemedicine services
- advances in biotechnology
- evolving partnerships for health that include the private and public sectors and civil society
- globalisation of trade, travel and the spread of values and ideas

Figure 1. New trends influencing health in the 21st century.

The *Jakarta Conference* (1997) was the first of the international conferences to be held in a developing region of the world. The Jakarta Conference on Leading Health Promotion into the 21st Century acted as a catalyst for health promotion action, nationally, internationally and globally. It was held against the background of major global changes, including the widening gap between rich and poor, demographic changes, the communication revolution, the globalisation of markets and the double burden of disease.

These changes shape people's values, their lifestyles throughout the lifespan, and living conditions across the world. Some have great potential for health while others have a major negative impact. The challenge is to bend the trends, to exploit developments for health promotion and development.

The Jakarta Declaration identifies the need to break through traditional boundaries and for the creation of partnerships for health between the different sectors at all levels of governance in societies. As such, it is relevant for both developed and developing countries. The WHO Health for All (HFA) in the 21st Century policy document, passed at the WHA in May 1998, identifies actions by all Member States of WHO to realise the goal of HFA, guided by two policy objectives: making health central to human - development, and developing sustainable health systems to meet the needs of people. Good health is both a resource for, and an aim for, health development. The Jakarta Declaration places health promotion firmly at the centre of health development.

THE JAKARTA CONFERENCE OBJECTIVES

- to review and evaluate the impact of health promotion
- to identify innovative strategies to achieve success in health promotion
- to facilitate the development of partnerships to meet global challenges

The conference not only endorsed the results of the previous international conferences on health promotion, but also confirmed the relevance for both developing and developed countries of placing health promotion firmly at the centre of health development. The five action areas set out in the Ottawa Charter remain essential for successful health promotion. The Jakarta Declaration states that there is clear evidence that comprehensive approaches to health development are the most effective, and that combined strategies are more effective than single-track approaches; particular settings offer practical opportunities for the implementation of comprehensive strategies, for example health-promoting schools, cities, workplaces, municipalities, cities and so on.

Participation is essential to sustain efforts. People have to be at the centre of health promotion action, and access to education and information is essential to achieve effective participation and empowerment of the people and communities (*cf.* Jakarta Declaration). One of the major outcomes of the Jakarta Conference is the promotion of partnerships, to include the public as well as the private sector, together with NGOs in networks and alliances for health and development. The Jakarta Declaration calls for the formation of a global health promotion alliance.

The Jakarta Declaration identified five priorities for health promotion in the 21st century:

- to promote social responsibility for health
- to increase investment for health development
- to consolidate and expand partnerships for health
- to increase community capacity and 'empower' the individual in matters of health
- to secure an infrastructure for health promotion

The time is right for a shift to action on these priorities.

- raise awareness of the changing determinants of health
- support the development of collaboration and networking for health development
- mobilise resources for health promotion
- accumulate knowledge on best practices
- enable shared learning
- promote solidarity in action
- foster transparency and public accountability in health promotion.

Figure 2. CALL FOR ACTION (Jakarta Declaration).

The future of health promotion calls for responses now in promoting social responsibility; it needs new policy styles and ethical boundaries. Expanding partnerships directs us to new forms of intersectoral co-operation; an increase in community capacity and the empowerment of the individual requires the advancement of health promotion methods; and, in securing an infrastructure for health promotion, we raise various questions of management. Increasing investment for health is based on transparency and accountability.

To realise its full potential and to fulfil its key role in health development, greater attention must also be given to an *evidence-based* approach to health promotion policy and practice, using the full range of quantitative and qualitative methodologies (*cf.* World Health Resolution on Health Promotion – WHA51.12).

Attention is drawn to the reference in the WHA resolution to qualitative as well as quantitative methodologies. It is a major challenge for health promotion to communicate to the policy- and decision-makers not only the nature of health promotion but also the *time factors* involved. It is important to be able to win the understanding of those concerned with health, in particular that of political audiences who work within a very tight time-frame – three to four years or less, depending on their respective times in office or durations of parliament.

Health has multiple determinants that impact over time. How can we explain the 'time factor' between health promotion inputs and the eventual outcomes, which will have numerous influences and which may not be apparent for some five, ten, or even twenty years, to an audience expecting quick results?

By stressing the difficulties of ascribing a monetary value to enhancing health, we do not do ourselves justice. We fail to recognise the 'spiritual' factors involved and the increased quality of life which results from health promotion.

Yet health economists and politicians need to be given an extremely tight monetary value for these qualitative issues. Only then will they recognise that if they apply their usual discounting techniques to adjust future values to today's values, the costs of health promotion are shown to be small in comparison with future returns. It involves an extremely favourable return on investment.

In follow-up to the Jakarta Declaration and the WHA Health Promotion Resolution, WHO is focusing on three broad areas:

- promoting the development of a global health promotion alliance
- promoting health in priority settings, including the school, through the Global School Health Initiative; the city, through its Healthy

City network; and the workplace, through its Workplace Health Promotion initiative; also healthy communities, municipalities, islands, and so on

* health promotion through the network of most populous countries, countries with populations of 100 million people or more (Mega Country network)

Health promotion uses three main entry points for action: settings, populations and health issues. The challenge is to apply the health promotion concepts, principles and approaches to each of the entry points to reflect the five action areas of the Ottawa Charter. These are the main 'entry points' for health promotion actions through advocacy, enabling and mediating.

To maintain the momentum brought about by the Jakarta Conference and Declaration as well as the Resolution on Health Promotion, and to stimulate action at country, intercountry and global levels, it has been decided to hold the next Global Health Promotion Conference in Mexico City in June 2000. This will follow up on the progress made since Jakarta and prepare to launch the global alliance for health promotion into the new millennium.

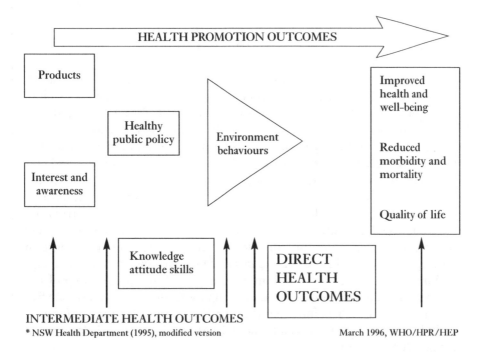

Figure 3. Health Promotion Outcomes.

Entry points for Health Promotion Action

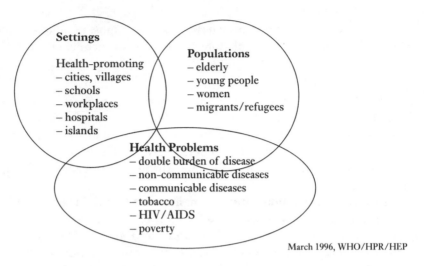

Settings

Health-promoting
– cities, villages
– schools
– workplaces
– hospitals
– islands

Populations
– elderly
– young people
– women
– migrants/refugees

Health Problems
– double burden of disease
– non-communicable diseases
– communicable diseases
– tobacco
– HIV/AIDS
– poverty

March 1996, WHO/HPR/HEP

Figure 4. Health Promotion entry points.

5TH GLOBAL CONFERENCE ON HEALTH PROMOTION (5GCHP)

The overall goal of the 5GCHP is to address the priorities for health promotion in the twenty-first century, to promote more social responsibility for health and for increased investment for health development, and to expand and consolidate partnerships for health. Conference papers will be prepared around the five priority areas for health promotion as outlined in the Jakarta Declaration. Each paper will review the 'state of the art' and best practices, and identify the global actions required for advancement into the next century. Examples will refer to issues of global concern such as tobacco, ageing, violence, lifestyles, changes in employment and family structure. Migration and urbanisation will also be addressed. The conference papers will set the scene and outline the global nature of the issue, its impact on health, and proposed actions to be taken. Through consultations, meetings and discussions at country and intercountry level, the preparation of the papers will help to stimulate discussion and motivate action around the five interrelated areas. It is intended that the preparation for the conference, including conference papers and other related activities, will galvanise action for health promotion.

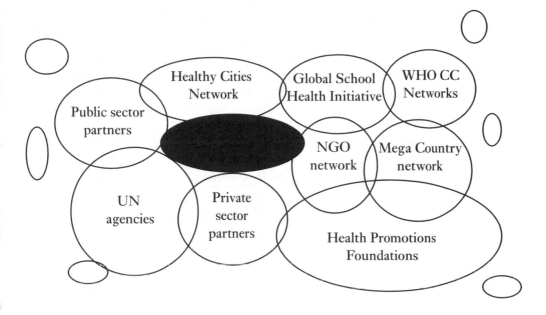

Figure 5. The Global Alliance for Health Promotion; draft model illustrating the dynamic, interactive nature of the coalition.

CONFERENCE OBJECTIVES

- to promote 'state of the art' and best practice within the five priority areas for health promotion, and to identify global actions for the advancement of health promotion into the next century
- to promote the role of health promotion in world health development and social change and in the political agendas of the UN, public agencies, health and other ministries, NGOs and the private sector
- to accelerate the development/progress of the Global Alliance for Health Promotion, and to pave the way for future developments

The conference programme will be innovative and interactive and will be open in format. It will use the latest leading-edge techniques of information technology, including an Internet website and satellite links to various regions of the world. The future of health promotion will depend on the ongoing advocacy and commitment of all those interested in the health and well-being of all people everywhere throughout the world. Tremendous progress and successes have been achieved but these must be continually re-won and reinforced in order to maintain sustainable growth and development in health promotion and health development. It remains an uphill and continual effort both to maintain progress gain and to make further advances. That is why it is essential to build new partnerships, to outreach to all sectors of society, academic, public and private sectors, NGOs, to expand our database best practices and appropriate evidence, to be creative and innovative. The rapidly changing world offers both challenges and opportunities. The development of a health promotion global alliance, virtual or otherwise, will, it is hoped, be one way of tapping this rich potential for health promotion. The future for health promotion is what we make it.

FIVE

Theories, Values and Paradigms: Reflections on the Fourth World Conference on Health Promotion in Jakarta

CECILY KELLEHER

INTRODUCTION

Whatever one's disciplinary background, anyone seriously involved in the field of health promotion today as either a practitioner or academic would acknowledge that the first World Health Organisation sponsored international conference at Ottawa (1986) was widely influential in the decade that followed. Its declaration formulated the five principles that became known as the Ottawa Charter: to build healthy public policy, re-orientate health services, create supportive environments, encourage community participation and develop personal skills. The second meeting in Adelaide (1988) focused more fully on means to promote healthy public policy and the third, in Sundsvall in Sweden (1991), focused on the creation of supportive environments. From this time on the settings-based approach to health promotion was more fully developed world-wide and since then we have seen a further highly influential change in health promotion practice, much of it in collaboration with the European Commission in the European region. This includes programmes for schools, workplaces, cities, hospitals, prisons and now ever more expansion into territorial or ecological approaches, including islands. More recently the movement has addressed the needs of mega-cities and mega-countries. All of these initiatives acknowledge the importance of the context in which individuals make choices and seek to provide a framework for action at individual and community level to facilitate change. These developments are described more fully by Des O'Byrne of the World Health Organisation in the previous chapter. While some readers may be sceptical about the relevance to serious research and practice of yet another international conference, in the case of health promotion the influence of such meetings has been important.

   In effect, over the last decade established health education and health promotion agencies have been moving away from a disease- or topic-specific approach to work practice, and significant if relatively modest resources have been directed towards these developments. In the main in most countries those resources have come from ear-marked health care and education budgets with little explicit contribution from other sectors. A major question now is what theory or theories underlie health promotion practice to justify such a profound paradigm shift (or indeed whether any single unifying theory exists) and how such practice is informed for the global movement now coined as health promotion. In recent years more attention has come to be paid to issues of quality, evidence and effectiveness (see for instance the text edited by Davies and MacDonald 1998), though much of this attention concerns models of practice and their evaluation rather than more fundamental questions about the nature and purpose of health promotion. There are trenchant critics of the health promotion movement, who feel that it is a composite of diverse social, political and biomedical concepts resting on a series of conclusions that cannot be justified. In recent years in health care generally, evidence-based practice has become a by-word, together with the use of outcome measures, particularly the randomised controlled trial, the so-called 'gold standard'. Protests by health promoters that this is an inappropriate paradigm have been received with scepticism, particularly where the focus has been on the explanation of negative study outcomes. It may be, therefore, that we need to re-trace the history of health promotion at this critical juncture to disentangle some of these composite ideas that have gained such currency within it.

Health promotion is indisputably an emerging field, one which is certainly not primarily an academic or even a professional movement. Whatever else may be said of health promotion, it is novel in that it is firmly rooted in the belief that health is determined by social and political forces and that therefore relevant players include policy-makers and a range of contributors to society whose function is not primarily to influence health status. This has translated in some instances into a rough and ready approach to policy which is assimilated in sometimes procrustean fashion into a diverse range of situations. Criticism of health promotion may thus be well founded in querying the basis of the approach, but the modern health promotion movement receives virtually no credit for the scale of its ambition. It is possible that this is in part because its critics are not equipped to appraise its success or otherwise. Commentators trained in any of the professions in the modern health-care sector are rarely competent to assess effectiveness using political or socio-historical paradigms. The intellectual equivalent is like asking a biochemist or an epidemiologist coherently to explain the rise or demise of Stalinism, Thatcherism or Buddhism within the confines of their own disciplinary paradigm. We may be able to appraise the health impact but not the process of making that impact. Like poor craftsmen we then blame our tools (Kelleher 1995, 1996). A positive impact on health status is declared unproven and a negative impact is hailed as evidence of ineffectiveness. This situation is compounded by the fact that those of us involved in health promotion come from a diversity of disciplinary backgrounds and tend to solve problems as our skills rather than as the problem dictates.

WHAT WAS THE JAKARTA CONFERENCE ABOUT?

It is worthwhile therefore to devote an academic paper to the proceedings of an international conference because it provided focus for this emerging movement at a critical stage. The fourth International Conference on Health Promotion was held in Jakarta from 21 to 25 July 1997. The meeting was organised by the Geneva office of the World Health Organisation and was hosted locally by the Ministry of Health of the Republic of Indonesia. It was intended to build on the three previous such conferences. Indeed, meetings like that in Jakarta that represent such a wide range of interests, whether they reflect current thinking or lead debate, can be highly influential at regional and country level, depending on how they are interpreted and acted upon. The theme for the Jakarta Conference was *New Partners for a New Era*. In essence the objective was to explore how a wide variety of hitherto not explicitly involved sectors could influence health and hence prepare us for the new millennium. Old concepts and boundaries are ceasing to apply in a rapidly changing planet. Partners include governmental and non governmental organisations across sectors in every country but also the private sector (particularly those involved in wealth creation) and players in related areas such as the mass media. It was also, significantly, the first conference held in the so-called developing world and was sited in an emerging mega-country, Indonesia, with a population of over 200 million people and a controversial political history. The Jakarta Conference, as we shall see, was dominated by a sociological, community-development paradigm (Baum 1998; Labonte 1989) with much emphasis being placed on the concept of social capital (Gillies 1998; Hawe 1998; Nutbeam 1998a, 1998b). Some individuals at least focused on the need for conceptually positive models of health, including salutogenesis (Antonovsky 1993, 1996). There were broadly three strands to the meeting, which represented invited persons from 78 countries who were all in one way or another involved in these issues in their own countries. The three strands were Setting of the Challenges, Leading Change and Partnerships in Action.

THE FINAL JAKARTA DECLARATION

The Jakarta Declaration (World Health Organisation 1997) reiterated that health was a basic human right and stressed that recognition of this, together with a reduction in inequities and the building of social capital, were important contributors to health gain. Health should be seen as a key investment by societies, it stated, with a goal of increasing health expectancy and narrowing the gap in health expectancy between countries and groups. The declaration stressed the new challenges posed by urbanisation, increase in the number of old people and the high prevalence of chronic disease. It indicated that evidence implies now that health promotion strategies can be effective but comprehensive, settings-based and participative approaches provide the best likelihood of success.

The declaration also stressed that new responses were needed to break down traditional boundaries, and identified five priority areas for action: (1) the promotion of social responsibility for health by all interests concerned, (2) increased investments for health development, (3) the consolidation and expansion of existing partnerships, (4) an increase in community capacity and individual empowerment and (5) securing an infrastructure for health promotion. Finally the declaration called for action by means of the formation of a global health promotion alliance with a series of priorities arising from the issues addressed earlier. These included raising awareness of the changing determinants of health, supporting collaborations and networks, mobilising resources, accumulating knowledge on best practice, enabling shared learning, promoting solidarity in action and fostering transparency and accountability in health promotion.

In the multi-disciplinary Tower of Babel that is health promotion (Kelleher 1996), many people have addressed these issues in different ways but have not necessarily reached robust conclusions, let alone a central definition or a defining theory. It is clear that health promotion is a political movement, but is it also a new discipline or a multi-discipline – and should it be? It is appropriate in this context to review the implications for the health promotion movement of the five recommended key areas for action.

SOCIAL RESPONSIBILITY, ALLIANCES AND FRAMEWORKS

Who has responsibility for the health of individuals and populations? A recent review reminded us that a handful of people enjoy enormous global influence generally (Kickbusch 1996). Those who control the media and communications wield power on a scale beyond the comprehension of most people (Catford 1995). Great trepidation has been generated by the question of whether an elementary coding error in computer date systems, for which no-one has any apparent accountability to society, could paralyse the planet or ludicrously divert resources on an uncountable scale to rectify the problem. Across Europe over the next two years the currency systems will alter irrevocably, perhaps with profound economic implications. Individuals everywhere are dependent on each other and on mutually shared resources. In the case of food supply as an example, in Ireland a small number of people purchase food for supermarket supply and distribution which in effect limits the choice and access of an entire population (Kelleher and Friel 1996). On the one hand we are seeing tighter central regulation at federal level in both the United States and the European Union, but there also remain huge issues of public accountability on the part of agencies at statutory level and an ever-increasing need to provide for explicit consumer representative voices. How is this to be achieved in an equitable fashion and how will health impact become a part of it? As a start there needs to be a cross-sectoral review of public policy to assess likely health impact.

The conference in Jakarta was opened by the then President Soeharto. Indonesia is a diverse island archipelago in the tropics which was governed by the same regime over many years and made considerable economic progress during that time. Its importance to the region was subsequently seen in the economic crisis which struck South-east Asia at the end of 1997. However, charges of corruption had been levelled repeatedly at the government, the election system had been criticised and most controversially its invasion of neighbouring East Timor in the 1970s was a cause of international criticism and local dissent. Soeharto spoke of Unity in Diversity, his country's national motto, expressing tolerance for its ethnic and religious minorities, and of its five-part holistic value system. (It is certainly very evident that religious symbols contribute prominently to public expressions of meaning in Indonesian society.) The speech presented Indonesia's socio-economic and health service achievements in the holistic language of health promotion. There were striking figures quoted in terms of health gain, but also disappointments for a family-oriented society in that maternal mortality was still 390/100,000 births (see Furedi's contribution to this book for further discussion on issues of reproductive health or population control). The address highlighted a paradox. I can imagine no leader of the democratic Western world delivering a speech with an equivalent concept of what constitutes health and well-being or a public policy more apparently oriented towards health-promotion development, yet the principles of democratic government we believe we have achieved in our own region appear to be nothing like as well developed in Indonesia. This is not to say that politicians here do not accept the social principles common to health promotion. A former premier of the Republic of Ireland, Dr Garret FitzGerald, indicated four advances that made him proud to be European: the Council of Europe concept of human rights, the conviction that the rich North is under an obligation to aid the poor South, a profound and total rejection of war as an instrument of policy and the growth of ecological consciousness (FitzGerald, *Irish Times* 3 July 1998). These themes are all reiterated in the European WHO targets for the year 2000 (1985), the only difference being that they are explicitly linked to health status in the latter document. For politicians in the main, however, these are social values not explicitly driven by health impact. In Ireland we have had a policy of cross-sectoral collaboration on health matters over six administrations but little explicit utilisation of the mechanism to drive public policy on health-related matters (Department of Health 1994; Kelleher 1993, 1996).

In Jakarta we heard of health challenges as seen by the representatives of four continents. The Hungarian Minister for Health, Dr Kokeny, described the changes in his society in terms of the traditional chronic diseases, like cancer and cardiovascular disease, which are now emerging, but also the change in social and political thinking in the last decade. Later in the conference his compatriot Dr Peter Makara would describe the experience of delivering health care to the migrant minority of gypsies. As we are well aware, Eastern Europe as a whole has seen profound socio-political changes in health status in recent years and the impact on population health is potentially considerable (Bobak and Marmot 1995). We also heard of the health-care delivery problems posed by huge distance and low population density in the Polynesian Islands. Dr Manguyu, president of the Medical Women's International Association, described the post-colonial legacy in Africa. Foreigners can have little appreciation of the diversity of peoples on the continent and the struggles for change in the face of enormous economic hardship and an unprecedented clash of cultures. This was also echoed later by another delegate from Nigeria, describing the struggle to move away from hospital-based élite services for a minority to primary care-based services for a majority that accept, respect and assimilate millennia-old systems of traditional health care (*cf.* Allen in this volume). In his book on the development of the primary health-care system in Nigeria, Professor Egwu (1996) states that policy-makers should take cognisance of the fact that traditional practices are ingrained, have predated Western medicine and remain the alternative sources of care for about 80% of rural people in Nigeria who have no access to orthodox health care. He adds that coverage of the general population with health services was never the objective of colonial or early post-colonial services, which were selective and for the privileged few. Professor David Mc Queen of the Centre for Disease Control in Atlanta reminded us of the complex socio-political and cultural environments in which we were attempting to forge change and of the geo-political singularity of large areas of the world – a mega-country like the United States being rather different from the mega-country of Indonesia.

There was concern at the conference to ensure a strong political affirmation while at the same time recognising the diversity of cultures. For those from a 'developed', northern hemisphere perspective a reiteration of human rights and the free participation of individuals in society were crucial starting points. Yet at another level it was asserted by other participants that much could be achieved with political will, without necessarily starting from the same ideological base. Is this a question of semantics? Is there a significant difference for the purposes of promoting population health, as opposed to promoting social well-being, whether the prevailing political structure could be defined as a democracy, a participative government structure or a supportive structure? When public health and health promotion moved beyond the so-called reductionist biomedical paradigm such questions became fundamental, but the in-depth research to examine them has not necessarily followed. One articulate participant reminded us from the floor that this century will probably be remembered for three social developments: the fall in colonialism, the challenge to racialist thinking and the empowerment of women, all three, she believed, being fundamental to the determination of health in societies. I myself chaired a session on the role of international conventions in promoting health. What emerged chiefly from the discussion was the diversity of interpretation from country to country, the lack of any explicit sanction for violations and the range of responses involved – from countries who were prepared to sign up to such conventions without any intention of acting upon them to others who refused to sign as a matter of principle because they knew they were incapable of operationalising them at any practical level.

So much for traditional geographical boundaries. What about organisations whose influence reaches across such divides, and what obligations do they have? The chairman of a body called Private Sector for Health Promotion stressed the resources, goodwill and existing record of philanthropy of the private industrial sector. This triggered widespread informal debate among various participants over the next two days, which culminated in a discussion in one of the networking sessions on the complex ethics involved in such partnerships. On the one hand we know that such resources could be crucial and that public service inclinations should be tapped if at all possible for the common good. However, this benign capitalist vision did not appeal to everyone present. There were those who believe that industrial conglomerates wield too much power and influence in product-dissemination or are concerned about the impact of some industries on the environment. There are also unresolved conflicts of interest such as the widespread problem with the supply of basic generic medicines, the competition of baby formula products against breastfeeding, or the mass production and supply of so-called health demoting dietary products. These socio-political questions highlight another paradox. Channelling resources of private enterprise into some aspects of health care can be highly beneficial for some. In America, for instance, workplace health promotion based on education for personal lifestyle and health care has been effective (O'Donnell 1996), though undoubtedly driven by the imperatives of private insurance health care (Pelletier 1996). As another example, the lobbying power of those with acquired immuno-deficiency syndrome in the United States over the last two decades has meant the development of effective if highly expensive multiple drug therapy; new treatments such as protease inhibitors would not have been developed without adequate investment (Hirshell and Francioli 1998). Meanwhile in sub-Saharan Africa the death toll continues unabated in the absence of comparable resources. Would it be appropriate for the health promotion movement to provide sustained, united advocacy on the potential public health impact of *laissez-faire* capitalism or should we work to maximise pragmatic alliances to accept health-care benefits as they arise, even if in the main they are highly selective? These are not new debates but they are becoming more pressing and more mainstream all the time.

INCREASED INVESTMENTS FOR HEALTH DEVELOPMENT

There is at present no obligation on any country to invest for health and well-being. Some countries, like Canada, have invested in such initiatives over a twenty-year period, harnessing the various agencies involved and attempting to earmark and ringfence resources (Health Canada/Sante Canada 1998). For the most part, health expenditure in most countries goes on care of the sick and there is relatively little expenditure on health promotion. Economic analysis has been confined to cost-effectiveness assessments of particular intervention programmes with little focus on a much more ambitious social or opportunity-cost analysis (Phillips 1997).

Dr Illona Kickbusch, Director at the time of the meeting of Health Promotion at the World Health Organisation, whose influence in the field has been far-reaching in the last decade, stressed at the outset the lack of political will world-wide really to tackle poverty or health inequality and the widespread inequity in income distribution (Kickbusch 1997). On the positive side she emphasised that health was on the political agenda in a way unforeseen a decade ago, and she stressed the need to emphasise health gain for populations and individuals as a social investment. She returned to a previous theme in suggesting we focus on salutogenic strategies (Antonovsky 1996), that is those things that promote or maintain health rather than a perpetual emphasis on the recording and monitoring of what reduces health. She stressed investment in health gain and a socio-political per-spective on solutions to global problems, which would mean tackling the conflicts that will arise when economic growth turns into unsustainable consumption. She cited the emergence of global networks of travel, transport and communication and the need critically to evaluate ways of using mass media to promote health (Kickbusch 1996).

Throughout these sessions the likely health issues in the next century were stressed: the massive population expansion, the mass growth of young people, the emergence of new epidemics of potentially manageable or even preventable conditions like diabetes and epilepsy. On the other side was the enormous potential influence of literacy and its impact, particularly on female independence. The potential impact of new media and technologies was also explored. The proposed designed use of soap opera as an educational tool was asserted by Sammy Fox, a television executive from the United States, who stressed the high-reach power, emotional impact and credibility of specific story lines as in the AIDS victim in a popular US hospital soap. We also heard about use of radio networks in Tanzania, an adult education initiative using both printed and television materials in Africa and most effectively the use of a mainstream prime-time soap to promote the predicament of a young married Indian woman. There were also a series of workshops over the week on examples of health promotion in action, in the range of settings, in relation to specific issues like tobacco control and women's health and examples of primary-care development in various parts of Indonesia itself.

HOW DO WE INCREASE COMMUNITY CAPACITY AND INDIVIDUAL EMPOWERMENT?

This is an issue of prime importance to health promotion since it goes to the heart of its methodological approach. The concepts of salutogenesis and social capital were repeatedly emphasised at the meeting. In essence this means that positive characteristics of both individuals and communities exist and could be expanded. Social capital was recently defined as the degree of social cohesion which exists in communities. It refers to the processes between people which establish networks, norms and social trust and facilitate co-ordination and co-operation for mutual benefit (Nutbeam 1998b). What is the evidence that social capital is health-promoting and how might it be exploited? First we need to have a concept of positive health that stands up to scrutiny. Individuals who are autonomous, who function in day-to-day life or who feel well may all be in a state of health or not, but it is difficult to measure what these states connote, how they are preserved and how they translate into long-term protection from disease-specific onslaughts. For instance a person with good mental health may not succumb to depression even in adverse social circumstances but will he or she avoid cancer or heart disease? Salutogenesis-based scales have been shown to vary in usefulness in predicting different disease patterns (Davey Smith and Egger 1997; Siegrist 1993). The advocate of holism might dismiss such a reductionist approach but the basic issue is whether personal development is designed to promote individual well-being (a subjective state related inextricably to inter-personal relationships and life satisfaction) as an end in itself, whether such personal development is a means to empower individuals to exert their own choices or finally whether it is a process of intervention that increases the probability of pre-defined health choices that may reduce the risk of specific diseases.

As is fairly self-evident, whatever model of social or community development is promoted, over the last twenty years we have seen a movement in three phases, from traditional preventive medicine strategies to identify and modify risk factors at individual and community level, through to quasi-experimental community studies of ever-increasing design complexity (Commit Research Group 1995; Elliott *et al.* 1998), to more holistic community-development interventions (Baum 1998; Gillies 1998). Reductionist, mechanistic approaches have given way to more constructionist approaches that seek to build on individual experience and capacity and to understand qualitatively what such life experiences mean. Social capital or capacity-building approaches make the assumption that communities with good communication networks and supports and a positive cultural identity will enhance both individual and community well-being and hence promote health. As in the case of salutogenesis there remain questions and paradoxes however. It is likely that such initiatives might be mediated in various ways. First, the creation of social norms for certain types of health behaviours might be influential. This is well supported by traditional biomedical and community psychology literature. It also raises questions about the ethics and motivation for such social engineering (Seedhouse 1997). Secondly, it may enhance social support for vulnerable individuals, particularly by extended family networks. In turn those satisfied with their social circumstances might well be more amenable to novel health messages. The well-established reality that the affluent tend to change lifestyles more readily than the less well off may be explained in part because they identify with the message-givers better and have the resources to act upon new information.

Whatever the explanation, recent studies do demonstrate benefits for individuals which are apparently attributable to their social circumstances (Hawe 1998; Putnam 1993). This ecological approach to health promotion (Green *et al.* 1996) finds echoes in traditional ecological epidemiology too (Marmot 1996). However, if it has already proven difficult to show meaningful health gains in more traditional models of community intervention, then it is likely to be even more complex using this approach. For this reason a range of new methodological approaches are advocated, as well as the explicit development of intermediate markers. Tones, Edmondson and Labonte (see their contributions in this volume), like Nutbeam (1998a) and Gillies (1998) at the Jakarta Conference, have all raised these issues. Nutbeam suggests a six-stage development model for the evaluation of health-promotion programmes and a new approach to outcome measures which would include specific health-promotion measures such as health literacy, evidence of social influence and action, and indicators of public policy change and organisational practice. Gillies reviewed a wide range of case studies from different cultures and contexts using health-promotion parameters. In recent times within the epidemiology field there has been increasing debate about the use of mechanistic, individual-level versus more ecological approaches (Shy 1997) and the possibility that important effects may be missed by focusing exclusively on individuals rather than on other factors at a social or group level. Within this book there are several contributions at a quantitative level to this debate (See Davey Smith *et al.*, McPherson and Dean). However, the precise relationship between individuals' constitutions and inclinations, their societal circumstances and their health behaviours will remain extraordinarily complex to delineate. The fundamental policy question of when to intervene and for what purpose remains. There will continue to be criticism for what some scientists in particular see as hasty and ill-founded advocacy for social reform without adequate scientific data to support the case (Feinstein 1997).

Perhaps some of the difficulties are even more basic. As Seedhouse (1997) has recently pointed out, our definition of health itself, as being in effect synonymous with well-being, is problematic and may have to be reviewed if we are to remain coherent. Biomedicine assumes a basic measurable reality and is certainly driven by a centuries-old code of ethics which begins with the age-old aphorism of *Primum non nocere*, or First do not harm. Further, when intervention is planned, individual explanation and consent is normally sought. When we extend this concept to a much wider range of determinants the issue is not whether we use a reductionist or a construc-tionist approach but whether we are value-driven or not and how those values might be formulated.

Those who assert the relativism of knowledge and the impossibility of a value-free assessment of a research question would contend that there are therefore no objective reasons for promoting health or indeed any objective definition of health but instead that there are only competing agendas whose benefits are a matter of interpretation. This has proved highly creative in exploring motivation, attitudes and beliefs but it can foster remarkable confusion in day-to-day health-promotion practice. The move from observation to intervention requires ethical clarification of motivation and as an active process health promotion is invariably a political statement of some kind. Seedhouse asserts that values drive health promotion but that moral philosophy indicates that not all values are equal. He outlines three main types of health promotion: 'medical', 'social' and 'good life'. Medical health promotion is characterised by prudence, utilitarianism and a conservative interpretation of the *status quo*. Social health promotion is informed by egalitarianism, social democracy and socialist or Marxist-type politics. Good life health promotion implies well-being and its attainment as a goal, but it is not primarily about health directly, rather one's conception of the conditions required for a good life. Wörner expands on this issue in this volume also. While Seedhouse deconstructs much theoretical thinking about health-promotion philosophy and practice, his own suggested 'foundations' model is, for this reader at least, an unsatisfactory anti-climax. Nonetheless it will be interesting to see where the debate takes us over the next decade of health promotion. However, the arid discussion about quantitative and qualitative methodologies must move on. Both approaches have become more sophisticated in recent years and now, I believe, share much in common. We must address the question, based on our needs, and assume that some things work and some things do not. Perhaps the most obvious sign of the coming-of-age of any field of activity is being able to say occasionally, or even often, that we got it wrong, and even better to agree when we get it right.

Meanwhile, is health promotion a movement, a discipline or a multi-discpline activity? All the signs are that health promotion as a concept is now on a sound footing at policy level; the framework provided by the Ottawa Charter has provided a means of interpretation across countries and continents, as witnessed by the reports at Jakarta. Within the health care and education sectors there is support for a cadre of workers whose primary purpose is public education and personal skills development, the provision of support and models of good practice for others whose work contains some health-promoting function, and social advocacy related to health-demoting activities. It might be more coherent to organise such departments by function, according to the five components of the Ottawa framework, rather than around topics or settings as at present. However, there is also a huge gap in health promotion policy skills which needs to be filled by political scientists and economists and which must develop over the next decade. There are too few people in public bodies who understand these macro-issues and who also have health promotion as a part of their priority or work-brief. We have moved beyond the skills of scientists and traditional health professionals and we need to foster the appropriate expertise. It remains to be seen how explicitly community projects need to be developed for the purposes of health promotion or whether these should be assumed into the normal provisions of public amenities and services. Good mending should be invisible. As Curtin (1999) points out, while health promotion is currently shifting towards a community development paradigm, such strategies have been part of social policy for decades and in Ireland there is a long history of such approaches since the foundation of the new state. This is tremendously exciting innovative research, but its challenges are immense.

CONCLUSIONS

Were the objectives of the meeting met? Clearly for the European delegation there was a reminder that the challenges to health truly are global. If we see reproduced in the Asian countries the chronic disease patterns of the Western world (as there is every reason to believe) there will be major need to address such health problems in the next century. The scope for global communication through media is considerable but there will be tensions between the entertainment/private enterprise ethic and the public service/ education ethic which have not yet been addressed in any depth. Nor were issues of financing broached. The meeting also touched upon, but did not resolve, some of the problems about health–promotion definition and implementation, both from an academic and a practical level. The final Jakarta Declaration re-endorsed the principles of the Ottawa Charter and was more explicit than previously on the need to foster partnerships and alliances to address the health agenda it summarised. A potential tension exists between disease-specific, reductionist public-health policies (which tackle individual lifestyle factors such as smoking or alcohol abuse) as opposed to the more holistic social capital approach, which stresses that successful changes in lifestyle patterns will only be resolved by more profound public policy reforms in areas which impact on health behaviours. It is likely that these issues will need to be addressed in the coming few years and existing infrastructures, both for funding and implementing health–promotion initiatives, will need to be reviewed in this light. The theoretical and academic basis for newer approaches, particularly of positive health and social capital, is under-developed in this specific field as yet and this problem may, if neglected, undermine the political strategy presently in train. There is a formidable operational task ahead for those charged with implementing the aspirations of the Jakarta Declaration and, more significantly perhaps, for those charged with evaluating its long-term impact.

ACKNOWLEDGEMENTS

Cecily Kelleher was funded to attend the meeting in Jakarta in part by the European Commission and was invited to attend in a personal capacity by the World Health Organisation. The views are the author's personal reflections.

REFERENCES

Antonovsky, A., 1993. 'The Sense of Coherence as a Determinant of Health', in Beattie *et al.*, eds., *Health and Wellbeing: A Reader*. London: Macmillan.

Antonovsky, A., 1996. 'The Salutogenic Model as Theory to Guide Health Promotion', *Health Promotion International*, 11: pp. 11–19.

Baum, F., 1998. 'Measuring Effectiveness in Community-Based Health Promotion', in J.K. Davies and G. MacDonald, eds., *Quality, Evidence and Effectiveness in Health Promotion: Striving for Certainties*. London: Routledge.

Bobak, M., and Marmot, M.G., 1995. 'The East/West Mortality Divide and Its Potential Explanations: Proposed Research Agenda', *British Medical Journal*, 312: pp. 421–5.

Catford, J., 1995. 'The Mass Media is Dead: Long Live the Multimedia', *Health Promotion International*, 10: pp. 247–53.

Catford, J., 1998. 'Social Entrepreneurs Are Vital for Health Promotion – but They Need Supportive Environments too', *Health Promotion International*, 13: pp. 95–8.

Commit Research Group, 1995. Community Intervention Trial for Smoking Cessation (Commit). II: Changes in Adult Smoking Prevalence', *American Journal of Public Health*, 85: pp. 193–200.

Curtin, C., 1999. 'Evolution, Current Trends and Future Issues for Community Development in the Irish Republic'. Paper presented to Health Promotion Winter School, North-Eastern Health Board, Dundalk.

Davey Smith, G., and Egger, M., 1997. 'Changes in Population Distribution in Sense of Coherence Do not Explain Changes in Overall Mortality' *British Medical Journal*: pp. 315, 490.

Davies, J.K., and MacDonald, G., 1998. *Quality Evidence and Effectiveness in Health Promotion: Striving for Certainties*. London: Routledge.

Department of Health and Children, 1994. *Shaping a Healthier Future: A Strategy for Health Care in the 1990s*. Dublin: Government Publications Office.

Elliott, S.J., Taylor, S.M.N., Cameron, R., and Schabas, R., 1998. 'Assessing Public Health Capacity to Support Community-Based Heart Health Promotion: The Canadian Heart Health Initiative Ontario Project (CHHIOP)', *Health Education Research*, 13: pp. 607–23.

Egwu, I.N., 1996. *Primary Health Care System in Nigeria: Theory, Practice and Perspectives*. Surelere, Lagos: Elmore.

Feinstein, A.R., 1997. 'Biases Introduced by Confounding and Imperfect Retrospective and Prospective Exposure Assessments', in B.R. Butterworth, ed., *What Risk? Science, Politics and Health*. Oxford: Heinemann.

Gillies, P., 1998. 'Effectiveness of Alliances and Partnerships for Health Promotion', *Health Promotion International*, 13: pp. 99–120.

Green, L.W., Richard, L., and Potvin, L., and 1996. 'Ecological Foundations of Health Promotion', *Health Promotion*, 16: pp. 270–82.

Hawe, P., 1998. 'Making Sense of Context-Level Influences on Health', *Health Education Research*, 13: p. iii.

Health Canada/Sante Canada, 1998. 'Health Promotion in Canada: A Case Study', *Health Promotion International*, 13: p. 27.

Hirshell, B., and Francioli, P., 1998. 'Progress and Problems in the Fight against AIDS', *New England Journal of Medicine*, 13: pp. 906–8.

Kelleher, C., 1993. *Measures to Promote Health and Autonomy for Older People: A Position Paper*. Dublin: National Council for the Elderly, publication no. 26.

Kelleher, C., 1995. 'Health Promotion: Shades of Lewis Carroll', *Journal of Epidemiology and Community Health*, 49: p. 4.

Kelleher, C., 1996. 'Education and Training in Health Promotion: Theory and Methods', *Health Promotion International*, 11: pp. 47–55.

Kelleher, C., 1998. 'Evaluating Health Promotion in Four Key Settings', in J.K. Davies and G. MacDonald, eds., *Quality, Evidence and Effectiveness in Health Promotion: Striving for Certainties*. London: Routledge.

Kelleher, C., and Friel, S., 1996. Nutrition Surveillance in Ireland: *Proceedings of the Nutrition Society*, 55: pp. 689–97.

Kickbusch, I., 1996. 'New Players for a New Era: How up to Date is Health Promotion?', *Health Promotion International*, 11: pp. 259–63.

Kickbusch, I., 1997. 'Think Health: What Makes a Difference?' *Health Promotion International*, 12: pp. 265–73.

Labonte, R., 1989. 'Community Health Promotion Strategies', in C.J. Martin and D.V. McQueen, eds., *Readings for a New Public Health*. Edinburgh: Edinburgh University Press.

Marmot, M.G., 1996. 'Improvement of Social Environment to Improve Health', *Lancet*, 351: pp. 57–60.

Nutbeam, D., 1998a. 'Evaluating Health Promotion: Progress, Problems and Solutions', *Health Promotion International*, 13: pp. 27–45.

Nutbeam, D., 1998b. 'Health Promotion Glossary', *Health Promotion International*, 13: pp. 349–64.

O'Donnell, M., 1996. Editorial. *American Journal of Health Promotion*, 10: p. 424.

Pelletier, K.R, 1996. 'A Review and Analysis of the Cost Effective Outcome Studies of Comprehensive Health Promotion and Disease Prevention Programs at the Worksite: 1993–1995 Update', *American Journal of Health Promotion*, 10: pp. 380–9.

Phillips, C., 1997. *Economic Evaluation and Health Promotion*. Aldershot: Avebury.

Putnam, P., 1993. *Making Democracy Work*. Princeton, NJ: Princeton University Press.

Seedhouse, D., 1997. *Health Promotion: Philosophy, Prejudice and Practice*. Chichester: Wiley.

Shy, C.M., 1997. 'The Failure of Academic Epidemiology: Witness for the Prosecution', *American Journal of Epidemiology*, 145: pp. 479–84.

Siegrist, J., 1993. 'Sense of Coherence and Sociology of Emotions', *Social Science and Medicine*, 37: pp. 978–9.

World Health Organisation, 1985. *Targets for Health for All*. Copenhagen: World
    Health Organisation Regional Office for Europe.
World Health Organisation, 1986. *The Ottawa Charter on Health Promotion*. Ottawa:
    Canadian Public Health Association.
World Health Organisation, 1988. *Healthy Public Policy: Adelaide Recommendations*.
    Geneva: WHO Health Education and Promotion Unit.
World Health Organisation, 1991. *Supportive Environments for Health: The
    Sundsvall Statement*. Geneva: WHO Health Education and Promotion Unit.
World Health Organisation, 1997. 'The Jakarta Declaration on Leading health
    promotion into the 21st Century' *Health Promotion International*, 12: pp. 261–4.

SIX

Health Promotion and the Study of Cultural Practices

RICCA EDMONDSON

INTRODUCTION

In the field of health promotion, questions of health and health research are increasingly often being linked with questions of cultural attitudes and practices and their interdisciplinary study. Both health-related behaviour and patterns of illness vary according to cultural setting; there are strong cultural influences on what people feel they should do to keep healthy, on how they experience pain and on behaviour which contributes to getting sick. Neither individual nor societal life, nor even human physicality, can be fully understood without taking cultural factors into account (and in different ways most of the contributions to this collection respond to this fact). Hence it is inevitable that health promotion as an enterprise should seek to blend insights from different approaches to understanding cultures with knowledge from fields such as medicine, psychology, political science and sociology; but these are all fast-evolving areas in which canons of research are various and sometimes relatively fluid. One specificity of health promotion research consists, therefore, in its pressing need to establish some congruence between heterogeneous methods if it is to direct them to coherent ends. In other fields, political science or sociology for example, researchers are able to spend most of their lives in isolation from those of their peers who espouse rival philosophies of enquiry, agreeing to differ and not responding in great detail to each other's priorities and values. This cannot be the case in health promotion, which embodies unique pressures to interdisciplinary understanding. If health is *inherently* multi-dimensional, then a preoccupation with promoting health means that researchers must learn how to be open to all relevant fields, not just the congenial few, and they must be prepared to assess each in appropriate terms. But multi-disciplinarity, like multicultural living in other fields, brings with it clashes which are enormously difficult to overcome. The validity of unfamiliar methods, priorities and perspectives can be acknowledged in principle

71

without becoming intelligible when one is confronted with them in day-to-day practice, still less so when one is required to put one's trust in their results. This paper explores some concepts and methods required for studying health-relevant aspects of cultures. It argues too that some problems associated with a multidisciplinary research field can be confronted more constructively if we interrogate rarely-acknowledged problems in studying cultures themselves; that is, the paper is concerned with the cultures of health-related disciplines as well as with cultural aspects of health-related behaviour in everyday life.

Understanding cultural behaviour is currently widely equated with understanding *meaning* (Edmondson 1997; Geertz 1973; Hall 1997; Labonte *et al.* in this collection). An action, event or other phenomenon becomes part of social interaction in the course of processes which construe or interpret it in some way which attach meaning to it. This is far from implying that we can interpret events however we like, or that it does not matter how we interpret them (see the contribution by Tones in this volume). The content of any social interpretation derives largely from conventions which are shared in the settings inhabited by the individuals or groups doing the interpreting; shared conventions are not changeable at will, but involve criteria and practices which are established in such a way that they constitute more or less hard-and-fast conditions of public living. A patient cannot be a patient, a health visitor cannot be a health visitor, without engaging in practices which are intelligible in terms of the expectations attached to those positions. This does not mean that patients and health visitors have no choice about what they do, only that their behaviour needs to be generally comprehensible in terms of shared ideas about being a patient or being a health visitor; even when it contradicts these expectations, for example because the patient in question is herself also a doctor, people around can usually form an approximate idea of why it does. Most students of culture, at this point, leave some space in their analysis of such processes for the contribution to interpretation of the actor and of the agent doing the interpreting. But this already leads to clashes in the context of health promotion, for proponents of the 'harder' sciences characteristically describe themselves as seeking the 'determinants' of health behaviour, whereas for those emphasising the role of meanings this is conceptual anathema: it undercuts the entire process of enquiry into what, in the ebb and flow of public and private meanings, influences what, and what forms of influence are concerned.

In order to explore in more detail what is involved in cultural analysis, we need to recall that meaning itself can be conveyed both linguistically and non-linguistically; this accounts for the uneuphonious sociological expression 'attitudes and behaviour' when the interpretation of cultural conduct is concerned, for we need a wide range of types of access to the meanings people convey. Here I shall discuss health-related *communication*, underlining the fact that we find out what individuals (and groups, organisations and agencies) think and feel about health by explicating what they do as well as what they say. I want to emphasise, first, that explicating this communication presupposes a conception of what is meant by 'attitudes and behaviour' which responds to the fact that health-related communication, perhaps even more than communication in most other socio-cultural fields, is typically incomplete on a surface level. At least some feelings, ideals, fears and aspirations related to health are characteristically so deeply-rooted that their holders do not and cannot report on them exhaustively at an ordinary conversational level (some reasons for this are explored below). This has important practical implications for both qualitative and quantitative research. Nobody, not even the most sensitive of ethnographic interviewers, can generally expect to elicit from respondents sets of research sentences which in direct, complete and unproblematic fashion make their health-related views, feelings and conduct accessible to all third parties, whoever they may be. For reasons explained below, the expression of meaning is usually incomplete, especially where phenomena such as health are concerned, and is usually embedded in its context of origin. To make sense in a new context, it needs to undergo operations which make explicit for readers of the research what might have been obvious but unsaid among respondents, and it requires re-casting in a form which, in recipients' contexts (and these themselves will be various), communicate something as close as possible to what the original respondents were in effect (if not always intentionally) conveying. Hence there is always the need for an explication of meaning – hermeneutics – which mediates between the worlds of *particular* respondents, researchers and readers; qualitative research results may well need to be re-presented as their readers' worlds of meaning change (Edmondson 1984). This is clearly a monumental set of tasks, but it can hardly be avoided if cultural aspects of health-related behaviour are to be taken seriously. Decontextualised accounts of meaning, such as those produced in large-scale surveys, can be useful and suggestive, but by themselves they cannot make adequate (let alone complete) our understanding of what actors mean by their health-related communication and conduct; hence, they should not be offered by themselves but always require a hermeneutic setting.

But I shall argue here that hermeneutic methods themselves, in health-related research as elsewhere, need to embody more explicit procedures if they are to avoid the appearance of chaotic intuitivism and if they are to become intelligible to recipients with different research practices. In particular, I shall argue that they need to incorporate methods from the philosophy of language in order to address deep-level conceptual differences, and to be furnished with practices for combining these with ethnographic methods in a manner which responds to the context-relatedness of researchers', respondents' and recipients' interpretations without collapsing into relativism. I shall claim, then, that many health-related aspects of culture, many health-related aspects of group and individual attitudes and behaviour, belong to domains which are inadequately explicated by either action-level or conventionally theorised forms of communication. Action-level communication I take to be located around the world of objects and practices – building houses, buying cars, mending limbs; at a more theoretical level, the one on which academic disciplines such as engineering, sociology, medicine or biology are chiefly situated, we can study how and why these procedures take place. At another level still, we find philosophical explication of the concepts and practices used in engineering or biology – the philosophy of science – and the concepts and practices used in everyday life: what we mean by intention, decision, moral distinction and so on. Much current qualitative and quantitative research in the social sciences proceeds on the assumption that health-related behaviour can be accounted for in terms of discourse confined to the first two levels; it assumes that even if people do not always mean much the same thing by 'health', 'ageing', 'discomfort' and so on, what they do mean can be clarified in terms of everyday distinctions, supplemented by theoretical accounts of, for instance, the range and function of particular types of usage. On this view, different attitudes to health can be differentiated, like different forms of electric current or different preferences in constructing walls, without proceeding to meta-levels of enquiry. These research opinions – in my view, mistaken ones – have for the most part gone unchallenged by philosophers, for in philosophical enquiry, as in psychology, it has been assumed that accounts of what 'decisions', 'preferences' or 'beliefs' consist of are more or less culture- and context-invariant. Both Winch (1958) and Habermas (1981), for instance, take it that the latter areas of enquiry are purely the province of philosophy and that their results can be taken for granted in the explication of social behaviour. Neither of these sets of assumptions is correct. Much health-related communication cannot be understood unless we explicate notions of decision, intention, communication and relatedness to life at levels on which subjects themselves do not normally converse and do not wish to converse; and the items found on these levels precisely do vary between cultural and other contextual aspects of setting. Moreover, these hidden reaches matter: they inform and give coherence to 'attitudes and behaviour' on the other levels. If in the study of 'compliance', for example, we fail to appreciate that the behaviour of some groups of patients embodies conceptions of intention and decision-making which do not fit those of the model of the individual adopted in conventional medical discourse, these patients' behaviour will seem contradictory and incoherent, and methods intended to amend it will be inappropriate.

Thus the intricacies related to understanding and conveying the burden of respondents' communication about health have strong and definite implications for research methods. This applies to quantitative methods too; whatever operations quantitative researchers wish to use in order to study, for instance, the distribution of specific attitudes relating to health, they need first to establish how to understand communication about health, and whether questions about health can be devised which will function appropriately over settings where they may be interpreted differently by respondents. For health research, therefore, we need an approach to understanding communicative action which can respond to different levels of health-related talk and behaviour, which can do justice to the results of ethnographic methods and solve problems they raise, and which can also be made comprehensible in terms of the linguistic forms of non-qualitative approaches. Research methods in general should thus cease to be de-theoretised; theoretical understanding of the research object is part of the practical business of doing research.

In what follows I shall examine some grounds for these contentions in more detail. First, I shall look at the ways in which cultures work, and the implications these have for ways of understanding health-related communication. Then I shall turn to the ways in which individuals talk, and adumbrate some associated problems which need to be taken into account in ethnographic aspects of research in particular. Lastly, I shall try to draw some conclusions about how the resulting methodological strictures might impinge on health promotion as a discipline.

HOW CULTURES WORK

Questions about what cultures are and how their workings can be detected are fundamental to contemporary research not only in health promotion but in the humanities in general; yet twentieth-century views of culture have been ambiguous in the extreme. Cultures as such are repeatedly portrayed as both all-pervasive and ill-defined; the crucial importance of culture in public life is acknowledged, but it is hard to establish just how this importance takes effect. Perceived failures in contemporary culture are blamed for wide-ranging social problems; it is claimed, for example, that we live in a culture of greed or moral crisis or educational decay, or that the culture of contemporary capitalism makes people more inclined to become depressed and ill (James 1997); but unambiguous signs of these developments are difficult to establish – still more so their causes. Despite the enormous perceived significance of culture, systematic social-scientific analysis of just what cultures are and how they function is far from adequately advanced

(Alexander and Seidman 1990), and commentators characteristically proceed by selecting only those details of the contemporary setting which support their own cases. (Hence, Deutscher *et al.* went so far as to write in 1993 that in the course of this century we have actually grown worse at understanding 'qualitative' aspects of society, rather than better.) This chapter is predicated on the view that the root of these problems is a failure to come to grips with the operation of cultures.

Health promotion, therefore, is far from the only discipline to be inclined to lapse into an *ad-hoc* approach to cultural accounts. The types of evidence used in claims about culture are characterised throughout the social sciences by an eclectic mixture of society-wide generalisations and details of individual conduct; just what interrelations these are taken to have and how they might influence the inhabitants of the cultures concerned is left undecided. Thus it is taken for granted that macro-scale and micro-scale processes influence each other – but accounts which try to explain how this occurs, by linking the two directly, result in an implausible degree of determinism and can often be contradicted by empirical investigation. When we look on the meso-scale (Edmondson 1997b), we find that micro–macro interactions cannot be predicted *a priori*; the intervening processes are so complex that we cannot just read off one set from another. Starting from larger-scale accounts and trying to move downwards, we find that populations who seem to share broad cultural attitudes towards the environment, say, actually behave very differently in individual political settings (Aarts 1997; Rootes 1997); starting at a more personal level, we find that even when individuals do share given cultural attitudes – towards the politics of mine closures, for instance – behaviour based on those attitudes is shaped by responses to features of socio-political settings, some of which derive from larger-scale phenomena and whose actual forms can only be discovered empirically, not *a priori* (Beckwith 1997). It follows from this that cultural influences do not operate unchanged as between different scales of social phenomena – even though health promotion interventions, for instance those concerning 'healthy lifestyles', repeatedly assume that they do. Whole populations may well respond positively to endorsements of wholefood diets and plenty of exercise, in principle; what they find themselves doing in practice depends on interactions among an array of social phenomena which can hardly be conjectured but need to be discovered.

The development of research instruments to trace multi-layered social processes has been thwarted by the fluctuating nature of cultures themselves and of the perspectives on social action they afford: other people's behaviour can seem blindingly perspicuous, and it can (perhaps more often) appear fundamentally beyond comprehension. Moreover, though cultures can give the impression of being graspable in broad outline, and patches within these outlines may seem to be visible in detail – otherwise our social worlds would not make even what sense to us they do – they are capable of profound and rapid change. Even old hands at cultural manipulation – politicians or journalists – can find themselves astonished when what seemed to be insignificant items suddenly become important and those which used to be accepted as vital imperceptibly fade away. Like weather systems, cultures allow of a limited number of predictions, inspiring some confidence in observers until the unexpected occurrence of watersheds such as the year 1989; they eclipse the unruliness of the weather with their capacities for producing new phenomena and for eliminating old ones. It is not true that cultures can be understood just by looking at them or even just by living in them; familiarity with a culture can make its workings difficult to perceive because they come to seem inevitable, too obvious to account for. It is therefore not true that cultures consist of chaotic sets of individual actions which are basically incomprehensible, taken as wholes; but nor are they either rigid and oppressive determinants or systems of coherent regulations, clearly directing those who live within them.

When we consider the nature of the phenomena we are dealing with, these features of cultures and argument about cultures become explicable. Cultures and subcultures are clusters of habits, attitudes, behaviour and beliefs, both implicit and explicit, clusters which tend either to underscore or to discourage certain beliefs, feelings, assumptions and ways of life (any or all of which may be relevant to health-related behaviour); and it is inevitable that phenomena of this nature should be both highly significant and hard to track down. In order to persist as features structuring social worlds which contain ever new events and ever new combinations of members, cultures must be fluid and flexible. Virtually none of the components of culture, therefore, can be absolutely invariant or absolutely determining. Cultural routines require functional ambiguity: they need to be comprehensible in general terms, but also to accommodate adaptation and change by new actors in new settings. Intrinsically, therefore, they are incapable of exhaustive description. Lastly, it is neither necessary nor productive that knowledge of cultural routines should be complete or conscious. One achievement of cultural commonalities is to disguise or to render unimportant the extent of disagreement or misunderstanding among actors, a lack of cultural consensus which may not be important to a given piece of action in hand and whose acknowledgement would disrupt it. A health team, for example, functions by highlighting procedures and assumptions which the members have in common; each member may have separate views on the politics and psychology of health, and as long as these views are not relevant to the team's joint action they may be best unstated: revealing them tends either to be precipitated by a crisis or to cause one. Cultures work from day to day by seeming natural; *how* they work is not generally apparent to their inhabitants (and thus cannot be discovered merely by asking them). This cryptic nature has dysfunctional aspects, making cultures manipulable, deliberately and otherwise, for political or economic ends; but it is also inevitable, because even such daily activities as greeting, apologising, per-suading, reconciling, expressing affection or distance, are predicated precisely on the assumption that actors do not, normally, consciously manipulate the cultural means of achieving them.

This may appear to be a devastating scenario as far as empirical investigation is concerned. Many qualitative researchers do, apparently, survive by ignoring the complexities pointed to here, and one common research strategy, in which investigators strive to feel relaxed in their research contexts and simply record their impressions, might be termed the *faux-naïf*. Depending on the investigator's capacity for empathy with collective settings, this approach does on occasion yield useful work, though *demonstrating* that it is useful provides a bigger problem, since the method depends on not formulating any criteria it may satisfy. (The 1980 text *Alltag in der Anstalt*, by Fengler and Fengler, won prizes for describing the life of ward assistants in a mental hospital; its methodological apology remarked, with *chutzpah*, that no doubt the setting would have looked rather different to different observers.) In fact, though, many advances have been made in the qualitative investigation of cultures; much more attention is being paid, both in qualitative approaches in general and in health-related research in particular, to ethical and interpersonal interactions between what are (chiefly for the sake of brevity) still termed researchers and respondents, or to the problems of recording and communicating research (Denzin and Lincoln 1994; Gubrium and Sankar 1994). The most urgent need now is for an adequate theoretical conceptualisation of the methods being used, for their systematic implications have remained far from clear. And here, for all the emphasis we need to put on behaviour, central to conclusions about the study of meaning must be an appreciation of how language works and how it is used to communicate.

HOW PEOPLE SPEAK

Both on the parts of individuals and on the parts of agencies or governments, attitudes related to health may be expressed metaphorically, allusively, indirectly, incompletely; they are very likely to be expressed in ways which indicate that their bearers are unconscious of them. This does not mean that there is no place in health research for language which is as clear and explicit as its context allows; but this is a secondary, specialised communicative form, predicated on understanding the first. Here particular *words* – 'healthy' or 'unhealthy', 'old' or 'young', for example – may mean different things to different people; but (as Antonovsky (1996), for instance, emphasises) this is not so much a *terminological* problem, a problem of definition, as one symptomatic of entirely different *approaches* to *conceptualising* sickness, health and their human contexts. Differing national and subcultural attitudes to health and ageing are marked by the facts that people count each other as 'healthy', 'young' or otherwise in relation, among other things, to their capacities to perform very different sets of activities in very different ways (Williams 1983). People asked to assess personal relationships which have a bearing on health or on generational relations, even mothers and daughters who describe themselves as very close, show divergent conceptions about what these relationships amount to (O'Connor 1994). Carers for older people may be prepared to say that they have a 'good relationship' with an older person more often than they would confide in them or claim to share worldviews, approaches to living, or philosophies of life (O'Connor and Ruddle 1988); this raises questions about the diverse meanings of 'good relationship' which cannot be addressed without considering meta-levels with a bearing on interpretations of 'people', 'confiding' or 'relationships' in the different settings concerned.

Moving from public attitudes to public policy, we find that the aims of the latter may be expressed in terms of states of affairs which may be understood highly discrepantly among both policy-makers and the public. From the Ottawa Charter to policies for promoting healthy older age, where 'independence' and 'dignity' are repeatedly cited as *aims* of public policy (Eastern Health Board 1995), health policy is couched in terms which leave it far from clear how the success of these aims can be assessed. Either they are expressed in terms with incommensurate meanings at a variety of levels, or else measurable policy 'targets' – beds (un)occupied, phone alarms distributed – neglect sweeping aspects of the question in hand. Principles of community care have aroused major contemporary disputes centring on data connected with attitudes, habits, relationships and feelings, as well as with the opportunities, choices and constraints which policies allow or prohibit (Dalley 1988). Community care, moreover, is a case which illustrates the bearing of socio-political context on the understanding of policy. The arguments in connection with community care have not changed radically in the last twenty years; but community care is coming to be regarded with more scepticism in official circles in recent times, together with changes in shared habits of assigning priority and of estimating what it is reasonable to expect in public life. It is therefore not only the public whose language and attitudes need to be interpreted in their contexts, but policy-makers and professionals also.

Two important sets of problems arise here in connection with interpreting health-related attitudes. The first is connected with *what can be said*, and the second with *the way language is used*; both have considerable implications both for methodology and for theory (and have parallels in terms of non-linguistic communication also). It may be, first of all, that the language for a given set of attitudes has not (yet) been formulated in widely accepted terms. Some phenomena are too basic to be easily discussed; this may be one reason why we do not yet know enough about attitudes involved in family relationships (Finch 1989). Others do not happen to fit easily with dominant worldviews in their cultures and are thus seldom broached directly, though they may have profound effects throughout their settings, as in the case of attitudes to death or to visualising life-courses; it may even be that the dominant world-views of late industrial capitalism have had inhibiting effects on language about health itself. Then, some items or attitudes are verbalised in certain settings but not in others; one of the distinguishing features of 'subcultures' based on class, age, gender, ideology, ethnic attachment or lifestyle is that they verbalise particular selections of matters, and in particular ways. Physical states connected with the experience of drug-taking are extensively verbalised in some contexts but not in others; a distinguishing feature of the subculture associated with Alcoholics Anonymous may be the capacity it bestows on members to talk about things which might make little sense elsewhere (Mullarkey 1994).

It may be a socio-political question whether the appropriate public language for a particular feeling, attitude or belief has been developed in a given setting. One of the standard aims of political movements is to change the scope of accepted verbalisation, as in the case of feminism, environmentalism or the discipline of health promotion itself. All these movements have had extensive impacts on what can and cannot meaningfully be said, in contrast to the situation some decades ago. It is now possible to discuss the issue of women's empowerment in giving birth or in gynaecological examinations, or women's attitudes to their bodies (O'Connor 1995); to discuss the effects on health of noise or light pollution or of 'the quality' of the environment. The contemporary *Zeitgeist* allows us to see physical injuries and mishaps as matters for public compensation, and defines human motivation as a matter for which collectivities and states can be expected to take responsibility. Thus, accepted public languages affect what people can and do think, feel and say, shaping their self-expression. This does not imply that conceptual change in some regions of society will be reflected consistently everywhere. Despite developments in some aspects of conceptual climate, many respondents may continue to clothe their views in terms which were conventional in former settings, all the while *behaving* in ways at variance with what their language might imply. (Gender relationships offer a variety of such examples.)

Language *as such* is also used for very different reasons and in different ways. Experience of empirical research confronts one with the fact that for many respondents it may be more common to use language for negotiating, threatening or imagining than for the neutral expression of the contents of their minds – even though it is the latter function which is taken to be dominant in most quantitative and some qualitative methods of determining attitudes. In some social settings, certainly, it may be counted as 'natural' to see language as a means to self-revelation, a means by which one person can express feelings primarily in order that they should be understood by another. People who use, or try to use, language in this way tend to be unconscious of it as a specific attitude; but it is in fact a highly socially specific view of linguistic communication, one incrementally developed within European 'high culture' over the last two or three hundred years, with the Romantic movement as its high point. People located within rural cultures on the one hand, and those located in international bureaucracies on the other, tend to use language in very different ways, and serious misunderstandings can result from behaving as if they did not. Thus, using and understanding language itself differs between settings.

As far as research practice is concerned, these considerations demand that the researcher should not only try to learn how the people he or she is dealing with use language but should also try to meta-conceptualise these uses in ways respondents do not employ. Some questions cannot be asked at all, or can only be asked in certain ways, according to local usage – which will usually be influenced by patterns of social and political power and religious and traditional taboos, among other matters. In health studies, these apparently abstract considerations have immediate implications for both principles of policy and methods of interpretation. In relation to friendship and its relation to health in ageing, for instance, whether or not respondents' own relationships are premised on communication according to Romantic principles will have policy implications in terms of the inter-action available to residents of older people's homes. Will it be necessary to facilitate the continuance of long-established intimacies, or will residents prefer good-natured conversation on a more general level? A different, methodological, case relates to the attempt sometimes made in survey questions to elicit preferences by asking respondents what they *would* do in certain situations. In some cultural settings, there is little convention of using hypothetical statements to *report on* mental states; in settings where the main use of hypotheticals is to issue threats or promises, respondents react with discomfiture to hypotheticals used by researchers.

Descriptions of these different uses of language are almost never provided as meta-accounts by the people who employ them, even though in effect they help to constitute distinctive lifestyles and world-views. This too has practical research implications: these usages can only be accessed by accustoming oneself to the communicative practices of the group in question, learning both what the practices are and how to account for them (where there is, of course, no guarantee that all the members of a group being researched will share the same language-uses). It follows that there is no alternative to personal experience when interpreting responses; in this sense, hermeneutic and ethnographic methods are two sides of the same coin. Methods used in researching language can coincide with those which are appropriate for researching the attitudes prevalent in a shared setting, and both will entail learning what people do as well as what they say. For instance, rural language-uses often entail specific approaches to understanding what human beings are and how they function; this, by extension, casts light on the specificities of urban approaches. Attitudinal language itself may be less significant in rural cultures than in more individualistic, atomised, 'core' European cultures. Empirical research in the West of Ireland suggests that attitudes may be conceptualised in rural settings as largely *behavioural* matters; anyone wishing to express commitment, or kindness, say, is expected to demonstrate these through what is accepted as the appropriate behaviour – giving lifts, helping with daily tasks – over a considerable time-period (Edmondson 1994, 1996). Trying to convey them (i) instantly and (ii) by *verbalising* them may be considered puzzling or even destructive. By contrast, the accelerated time-frames of middle-class industrial cultures and the decline in regular, repeated contact between individuals has meant that, in other settings, speech has become accepted as *standing for* attitudes; this has altered the ontological status imputed to cognitive intentions (Edmondson 1997a). If health research to date has been, implicitly, more committed to the more academic and urban conceptualisation than to the rural one, it has created for itself problems in understanding the daily practices of a large proportion of its constituents, as well as omitting to consider the weaknesses in its own models of behaviour and behavioural change.

Understanding respondents' language, then, may require interaction in some form of 'participative' observation over an extended period spent in *acquiring respondents' communicative habits*. This furnishes not only the forms which respondents use for communication in general, but also their contents, and it has special advantages for health research; for far from being easily formulable in short-term interaction with strangers, many attitudes related to health or ageing may *best* be expressed indirectly, in a succession of settings. Some attitudes, indeed, can *only* be expressed indirectly; these may include attitudes to life and death, to one's body, to ageing, to physical well-being, or to the 'coherence' one perceives in the universe. This does not detract from the presumption that respondents and what they say should be at the centre of research. It does mean that health-related feelings, views and behaviour cannot necessarily be discovered by *eliciting propositions* purporting to describe respondents' inner lives. Many people are not in the habit of issuing such edicts about their internal selves; they may not wish to do so or enjoy doing so, and it may not be successful to try to distort their habitual forms of interaction by forcing them to do it.

This point underlines the intimate links between forms of behaviour and linguistic understanding, for meaning is frequently only perceptible during long sequences of interaction. An example relating to life-course decisions may be shown in the following.

> We used to have only four or five cows. People used to have several boys then, we had one. People were plentiful before the place got empty. They'd come at fifteen or sixteen with one shirt and a pair of socks wrapped up in newspaper and that's all they would have . . . There wouldn't be anything about paying him or anything, only that it was a fair day or something like that . . . Very many came from big families and they would be very glad to get their dinner anyway . . . There were a lot that used to make him eat in the scullery, you know. They were very conscious of their state in life that day, now. When he'd have a little money after a while he'd get a bicycle second-hand and he'd get a suit and he'd get a Woodbine and he'd be as good as any man at the dances . . . So he'd have a great time and after a couple of years a sister would send his passage to America and he'd go there . . . One of them, Sean Malley was his name and he had arrived at the stage when he had got quite stylish and his sister sent him the passage. He was sitting down eating breakfast and my mother said, 'Maybe, Sean, if you didn't go at all?' and he said, 'Well sure it couldn't be worse than this,' he said, and she was very offended with her two eggs and her brown bread . . . (transcript, 10.10.1995)

Narratives such as this, offered by respondents in rural Ireland in a variety of forms, have in common an intensely practical approach both to daily details which are remembered and recounted and to large ones, such as decisions to emigrate. Together these constitute an approach to life-course construction which emphasises *how* things were done rather than purporting to theorise (and such theories are anyway often spurious) about *why* they were done. Respondents prove highly resistant to discussing why they 'took decisions' (as an alternative approach would put it), preferring to concentrate on the way a whole context evolved. In meta-level terms, they evince scepticism about the entire concept of decision-taking as far as lifestyle decisions are concerned (note the compatibility between this observation and some made by Allen in this volume). For the purposes of this chapter, the crucial point is that such an attitude *could not be inferred by linguistic means* from *one* set of remarks such as the above, or even three or four. An *accumulation* of narratives with the same tenor is necessary in order for the researcher *to understand what the language is saying*; the researcher learns how to behave, how to communicate appropriately in his or her new setting. It is this, rather than the learning of new 'rules', that may be (or should have been) what Winch (1958) meant by 'learning how to go on' in social research.

Attitudes such as this approach to the life course, pervasive throughout a way of living, are highly relevant to health-related conduct; they suggest that certain approaches to inculcating habits connected with health or ageing (for instance, causal theoretical ones) might be found inappropriate by their audience. Implicitly, they are philosophically inappropriate. It may be theoretically problematical that this position is impossible to describe in the language used by respondents; *contra* the opinion espoused by Schutz (1962), Harre and Secord (1972) and, later, feminist researchers such as Oakley (1992), respondents may be (understandably) resistant to these accounts because they do not need or desire meta-descriptions of their own practices. More directly relevant here is the fact that the practice in question is not adequately characterised in terms of its use of identifiable, discrete *concepts* with determinate causal relations to what people do. (To this extent, incidentally, what might be termed a 'rural' approach to attitudes may be considered realistic rather than otherwise.) Attitudes are not cognitive items in respondents' minds which can be isolated, labelled and set out as elements in causal chains; they form aspects of *practices*, parts of living lives. Methods appropriate to discovering attitudes in cultural research, therefore, will not initially or standardly consist of once-off, briefly applied 'instruments', but will more often require elaboration located in processes of interaction with respondents themselves.

On completing such processes, in the nature of the case the researcher cannot offer *isolated* items of proof that they have been successful: this constitutes another problem in combining the language of quantitative and qualitative approaches, for the former aims to produce results which are communicable crisply and quickly, whereas with qualitative research it is not only the process of investigation which takes longer, but also the process of conveying results. Furthermore, the two methods differ even as regards some of their respective patterns of inference. Quotations such as the one above cannot *demonstrate* a conclusion; they can *illustrate* an attitude which the researcher will have learned as one learns any other system of communication – by methods which are partly unconscious. Their proper textual function is pedagogical rather than evidential (Edmondson 1984), interactive as much as logical: what they do is help the reader to conceptualise a general set of attitudes which the author claims, but cannot immediately prove conclusively, is current in the setting in question. (In the '*faux-naïf*' approach, the author's entire text tries to *exemplify* such attitudes.) This does not mean, of course, that qualitative authors' claims are immune to validation, for it can certainly be asked whether the writer in question can be judged to have followed methods and provided arguments which convincingly support the case being made, and it can be asked whether anyone else who visited the scene in question and was able to exemplify the attitudes described by the author would be considered by its indigenous population to be behaving intelligibly. This merely cannot usually be done *quickly*. (It is also likely that, if the account is a valid one, it will have determinable *corollaries* which can be sought empirically: some, perhaps, by non-qualitative means.) Communicative practices, therefore, must be studied using hermeneutic and ethnographic methods in order for the researcher to become a member of the communication community in question (even though, perhaps, an irritatingly self-conscious one); then, to the extent that concepts and practices in the new community differ from writers' and readers' native settings, methods which are partially philosophical must be used to analyse this communication. It is to this that we now turn.

THE ETHNOGRAPHIC AND PHILOSOPHICAL STUDY OF PRACTICES

It is generally unacknowledged in the methodology of qualitative sociology that some cultural habits and concepts need to be reconstructed at a meta-level, using specifically philosophical methods. Philosophers have been too incurious about how concepts are really used in the world around them to draw attention to this necessity, and they have also been too modest. Winch (1958), like others since, wrote that philosophers should not tell social scientists how to proceed; not only this, the original philosophers of language believed that they could gain access to a single public world by interrogating their own linguistic practices. But in fact there are many such public worlds, and several ways of communicating within them; we therefore require a wide range of empirical experience of actual usage, not only our own intuitions about what is correct. But here, sociologists for their parts need to be able to distinguish between levels of use, and this is rare in the contemporary setting (in which questions in epistemology and the sociology of knowledge are regularly confounded). We need not just gather 'information' about people's beliefs about health but, on a different epistemological level altogether, to reconstruct concepts relevant to health which are in use in specific settings. Reconstructing concepts means, in practice in the field, exposing oneself to considerable conceptual uncertainty; it means under-going, in interaction with others, the type of tentativeness, the retreat from taking anything for granted, which philosophers such as Austin or Urmson used in their non-interactive enquiries. The oft-suggested recourse of 'writing down everything' in qualitative fieldwork diaries is actually dangerous here; reconstructing concepts requires such radical uncertainty about what is going on that recording can be damaging, for in practice and in a hurry it reduces events to the investigator's original conceptual schema. In fact, he or she needs to break down this schema, to abandon it as far as humanly possible, so as to be able to acquire the patterning which is characteristic of respondents' practices. (Textual examples in the resulting publications often function to persuade the reader to reorganise his or her own conceptual habits, providing a bridge into a new world-order.)

This form of radical vulnerability demands, for example, that if researching practices concerning friendship, say, or loneliness, the researcher should refrain from looking at behaviour in the setting in question and assessing it according to his or her 'usual' conceptions of friendship or loneliness. The investigator needs first to acquire local habits of conversation and behaviour. Suppose he or she finds that people who come together often and apparently by choice in this setting do not exchange intimate details or discuss their feelings directly. What is happening? In linguistic philosophy, one would examine cases of sentence-use in relation to friendship or self-expression to try to discern what these ideas might involve; in the field, what one might term 'interactive philosophy' requires the investigator to join in specific examples of communicative behaviour, to become competent in the setting, before he or she can reconstruct the meanings attached to the ideas in a given context. Maybe there is a different concept of friendship being enacted here from the one the researcher is used to; to find out, it is necessary to respect and to reconstruct what local behaviour appears to presuppose, to test the reconstruction by acting it out, and thus to become exposed to the reactions of the inhabitants of the setting.

A case in point here is 'loneliness', a problem often imputed to older people by charitable organisations and the public at large (though Victor 1994, and Page in this collection, suggest that it is at least as frequently to be found among the young). Often, 'loneliness' is interpreted to mean that the person suffering from it needs to be among people more, or among friends more; it is taken for granted that loneliness primarily involves some form of isolation from other people. An activist for older people in Germany provided a quite different set of interpretations (Edmondson, field notes 1995). According to him, organisations which are politically content with the status quo find themselves emphasising 'loneliness' as an individual problem, because it is one whose solutions would not be expected to be politically disruptive. He himself – as a lay philosopher in the field – interprets 'loneliness' in highly socio-political terms, claiming that older people who complain of being lonely are often in fact made unhappy by their social powerlessness and their lack of acknowledged social roles (transcript 4.4.1995). This raises questions about the *meanings* of 'loneliness' presupposed by respondents' conduct, and clearly these are highly significant as far as health promotion research is concerned.

In the conduct of surveys into attitudes, particularly large-scale ones, such questions are typically avoided; indeed, the obligation to produce results which are comparable with earlier surveys often precludes examining them. Thus, batteries of standard questions roll like juggernauts through social-scientific history without serious interrogation of their rationales. This state of affairs is exacerbated, moreover, by impatience with the philosophical question as to what 'attitudes' actually are: a question on which social science researchers have an obligation to weigh up alternative opinions. Some commentators have suggested that attitudes should be seen as unitary, mental items – a notion which is congenial in the mental world of surveys, for it implies that attitudes can be uncovered by tracking degrees of assent or dissent to simple statements. Norms, for example, have been explicated as propositions entertained by their holders, such that if they do not follow their own normative attitudes they become uncomfortable (Eichner 1981). Even if it were the case that some attitudes could be conceptualised like this, significant types of attitude are clearly composed of *tendencies towards particular kinds of feeling and behaviour*, such as deferring to authority, or oscillating between wanting to be slim and eating too much. The view that an attitude is a 'hidden mechanism' causing or directing conduct (Kerry 1971) implies a model of human thought, feeling and action which envisages people as carrying identifiable items – attitudes – in their heads, items which subsequently cause behavioural responses. But it is an unrealistic picture of a human being, a misleading philosophical anthropology, to suppose that action always takes place on the basis that a person first entertains ideas and then acts upon them. Often, people discover their own views by noticing how they themselves behave (Ryle 1949); they may find themselves showing certain attitudes without having had any detectable *ideas* at all. Other 'attitudes' can be rendered as assumptions, preferences, beliefs, choices, priorities or principles; each of these may be related to thinking, feeling and behaving in different ways in different circumstances (*cf.* LaPiere 1935). Moreover, some real or apparent inconsistencies between attitudes can be accounted for if it is borne in mind that certain types of attitude should be understood as intrinsically shared, or as properties of *groups or settings*, rather than in the first place as individual phenomena (Edmondson 1993). These are not merely abstract debates but contain definite implications for research practice. First of all, many social attitudes take the form of habits and practices; here researchers may need to know what is generally done on a given type of occasion, rather than what any individual believes should be done. One such example concerns behaviour in relation to a death. In Ireland, practice dictates that if someone wishes to show sympathy (which is scarcely considered a matter for individual deliberation), this necessitates visiting the corpse, shaking the hand of the bereaved and expressing sympathy in terms falling within expected parameters, and attending either the removal of the corpse to church or the funeral. This practice constitutes a shared attitude to death and how to respond to it. The attitude is essentially a public one; its domain is the public sphere (Geertz 1973); it may or may not be reflected on or verbalised by participants, but it would not usually make sense in an Irish context to try to show sympathy by any other means. 'Attitudes' such as this may be given to us by social settings, and appropriately researched via participation in those settings.

This underscores the points that important health-related attitudes may be unknown to their holders, and that special methods are required to find out about them. Attitudes may consist of patterns underlying behaviour, feeling and thought which people indigenous to social settings may take so much for granted that they are unaware of their presence. Particular under-lying patterns may be fostered by institutions, for example, whose practices can amount to a specific ethos within which it makes sense for certain actions to be framed (and within which other actions simply would not make sense and are therefore not attempted). If one changes from working in a hospital with a competitive ethos to one with a co-operative ambience, one's former habits of conduct may not be found appropriate or even intelligible. This has practical implications not only for research but also for changing behaviour. In women's health centres, for example, some assumptions built into conventional hospital organisation were rejected – for instance, the assumption that appointment times should be set by administrators rather than 'patients'; 'attitudes' were to be changed by changing *practices*. Similarly, those wishing to make an impact on attitudes towards the dying form new institutions, hospices, in which it is intended that certain setting-dependent attitudes will not arise, but that positive and supportive approaches will make more sense.

In analysing such developments it is a step forward that qualitative researchers are turning to the notion of 'practices' (Bourdieu 1980). In the past century of attempts to account qualitatively for the existence and experience of cultural 'regularities', these have been dealt with primarily in terms of putative systems of 'norms' and 'rules'; in fact, examining texts purporting to interrogate such phenomena will show that in effect they very rarely actually do so (Edmondson 1987). Social phenomena unambiguously identifiable as rules can seldom be discovered outside school corridors; allegedly 'normative' systems are more likely to incorporate imaginings, self-images, tendencies, preferences and other items which cannot be adequately described in the theoretical terms conventional to this approach. Cultures are, indeed, sometimes experienced as external and compelling, but not usually because they straightforwardly impose on us strictures which we straightforwardly oppose. This complexity is more effectively captured by the looser, if more enigmatic, notion of practice (Edmondson 1996; Turner 1994): a blend of what people tend to do, think, feel and say, on the basis of expectations they share with each other and behaviours they engage in together.

Practices, or conventional groups of practice which might be termed routines, may be observed and acquired in ethnographic practice, but even here their existence (let alone their meta-construction) may not be appreciated until the occurrence of crises which lay them bare. For the reasons discussed above in connection with cultures, routines bestow social meaning and simultaneously conceal it, from the researcher as well as from everyday inhabitants of a setting; so the researcher often depends on the occurrence of some mishap in interaction which will make clear what expectations have been violated. This is most frequently necessary in health-related qualitative work, where practices and routines tend to be basic to the conduct of everyday life and hence depend for their working on not being over-conceptualised, on remaining opaque to indigenous actors and on resisting surface description. 'Mishaps' may sometimes occur, in these contexts, because actors themselves do not realise either that practices are involved or what these are. Thus, one West of Ireland couple disagreed vehemently because the husband could not understand his wife's habit of visiting a local holy well in cases of illness or other crisis; he wanted to elicit from her clear statements of belief, whereas her reiterated response was 'It helps you get by' (Edmondson, field notes, May 1990). They were in fact interacting in terms of two different forms of discourse: he presupposed that reasonable conduct should emanate from considered opinions, whereas she was alluding to a practice in which she engaged because it enabled her to take a more positive approach to the predicaments of everyday life. The husband was in effect taking a modernist, post-Baconian approach to individual behaviour, whereas, in his wife's terms, embeddedness in a local setting could itself be regarded as conferring intelligibility. In order to reconstruct how their respective arrays of concepts and practices succeeded in structuring the world for each, it would be necessary to excavate down to the basic assumptions underlying them. In such cases, it may not be the basic assumption – for instance, the one about social embeddedness – which the researcher finds hard to understand, but how someone could actually come to use it (Edmondson, forthcoming). Here again, entire sets of interrelating practice need to be worked out. A hermeneutic ethnography, or an interactive philosophy, are needed to reconstruct the ways in which crises and routines are negotiated from day to day, and the practices which are entailed in the communication they involve.

CONCLUSION

It follows from these arguments that qualitative work in health promotion studies must, first of all, be reflexive: it must avoid adopting without analysis the concepts, images, habitual feelings and attitudes dominant in any setting; and it must involve a continual struggle to evade at least some of the influences on the researcher of his or her conceptual context of origin. Interpretation is inevitably affected by the interpreter's perceptions of what is reasonable or intelligible, but constant vigilance is needed to destabilise these perceptions in one's own procedure. The need for this is easier to perceive in relation to the influence of cultural setting on others who believe themselves to be taking independent decisions. Policy framers, for example, in the past as in the present, inevitably make assumptions derived from their own moral or political commitments, from the intellectual fashions of the time, and from the expectations about human beings which are taken for granted as reasonable in their cultural contexts. Foucault among others has drawn attention to the fact that it seemed unassailably reasonable to the Victorians to relate public caring to economies of scale (1973). In recent times, this has given way to a more atomic, individualistic conception of society; but theoretical reflexivity underlines the dangers of assuming *a priori* that either approach is better founded. It does not require that the researcher permanently abandon allegiance to a particular philosophical anthropology, but it does require him or her to acquire the virtue of noticing what underlying concepts and structures constitute the approach in which he or she is operating at the time.

The arguments in this chapter do suggest practical expedients in doing research; many of those expedients concern enhancing the theoretical sensitivity of the researcher. It has been pointed out that, in order to exercise this sensitivity, it is necessary to learn to negotiate settings; this has the clear implication that participative, ethnographic approaches should generally take primary, not secondary, place in cultural and attitudinal health-related research. For the sake of clarity it may be useful to repeat that adopting more philosophically sensitive procedures does not mean that large-scale surveys should never be used in health promotion; but, especially the more closely concerned with cultural attitudes they are, they should be treated with extreme caution as approximate clues to a changing setting rather than as conclusive knowledge. Survey enquiries need to be based on some form of qualitative investigation into the nature of the central practices and concepts concerned, and the investigators involved should be trained to assess theoretically and culturally crucial aspects of interpretation in the field. Here it is simply destructive to make radical distinctions between theoretical reflections and practical research. Pressures exerted by practical issues, the demands of funders or the need for grants, can tempt sociologists to present cultural research as easier than it is: as a mode of acquiring propositional knowledge on which technical policy choices can be based, rather than as a source of reflections which can be used to inform decisions. Much as we need to refine the sensitivity of enquiry, the results of cultural research into health-related attitudes will never produce information of a type which makes policy decisions automatic, and nor should they do so. Decisions on health need to be taken in large part by those affected by them; participative means of making these decisions need refining every bit as much as do research methods.

The relation of reflexivity to participation has another dimension, important for ethical and political as well as methodological reasons. Enquiry which involves participating in other people's settings is both developmental and interactive, more a *process* than an *operation* conducted according to straightforward routines. Rather than regarding themselves as in charge of situations, seeking items in other people's heads which may subsequently be altered, researchers will be involved in longer-term interpretive processes. These may be more and less harmonious ones, but those which involve painful rebuffs may often be the more enlightening in the end. The 'ethnomethodological' method stresses that exposing mis-understandings is central to learning about a culture (Garfinkel 1967); and it is when respondents are in a position to harm the researcher that misunderstandings will most urgently be borne in on him or her as requiring explication. Far from leaving the researcher in charge, in the position of a manager, such processes may be expected to change him or her on a long-term basis. Aiming to achieve the creative melting of horizons endorsed by Gadamer (1960) means that researchers must prepare to be altered by their research. Hence the demands of research practice as far as culture and health are concerned have implications for daily life within health promotion studies too. As many have argued, the barriers enclosing areas of practice must be removed for the discipline to progress. Nonetheless, it is easy to underestimate the difficulties involved in removing them, for the different research practices in the field are based on radically divergent underlying assumptions and emotional habits as well as beliefs. Qualitative researchers not only study but use whole practices, rather than 'instruments'; they engage in routines rather than employing 'skills'; they try to allow themselves to be changed during processes of negotiation rather than being obsessed with changing the views and conduct of others. Such approaches are difficult for those trained in technical decision-making to understand; if health promotion is to be able to embrace both quantitative and qualitative approaches, more than merely cognitive channels must run between the two. New disciplinary practices must be fashioned, in which each can learn to live the life of the other, if they are to understand each other's results.

ACKNOWLEDGEMENTS

The research on which this article is partially founded was funded by the Centre for Health Promotion Studies and the Health Research Board, Ireland.

REFERENCES

Aarts, K., 1997. 'Soil Pollution, Community Action and Political Opportunities', in Ricca Edmondson, ed., *The Political Context of Collective Action*. London: Routledge.

Antonovsky, A., 1996. 'The Salutogenic Model as a Theory to Guide Health Promotion', *Health Promotion International*, 11 (1): 11–18.

Alexander, J., and Seidman, S., eds., 1990. *Culture and Society: Contemporary Debates*. Cambridge: Cambridge University Press.

Beckwith, K., 1997. 'Movement in Context: Women and Miners' Campaigns in Britain', in Ricca Edmondson, ed., *The Political Context of Collective Action*. London: Routledge.

Bourdieu, P., 1980. *The Logic of Practice*. Cambridge: Polity Press.

Dalley, G., 1988. *Ideologies of Caring*. London: Macmillan.

Denzin, N., and Lincoln, Y., 1994. *Handbook of Qualitative Research*. London: Sage.

Deutscher, I., Pestello, F.P., and Pestello, H.F.G., 1993. *Sentiments and Acts*. New York: Aldine de Gruyter.

Eastern Health Board, Dublin, 1995. *Review of Services for the Elderly and Four-Year Action Plan 1995–1998*.

Edmondson, R., 1984. *Rhetoric in Sociology*. London: Macmillan.

Edmondson, R., 1987. *Rules and Norms in the Sociology of Organisations*. Berlin: Max Planck Institute for Human Development.

Edmondson, R., 1993. 'Attitudes Among Older People: Why Do We Need to Know?' Paper to ISA Research Committee on Empirical Methods, Budapest.

Edmondson, R., 1994. 'Theory and Prejudice in Empirical Studies of Older People', International Sociological Association Congress, Bielefeld.

Edmondson, R., 1996. 'Uses of Empirical Data in the Sociology of Knowledge', ISA Research Committee for the History of Empirical Methods, Amsterdam.

Edmondson, R., 1997a. 'Older People and Life-Course Construction in Ireland', in A. Cleary and M. Treacy, eds., *The Sociology of Health and Illness in Ireland*. Dublin: UCD Press.

Edmondson, R., ed., 1997b. *The Political Context of Collective Action: Argumentation, Power and Democracy*. London: Routledge.

Edmondson, R., 1998. *Ireland: Society and Culture*. Hagen: Distance University.

Edmondson, R., forthcoming. *How Cultures Work: Crises and Routines*.

Eichner, K., 1981. *Die Entstehung Sozialer Normen*. Opladen: Westdeutscher Verlag.

Fengler, C., and Fengler, T., 1980. *Alltag in der Anstalt*. Rehburg-Loccum: Psychiatrie Verlag.

Finch, J., 1989. *Family Obligations and Social Change*. Cambridge: Polity Press.

Foucault, M., 1973. *Madness and Civilisation: A History of Insanity in the Age of Reason*. New York: Vintage.

Gadamer, H.-G., 1960. *Wahrheit und Methode*. Tübingen: J.C.B. Mohr (Paul Siebeck).

Garfinkel, H., 1967. *Studies in Ethnomethodology*. Englewood Cliffs, NJ: Prentice-Hall.

Geertz, C., 1973. *The Interpretation of Cultures*. New York: Basic Books.

Gubrium, J.F., and Sankar, A., eds., 1994. *Qualitative Methods in Aging Research*. London: Sage.

Habermas, J., 1985. 'Remarks on the Concept of Communicative Action', in G. Seebaß and R. Tuomela., eds., *Social Action*. Dordrecht: Reidl.

Habermas, J., 1981. *Theorie des Kommunikativen Handelns*. Frankfurt am Main Suhrkamp.

Hall, S., 1997. *Cultural Representations*. London: Sage.

Harre, R., and Secord, P., 1972. *The Explanation of Social Behaviour*. Oxford: Blackwell.

James, O., 1997. *Britain on the Couch*. London: Century Random House.

Kelleher, C., 1993. *Measures to Promote Health and Autonomy for Older People: A Position Paper*. Dublin: National Council for the Elderly, Publication No. 26.

Kerry, T., ed., 1971. *Attitudes and Behaviour*. Harmondsworth: Penguin.

LaPiere, R.T., 1935. 'Type-Rationalizations of Group Antipathy', *Social Forces*, 15: pp. 232–7.

Mullarkey, J., 1994. *Alcohol to Alcoholism to Alcoholics Anonymous: An Ethnographic Study of Alcoholics Anonymous in Ireland*. MA thesis, University College Galway.

Oakley, A., 1992. *Social Support and Motherhood: The Natural History of a Research Project*. Oxford: Blackwell.

O'Connor, J., and Ruddle, D., 1988. *Caring for the Elderly, Part II: The Caring Process: A Study of Carers in the Home*. Dublin: National Council for the Aged.

O'Connor, M., 1995. *Birth Tides: Turning Towards Home Birth*. London: Harper Collins.

O'Connor, P., 1994. 'Very Close Parent/Child Relationships: The Perspective of the Elderly Person', *Journal of Cross-Cultural Gerontology*, 9: pp. 53–76.

Rootes, C., 1997. 'Shaping Collective Action: Structure, Contingency and Knowledge', in Ricca Edmondson, ed., *The Political Context of Collective Action*. London: Routledge.

Ryle, G., 1949. *The Concept of Mind*. Harmondsworth: Peregrine.

Schutz, A., 1962. *Collected Papers*, ed. Maurice Natanson. The Hague: Nijhoff.

Turner, S., 1994. *The Social Theory of Practices: Tradition, Tacit Knowledge and Presupposition*. Cambridge: Polity Press.

Victor, C., 1994. *Old Age in Modern Society*. 2nd edn. London: Chapman and Hall.

Williams, R.G.A., 1983. 'Concepts of Health: An Analysis of Lay Logic', *Sociology*, 17, pp. 185–205.

Winch, P., 1958. *The Idea of a Social Science and its Relation to Philosophy*. London: Routledge and Kegan Paul.

SEVEN

A Story/Dialogue Method for Health Promotion Knowledge Development and Evaluation

RONALD LABONTE, JOAN FEATHER
AND MARCIA HILLS

INTRODUCTION

This paper introduces one of a number of possible postpositivist approaches to the development of knowledge and the evaluation and planning of programmes in health promotion. It is not intended to replace all other methods, but it does possess special advantages derived from its use of age-old techniques related to the structure of dialogue and the generation of theory based on practice. These techniques are currently being adapted across a varied range of programme evaluation questions; they are particularly well suited to analysing health promotion strategies and activities, for they can be used by practitioners, health promotion agencies or community members.

There is growing argument that conventional (positivist) science norms are insufficient to make sense of what health promotion is, and how its effects should be evaluated (Baum 1995; Dixon 1995; Dixon and Sindall 1994; Fawcett et al. 1995; Labonte and Robertson 1996). At the same time, health promotion has been challenged as being more ideological than theoretical, often little more than a series of normative claims (Labonte and Robertson 1996). This article describes a 'story/dialogue method' (S/D-M) that attempts to bridge the gap between descriptive stories and rigorous explanation, and so points towards accountability norms that are more in keeping with what health promotion practice attempts to accomplish. The S/D-M was developed in a partnership between practitioners and researchers who were frustrated equally with researchers whose positivist assumptions (e.g. 'objective' truth) and methods (e.g. randomised controlled trials or quasi-experimental designs) often did not fit the 'reality' of practice, and

95

with practitioners who risked losing resources for their work by failing to articulate better practice-based theory. Lewin's famous aphorism, 'There's nothing so practical as a good theory,' can be turned on its head; there's nothing so theoretical as a good practice. The development of the S/D-M was prompted by a desire to assist practitioners to make explicit their assumptions (theories) about their work, and to subject them to some critically respectful scrutiny with their peers. The product of this scrutiny is a generalised description of what health promotion is and seeks to accomplish, useful for and usable by other health promoters in other practice situations. Rather than generalised theory being privileged over particular experiences, particular experiences become the necessary components in the continual development of generalised theory.

This article begins with a discussion of why interest in the use of stories, or narratives, for knowledge development has increased in recent years. The S/D-M is then described briefly and illustrated with examples from some of the uses to which it has been put. (A more detailed account of the method can be found in Labonte and Feather 1996.) This article focuses on the method's use in knowledge development, as other method applications are still underway and not yet properly documented.

BACKGROUND TO THE STORY/DIALOGUE METHOD

The systematic use of stories in programme planning and evaluation first began in international development work. Aid workers realised that they needed to respect the oral culture of many poor communities, and discovered that local people had an amazing knowledge about their lives and their environments that conventional (positivist) research was unable to tap (Slim and Thompson 1995). Because researchers were not members of that community, they often did not know the right questions to ask, the right way to ask them or how to use the results. The contemporary women's movement was another impetus for renewed scholarly interest in the use of stories to create knowledge, and for similar reasons. Feminists criticised many of the theories about human behaviour because the science that generated them had ignored women's voices (Gilligan 1982; Tronto 1993). Early consciousness-raising circles emphasised the value of women speaking from their own experience. This emphasis on personal experience and voice is also found in empowering approaches to education, including health education (Wallerstein and Bernstein 1988). As Freire and Macedo (1987) argue, the first act of power people can take in managing their own lives is 'speaking the world', naming their experiences in their own words under conditions where their stories are listened to and respected by others. As stories are shared between people, they become 'generative themes' for group reflection, analysis and action planning. Stories, in the form of personal narratives, traditionally have formed an important database for qualitative studies. While some qualitative researchers claim the same objectivity and detachment as conventional researchers (Labonte and Robertson 1996), many align more closely with action research tenets (Argyris, Putnam and McLain-Smith 1985) and their emphasis on contingent and practical knowledge. Such researchers maintain that only in analysing with people how they 'speak their world' can they, and the people with whom they research or evaluate, understand the practical significance of their experiences (Guba and Lincoln 1989). It is precisely this element of reflection on meaning that is absent from most conventional scientific research. In many of the social sciences, there is renewed interest 'in narratives, in the telling of stories' as an important means of understanding this meaning-saturated quality of social life (Kvale 1995).

Health promoters themselves recognise the importance of stories in researching, learning, evaluating and planning their work (Centre for Development and Initiative in Health 1993; Dixon 1995; Feather and Labonte 1995). Many health promoters, however, feel defensive because stories do not fit into the conventional scientific method. Dixon (1995) argues that a distinction should be made between conventional methods for institutional evaluations and 'community stories' for community-controlled evaluations, although this still risks institutional funders demanding evaluation using methodologies inappropriate to community-based programmes. Even when stories are used in knowledge development and evaluation, an important issue remains of using stories more rigorously. Stories are not accepted simply as presented, but are used as a grounding base against which probing questions can be asked about what was done, why it was done and what it accomplished.

THE STORY/DIALOGUE METHOD

There are different ways to use stories in knowledge work. One method is simply to listen to a story and reflect upon it personally, which is the way most people read stories or enjoy the oral craft of story-tellers. Another way is to engage with others, including the story-teller, in a dialogue about the story, which is how the S/D-M works (see Figure 1). At the heart of this method is the reflective practitioner – the story-teller and those participating in the dialogue. At every stage in the method, participants are encouraged to reflect on how what they hear and learn from others has meaning for them personally. This requires organisational commitments to this type of inquiry (the learning organisation) and supportive peer relationships (the learning practice community) (Labonte 1996).

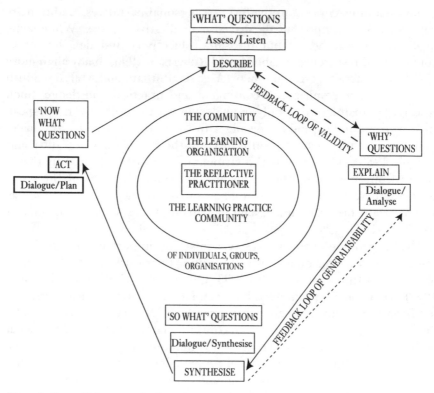

Figure 1. Story dialogue method.

The notion of reflective practice derives from Schon's (1983, 1990) work, in which he proposes a 'transformative' option to the adversarial construction of the professional/client relationship. In a 'reflective contract' the professional slowly gives up an initial claim to authority and begins to negotiate a shared understanding with the person or group with whom she or he is working. The professional's unconscious assumptions about what is effective in his or her own work become conscious and negotiable. In health promotion and community development, this is often characterised as a 'problem-posing' approach to programme work, in which neither the issues nor their resolution are taken for granted but are analysed against a repertoire of experience and knowledge from both professionals and community members.

STORY/DIALOGUE METHOD WORKSHOPS

Over 2,500 practitioners, researchers and programme managers in seven countries have participated in workshops on this method. Most of these

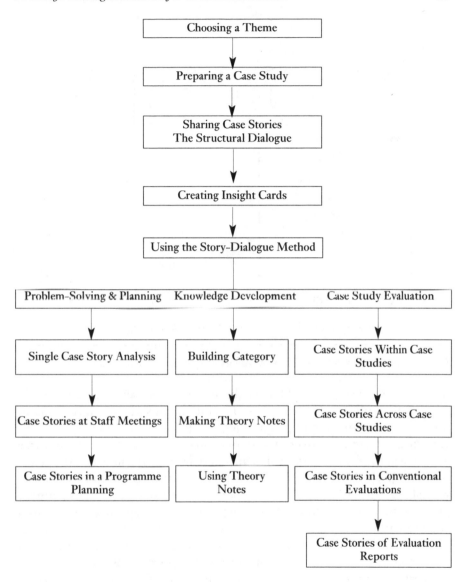

Figure 2. Steps in the story-dialogue method and its uses.

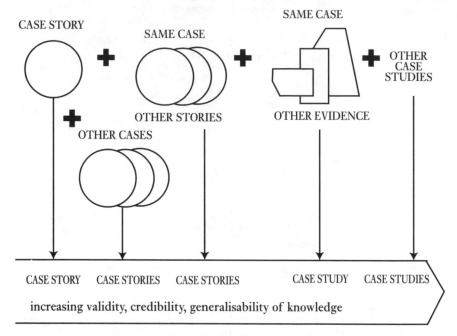

Figure 3. Improving validity and generalisability of practice-based lessons.

workshops have emphasised knowledge development, although some post-workshop applications include staff and organisational development, programme planning, and programme and policy evaluation. Workshops vary in size from 20 to over 200 participants, and range from one to three days in length. While most participants have been 'front-line' health agency staff (e.g. health promoters, community health nurses, social workers), many workshops attract academic researchers, policy workers and government programme managers interested in the method as an approach to research and evaluation. S/D-M workshops always have two goals: training in the method itself, including some discussion of other uses of stories in health promotion (e.g. stories as testimony in advocacy work, or as means to create solidarity within self-help groups), and application of the method to specific problems or issues important to participants attending the workshop. All workshops include at least one full day in which small *story groups* of 5 to 9 participants analyse two or more *case stories* constructed around a *generative theme using a structured dialogue* intended to assist participants in creating generalisable knowledge, or *theory notes*, about practice. (Italicised terms are explained later in this article.) Longer workshops use theory notes to develop evaluation indicators or logic models of practice, or to identify skills training needs. The different steps and applications of the method are outlined in Figure 2, and the relationship of case stories to case studies outlined in Figure 3.

THE GENERATIVE THEME

An S/D-M workshop begins with determining one or more generative themes. A good theme is one that identifies 'tensions' or strained relations that exist within and between the people who are part of it. A generative theme speaks to power relations in health promotion practice (e.g. between practitioners and community members, state institutions and community groups, front-line workers and senior managers), rather than to content issues of health promotion work (e.g. heart health, tobacco, injury prevention). An assumption behind the S/D-M is that an important element of health promotion work is empowerment, in which power relations between different actors and groups involved in activities around a specific issue become more equitable. (For discussions on the relationship between power, empowerment and health, see Labonte 1997; Wallerstein 1992; Wallerstein and Bernstein 1994). Generative themes are selected by workshop organisers (usually a health department, health non-governmental organisation or university), based upon their knowledge of important practice tensions experienced by health promoters in their area. Themes are written up in paragraph form and distributed in advance to all workshop participants (see Appendix 1).

CASE STORIES

Workshop participants are invited to prepare a case story around the generative theme. In longer workshops, all participants have an opportunity to be story-tellers, where their experience becomes a 'trigger' for a deeper analysis of the theme. More commonly, and depending on the number attending a workshop, about one-third of participants will prepare case stories in advance. A case story describes the practitioner's experience with the tensions summarised in the generative theme. It is a first-person account of how the practitioner dealt with the tensions, what was happening in the context of his or her practice and what happened as a result of the actions taken. Story-tellers, who are provided with briefing notes to help them prepare case stories, are encouraged to problem-pose their experience, rather than problem-solve it. Story-tellers are also encouraged to write down their story in narrative or point form, which typically runs one to three pages in length (see Appendix 1).

Workshop evaluations indicate that the more reflective time the practitioner takes in preparing a case story, and the more the story poses the tension rather than resolves it, the richer becomes the structured dialogue around it. Many persons who have been story-tellers in these workshops also comment that:

- the process of preparing the story itself led them towards new insights about their practice
- reflecting on their practice is rarely encouraged or supported in their own workplaces (but could be)
- preparing 'good' case stories was a new skill that could be developed with practice

STORY GROUPS

Once in the workshop setting, participants form story groups. Story groups typically average five to nine participants, who work through two or three separate rounds of story-telling, each round lasting between ninety minutes and two hours. In each round, one person is a story-teller, four persons volunteer for the dual role of story-recorders/story-listeners and the rest are story-listeners. Story-recorders are asked to listen for significant comments in the dialogue made under each of the four question categories (described below) and to note them in point form. The purpose of recording the dialogue in this way is twofold: to provide participants with a practice opportunity in a participant/observation technique, and to ensure that the dialogue remains the database for later 'second-level synthesis' (also described below). Workshop evaluations indicate that when participants have responsibility for recording key dialogue points, the quality of their listening becomes more intense and they understand better the distinctions between descriptive and explanatory modes of questioning. Story groups begin with a verbal telling of the story. This is followed by a 'reflection circle', in which other group members, one at a time and without dialogue, reflect upon and speak of how the story and the issues it addresses are similar to (or different from) their own experience. These reflection circles have proved useful in shifting story group members' thinking away from the descriptive content of the story-teller's experience and towards the organisational and social contexts in which health promoters work, which constitute the terrain in which empowerment occurs.

THE STRUCTURED DIALOGUE

After the reflection circle, story group members begin a structured dialogue around the story. A structured dialogue is intentionally designed to move discussion from a description of what happened, to one or more explanations for why it happened, a synthesis of key lessons derived from the case-story and similar experiences and some articulation of new actions. The structured dialogue, and its use, are fashioned after Habermas' (1984) notion of 'ideal speech situations'. Habermas' complex theory of power relations in society hinges on the role communication plays in maintaining or transforming social systems of dominance. Transformative communication occurs under ideal speech situations, in which participants search for a better understanding of particular events in the world. The rules for ideal speech are that people's claims be 'comprehensible' (understandable to others), 'true' (they are not logically or rationally false, and can be defended by argument or data), 'appropriate' (justified by a shared purpose among participants) and 'sincere' (people state what they mean). Truth and appropriateness can only be defended in open dialogue. An open dialogue, in turn, is facilitated by using open questions which invite reflection. Four categories of open questions are used to generate a structured dialogue:

1. *What* do you see happening here? (Description)
   'What' questions invite people to describe what is happening in their case story from their own vantage point. They ground the explanation in experience.
2. *Why* do you think it happens? (Explanation)
   'Why' questions invite a discussion on causes, where participants begin to interpret or make sense of what has been described.
3. *So what* have we learned from our own experiences? (Synthesis)
   'So what' questions invite a synthesis, or distillation, of new knowledge.
4. *Now what* can we do about it? (Action) (adapted from Vella 1989, and Wallerstein and Sanchez-Merki 1994)
   'Now what' questions translate this new knowledge into normative claims of what health promotion practice ought to do.

A number of prompts exist for each question category, and are often tailored to the specific generative theme. Although the four questions and their prompts are not intended to be used in a linear fashion, providing time for each question category helps to prevent discussion from bogging down in description. While some practitioners initially find the structure awkward, workshop evaluations note its importance in moving practitioners to a deeper understanding of their work experiences. Story-tellers frequently note that the structure of the questioning surfaces a different and more generalised quality of insights about practice than they normally encounter in peer exchanges or conference presentations. Often, case stories shared in the same story group concern quite different health 'content', for instance one story on environmental activism, another on smoking control programmes, a third on community gardens, causing some initial scepticism among participants about what they might learn from one another. But as was expressed in a recent workshop, 'We were surprised by how much our work had in common, once we got beneath the superficial differences of the issues themselves.'

Each story-telling round concludes with the generation of insight cards. Insights represent key points taken from the structured dialogue on the story that story group members think is significant enough to be shared with other practitioners. Insights are written as full statements, naming an actor and an action, for example 'The leader needs to be able to unpack the differing agendas of the partners' (an insight card from the case story in Appendix 1). This is the point where story-recorders' notes play a role, to obviate the risk of some persons reaching personal conclusions ungrounded in discussion points on the actual case-story experience. Between 10 and 15 insight cards are generated for each story and posted on a wall.

VALIDITY AND GENERALISABILITY

An important issue in using the S/D-M is the validity of the knowledge gained through analysis of the story. Validity here does not mean that the method generates 'truth' in a universal sense, but that its findings have 'the quality of being well-founded' on experience (Heron 1988), and represent a diversity of opinions that create 'saturated' categories (Strauss 1987) that are 'grounded' in the description of actual events (Glaser and Strauss 1967). Validity means that a good explanation is understandable, and that it reflects what happened, and not just what practitioners wanted to see happen (Razack 1993). In the S/D-M, this requires a return to the description of the story: what more details are needed to know that the explanations, or generalised lessons, are valid ones? Does the explanation cover all of the story details, or has it selected those that fit well and ignored others that do not? Validity is of particular concern when the S/D-M is used for case study or evaluation purposes. In one application currently underway, validity is being addressed by incorporating data from project records and files, individual interviews and case stories from many persons involved in the project during S/D-M workshops, thus triangulating data sources and practitioner perspectives.

Heron (1988) argues that postpositivist research findings should be generalisable or replicable. He does not mean this in the positivist sense, in which the same actions should be transferable to other locales with similar results. Rather, he argues for 'creative metamorphosis', in which the underlying 'wisdom' gained is shared with persons facing similar situations. This requires the knowledge claims to be of sufficient depth (specificity) and abstraction (generalised statements) that others in similar situations can make use of them. The S/D-M is designed to provide both. It begins with

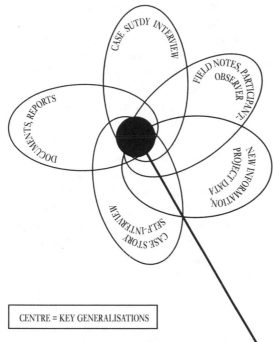

Figure 4. Case stories in case study evaluation.

specific practice experiences (the individual case story) and ensures that efforts are made to extract important lessons for all practitioners from the particular case, 'an in-depth analysis of an experience', as was expressed at one recent workshop. Generalisability is strengthened by analysing two or three different stories on the same theme in each story group during an S/D-M workshop (see Figure 4). If the method is used in peer-group meetings, in which instance the peer group becomes the story group, such stories can be analysed over a series of meetings. Participants in the story group then work up the results to a more abstract, or second-level synthesis of practice.

A SECOND-LEVEL SYNTHESIS

To move from insights from a particular story to more generalised lessons derived from several stories, a second-level synthesis of the insight cards occurs. There are two steps involved in a second-level synthesis, building categories from the insight cards and writing theory notes based on the categories. Categories allow participants to consolidate lessons from a range of stories. After the categories have been made, story groups write up a descriptive statement that links the statements on the insight cards, in effect writing a more abstract, or generalised, 'story' of the lessons learned from the particular case stories they have been analysing. This theory note is an attempt to explain what lessons the category of insights holds for other practitioners who may be in other practice situations. As one workshop participant stated, 'The theory notes allowed me to see how the case story was made useful.' After theory notes are written for each category, they are structured or linked together into a composite theory note (see Appendix 1).

Composite theory notes generally have a normative quality to them. The structure of the S/D-M leads to theory notes being written in an imperative mode, in which the subtleties of explanation and context present in the dialogue around the story are removed. This is intentional. People do not live as if each situation they encounter were completely novel. They bring to life a repertoire of analytical devices, strategies and other forms of knowledge built up from previous experiences. The same applies to health promotion work. The S/D-M is designed to make this health promotion repertoire more explicit and open to peer analysis. Resulting theory notes speak to practitioners in particular work contexts. These notes are not theory in the 'grand' sense in which some transhistorical understanding or statement of causal relations is sought (Giddens 1984), but neither are they simply the ungrounded ideological claims for which health promotion has been criticised. The difference lies in their connection to a group analysis of actual practice experience.

A theory note derived from a single case story may fail to identify lessons pertinent to a wider range of health promotion practice concerns. For this reason the S/D-M encourages the triangulation of at least two or more case stories in any given story group. In some instances, case stories and theory notes are published alongside one another following an S/D-M workshop, together with a synthesis of all of the different story groups' theory notes (e.g. Labonte 1997). This provides more contextual richness to the generalised lessons contained in the theory notes, and a more robust account of these lessons by drawing from a wider range of case stories.

USING THEORY NOTES

Theory notes are used by S/D-M workshop participants in a number of ways. In shorter workshops, they are often used to identify new practice tensions that become the focus for later workshops or peer-group meetings. In longer workshops, theory notes have been used to develop 'benchmarks' for good practice. Workshop participants examine their theory notes, extracting from them those actions or outcomes for which they believe health promoters should hold themselves accountable (see Appendix 1). Once these benchmarks are established, workshop participants develop an argument why achieving them will improve health. This additional reflexive step in S/D-M workshops returns practitioners to the larger issue: how does their work contribute to improved health?

STRENGTHS AND WEAKNESSES OF THE METHOD

The examples provided in Appendix 1 of results from the S/D-M come from workshops that were also training in the method itself. The potential usefulness of the method lies in its more continuous application and refinement within practice settings. 'One-off' S/D-M workshops generate some useful lessons, but the limitations of workshop settings preclude assuming that these lessons, in the absence of further reflection and analysis, represent 'good' practice-based theory. Rather, the lessons point the way towards such theory, and the S/D-M provides practitioners with a tool for participating actively in its generation. Triangulating several different stories on the same case increases the validity of the theory notes (conclusions) reached by story-group members, while triangulating several different cases on the same generative theme increases their generalisability.

Evaluations of S/D-M workshops indicate that the method's appeal to practitioners lies in the power of sharing stories, grounding the stories in first-person experiences, affirming that practitioners and community members have important knowledge, the story group process that, in one participant's words 'helped to make everyone work together as equals', and the logic of the structured dialogue. Weaknesses in the method do exist, and pertain primarily to differences in the ease with which practitioners are able to prepare 'good and revealing stories' (Feather and Labonte 1995), to move from the concreteness of description to the abstraction of explanation, to 'discover' or articulate insights and to search for patterns when creating categories. When practitioners encounter difficulties in these areas, there is a tendency to retreat into the personal stories and problem-solve the particular, rather than to move on into assessing and analysing the generalised knowledge the stories help to create.

The ability to document revealing experiences, to analyse and explain these experiences, to synthesise the analysis and to search for patterns and abstract from the particular to the general are all skills that can be acquired with practice. The S/D-M has evolved to assist practitioners in acquiring these skills, notably through briefing and support of story-tellers prior to their crafting of the case story, use of briefed facilitators in each story group, creation of a detailed handbook on the method and development of additional stages, such as 'benchmarking', that return the abstract theory notes to the particulars of practice.

CONCLUSION: THE METHOD'S RELEVANCE TO HEALTH
PROMOTION KNOWLEDGE DEVELOPMENT
AND EVALUATION

The S/D-M is one of many approaches to knowledge development, programme planning and evaluation. It is not intended to replace other methods, nor does the group approach to story analysis, synthesis and generalisation preclude the more traditional qualitative analysis of such 'texts' undertaken by individual researchers. The logic of the method – the structure of the dialogue, generation of practice-based theory and application of theory to the creation of evaluation indicators – represents one technique for postpositivist research that can be, and is being, adapted to a range of programme evaluation questions. It is particularly suited to analysis of health-promotion strategies and activities, whether from the vantage points of practitioners, their agencies or community members.

Expert knowledge in theorising and evaluating health-promotion practice is important, but often has overshadowed the knowledge of practitioners and community members. The S/D-M, by basing itself on the day-to-day experiences of these groups, moving from their particulars to a statement of more generalised or abstract knowledge and applying that knowledge to specific programme evaluations, can create a better balance between the knowledge and power of institutions and professionals, and the knowledge and power of communities.

ACKNOWLEDGEMENTS

This paper is reproduced with adaptations from an article published in *Health Education Research*, 14 (1999, pp. 39–50), with kind permission. Thanks are due to the hundreds of health-promotion practitioners who have participated in the various iterations of the method; Marcia Hills and Nina Wallerstein who worked with Ronald Labonte in several applications of the method; the project team which piloted the method: Nicole Dedobbeleer, Marcia Hills, Nancy Kotani, Heather Maclean, Karen Parent and Irving Rootman; to Health Canada, for funding various stages in the development of the method, and Nancy Hamilton of Health Canada for her support and insights; to Patricia Williams, Edmee Korsberg and Carmelle Thibodeau, who reviewed drafts of the handbook (Labonte and Feather 1996) on use of the method; and to Bonnie Sproat, who designed and produced many of the documents and graphics used in applications of the method.

Examples of a generative theme, case story, theory note and benchmarks

The following examples are taken from a two-day workshop in Melbourne, Australia (August 1996), on the topic, 'Creating Partnerships for Health Promotion'.

Generative theme

Everyone talks about the need to develop new partnerships or intersectoral collaboration. Our work should lead us beyond ourselves, to partnerships with like-minded groups, organisations and sectors. But territoriality, competition over resources, different language and concepts, different accounting structures and priorities, all seem to get in the way. Power differences/inequalities between partners are often large and are rarely talked about so that they might be resolved. This is particularly true in partnerships involving community people and groups, whose participation is often token, largely because the terms of participation remain largely with institutions. Despite recognition that supports for citizen participation are essential, they are often meagre or lacking. There is also a general participation exhaustion, with everyone running from one consultation meeting to another in the hopes of not missing something that just might be important, but often is not.

Case story

I am a medical graduate who has had a lifelong interest in involvement in community-based youth activities. I was recruited five years ago to establish an adolescent health programme – The Centre for Adolescent Health – which was the first clinical academic programme in adolescent health to be established in Australia. Those who came together to stimulate this initiative were three hospitals, a university and VicHealth (the Victoria Health Foundation, an Australian health non-governmental organisation funded through a special tobacco tax). What quickly became apparent was that these multiple agencies did not share one single vision, had many differing agendas and had chosen me for different reasons. The hospitals' agenda was largely focused on improving service delivery to young people in problem areas. The academic agenda was more to do with research excellence and education/training. VicHealth had a more politicised agenda informed by the release of a report on youth homelessness emphasising outreach and development work with youth in the most severe social circumstances. In a similar fashion the agencies valued me in different ways. The hospitals valued my physician status and my knowledge of health service delivery.

The university valued my academic achievements. VicHealth looked towards my non-professional commitment to young people as an indication of my understanding of the importance of a social view of health and the promotion of well-being as integral components of an adolescent health programme.

My initial attempts were to try and please the multiple constituencies by attending management meetings, faculty meetings, staff meetings and key committee meetings at all of these agencies. It quickly became apparent that this was not a good strategy. I was not keeping anyone happy and not achieving core objectives. I came to realise that the true constituency for the Centre for Adolescent Health was young people in the community and that addressing their needs was the key outcome. As I worked towards identifying and addressing these needs, I took a pragmatic decision to focus my partnership building attention on two of the agencies only, one hospital and VicHealth. By slowly building on the particular strengths of these agencies, we were able to begin to develop a common vision that helped us to then take on board other partnerships.

The things I learned during this process were, firstly, the need to keep a focus on the big picture and the true constituency for the work of the programme; secondly, that there was a need to create a vision around which to rally the partners, rather than to necessarily try to create a hybrid vision from all the different agencies involved; and thirdly, to build on partners' particular strengths and not to try to pursue too many concurrent relationships.

Theory note

Effective partnerships require the establishment of a clear vision of the role of the organisation and a definition of what future role the organisation will play. Having agreed on the vision, effective leadership requires working to ensure that the partners have a common goal and a commitment to share in a true partnership. Effective leadership must focus on the common goal for success, and not try to please all the partners.

Partners may be pre-determined, self-selected or chosen. As development and management of multiple partnerships is difficult, it is essential to identify key partners to ensure any long-term sustainability for the partnership. Key partners may be those who have certain forms of 'power-over' in relation to the issue, often through their control over funding relationships. Changes with partnerships and the external environment require monitoring of power bases – who has power, who has not, and how this changes over time. Introduction of new partners, or termination/repositioning of existing partners, may be needed to ensure their ongoing relevance to the issue around which the partnership formed, and their effective contribution to achieving partnership goals.

Good partnerships take time to develop. It takes time to develop a shared common goal, a sense of ownership of the project and an intellectual and emotional commitment to successful outcomes for the project. To accomplish this, the leader needs to be able to unpack the agendas of different partners (which are often hidden) and to understand fully their individual motivations, interests, goals and expectations. The leader may also need to expose the partners to the constituents (those benefiting through the partnership's activities) and the setting at the coalface (where the activities take place). The leader needs to develop and nurture current partnerships while recognising the need to identify potential new partnerships and train future partnership leaders. The leader also needs to be aware of his or her own personal limitations and be prepared to draw on others' skills to supplement his or her own.

Finally, partners from the constituency (those benefiting from the partnership's activities) need to be provided with opportunities to develop and use skills that empower them to play an active role in the project/ organisation.

Benchmarks

- The agendas of each partner are clearly stated and a common agenda reached, through agreement on one or more goals.
- The partners agree to a process that exposes managers of the partnership 'coalface' experiences.
- Partnerships establish a process to actively skill the constituency (those benefiting from the partners' activities) so that they are empowered to participate actively in the partnership itself.
- Partners agree on mechanisms to enable skilled constituents to partic-ipate in the partnership, and methods to monitor that participation.
- Partnerships are strategically managed through establishment of a clear, common vision formally documented and agreed to by all of the partners.

REFERENCES

Argyris, C., Putman, R., and McLaine-Smith, D., 1985. *Action Science*. San Francisco: Jossey-Bass.

Baum, F., 1995. 'Researching Public Health: Behind the Qualitative-Quantitative Methodological Debate', *Social Science and Medicine*, 40, 4; pp. 459–68.

Centre for Development and Initiative in Health, 1993. *Case Studies of Community Deveopment in Health*. Melbourne: CDIH.

Dixon, J., 1995. 'Community Stories and Indicators for Evaluating Community Development', *Community Development Journal*, 30, 4: pp. 327–36.

Dixon, J., and Sindall, C., 1994. 'Applying the Logics of Change to the Evaluation of Community Development in Health Promotion' *Health Promotion International*, 9, 4: pp. 297–39.

Fawcett, S., Paine-Andrews, A., Francisco, V., *et al.* 1995. 'Using Empowerment Theory in Collaborative Partnership for Community Health and Development' *American Journal of Community Psychology*, 23, 5: pp. 677–98.

Feather, J., and Labonte, R., 1995. *Sharing Knowledge from Health Promotion Practice: Final Report*. Sasatoon: University of Saskatchewan, Prairie Region Health Promotion Research Centre.

Freire, P., and Macedo, D., 1987. *Literacy: Reading the Word and the World*. Massachusetts: Bergin and Harvey.

Giddens, A., 1984. *The Constitution of Society*, Berkeley: University of California Press.

Gilligan, C., 1982. *In a Different Voice: Psychological Theory and Women's Development*. Cambridge: Harvard University Press.

Glaser, B., and Strauss, A., 1967. *The Development of Grounded Theory: Strategies for Qualitative Research*. Chicago: Aldine Atheron.

Guba, E., and Lincon, Y., 1989. *Fourth Generation Evaluation*. London: Sage.

Habermas, J., 1984. *The Theory of Communicative Action*. Volume 1. London: Heinemann.

Heron, J. 1988. 'Validity in Cooperative Inquiry', in P. Reasons *et al.*, *Human Inquiry in Action*. London: Sage.

Kvale, S., 1995. 'Theme of Postmodernity', in W.T. Anderson, ed., *The Truth about Truth*. New York: Putman

Labonte, R., 1996. *Community Development in the Public Health Sector: The Possibilities of an Empowering Relationship between State and Civil Society*. Toronto: York University (unpublished phD dissertation).

Labonte, R., 1997. *Power, Participation and Partnerships in Health Promotion*. Melbourne: Victoria Health Foundation.

Labonte, R., and Robertson, A., 1996. 'Health Promotion Research and Practice: The Case for the Constructivist Paradigm' *Health Education Quarterly*, 23, 4: pp. 431–47.

Labonte, R., and Feather, J., 1996. *Handbook on Using Stories in Health Promotion Practice*. Ottawa: Health Canada.

Razack, S., 1993. 'Story-telling for Social Change', *Gender and Education*, 5, 1: pp. 55–70.

Schon, D., 1983. *The Reflective Practitioner*. New York: Basic Books.

Schon, D., 1990. *Educating the Reflective Practioner*. New York: Basic Books.

Slim, H., and Thompson, P., 1995. *Listening for a Change: Oral Testimony and Community Development*. Gabriola Island, BC: New Society.

Society for Public Health Education and Centers for Disease Control and Prevention, 1994. *Creating Capacity: A Health Education Research Agenta.* Atlanta: CDC.

Strauss, A., 1987. *Qualitative Analysis for Social Scientists.* Cambridge: Cambridge University Press.

Tronto, J., 1993. *Moral Boundaries: A Political Argument for an Ethic of Care.* New York: Routledge.

Vella, J., 1989. *Learning to Teach: Training of Trainers for Community Development.* New York: International Save the Children.

Wallerstein, N., 1992. 'Powerlessness, Empowerment and Health: Implications for Health Promotion Programs', *American Journal of Health Promotion*, 6, 3: pp. 197–205.

Wallerstein, N., and Bernstein, E., eds., 1994. 'Special Issue: Community Empowerment, Participatory Education, and Health – Part I and Part II', *Health Education Quarterly*, 21, 3–4.

Wallerstein, N., and Bernstein, E., 1988. 'Empowerment Education. Freire's Ideas Adapted to Health Education', *Health Education Quarterly*, 15: pp. 379–94.

Wallerstein, N., and Sanchez-Merki, V., 1994. 'Freirian Praxis in Health Education: Research Results from an Adolescent Program', *Health Education Research*, 9, 1: pp. 105–18.

EIGHT

Building Sound Foundations: Measurement in Health Promotion Research

KATHRYN DEAN

INTRODUCTION

Research issues in the field of health promotion often focus on evaluation research rather than research conducted to provide the knowledge needed to develop sound and effective interventions. Health promotion evolved from a practice field drawing knowledge from research conducted in other disciplines. This may explain why weaknesses found in research conducted on population health (*Lancet* 1994; WHO 1992), and concerns about both methodological problems and how to face research challenges, are often not taken seriously. Indeed, recent critiques of the soundness of knowledge for applications to protect and improve health (Pearce 1996; Susser and Susser 1996a, 1996b; Taubes 1995) are considered by some to make much ado about issues of little importance. Attempts to face scientific challenges such as multiple causation in population health research have even been denigrated. In this perspective, methodological issues in the measurement of variables or the identification of causal pathways, while intellectually challenging and appealing to scientists, are diversions from taking action (Robertson 1998). Diverting resources and time from outcomes research to scientific efforts directed at understanding etiology, it is believed, creates unnecessary human suffering and loss.

RESEARCH OR ACTION: A FALSE DICHOTOMY

To support the perspective that facing research challenges creates diversions, Robertson develops an argument that is useful for considering the consequences of a false dichotomy pitting research to advance knowledge against intervention research. Maintaining that disease or injury can be eliminated simply by identifying and acting on single factors that are necessary components of specific health problems, Robertson uses the example that clogged coronary arteries account for most ischaemic heart disease. He maintains that if a substance, dietary or drug, could be found to eliminate blockage in coronary arteries without causing adverse side-effects in other systems, it could be added to the water supply to control the disease without having to know about the multiple genetic and lifestyle influences involved in the development of coronary disease. This is the type of thinking behind interventions in the 1980s to reduce cholesterol levels in general populations.

Based on well-documented relationships between cholesterol and the risk of death from coronary heart disease, interventions were conducted in many countries to lower blood cholesterol by diet and/or drugs. Only after extensive resources were used in these interventions did it become recognised that among those whose cholesterol had been lowered, mortality was not reduced, but was actually higher than in control groups that were not subjected to the interventions (Holme 1990; Muldoon *et al.* 1990; Strandberg *et al.* 1991). Alarmed by a U-shaped curve showing the greater mortality found among persons with both low and high cholesterol levels, experts from many countries were assembled to study the evidence. Examining findings involving 68,406 deaths, it was documented that higher mortality rates associated with low cholesterol held both across studies and for a diverse range of causes. Especially high excess death rates were found from digestive system conditions, but also cancer, respiratory system and injury deaths were associated with low cholesterol (Conference Report 1992). While these findings held for both men and women, a 'surprising observation' was reported that, for women, high blood cholesterol was not associated with mortality, not even cardiovascular mortality. Along with other major conclusions, it was recommended based on the findings presented at the expert conference that attempts to lower blood cholesterol levels in general populations should be reconsidered (Hulley *et al.* 1992).

The U-shaped mortality curve associated with blood cholesterol resulted in sharp debates about examining all-cause mortality as well as disease-specific mortality in intervention research. Parallel debates involved issues about high-risk versus population strategies of preventing disease (Davey Smith *et al.* 1993; Rose 1992). Illustrating the issues involved in choosing high-risk or population strategies of preventing disease, Rose (1992) used two other U-shaped curves, mortality associated with weight and symptoms associated with blood pressure, to point out that shifting whole population distributions could bring losses as well as gains. Rose concluded that preventive medicine must use both strategies, but that greater gains would be derived from population strategies.

The goal of lowering cholesterol in general populations to reduce cardiovascular disease is similar to Robertson's hypothetical example (1998, p. 54) of putting an additive in the water supply to eliminate blockage in coronary arteries. A serious weakness in this thinking is that single factors, acted upon with this type of magic bullet (or 'broom') approach to health promotion, are generally not distinct causes that can be readily separated from the complex causal processes in which they are embedded (Dean 1993; Susser and Susser 1996a). It is exactly the causal webs or chains characterised as intellectually interesting but not necessary to research that need to be understood to find out if single factors can be acted upon successfully. It must first be assured that factors considered necessary conditions are indeed determinants. It is knowledge about causal processes that allows the identification of correlations that can mislead, of deviations that are comorbidities rather than causes, of markers that result from interactions among variables that cannot be acted upon in isolation. The 'black box' paradigm behind magic bullet approaches to risk reduction looks only at factors and outcomes without consideration of parallel or intervening factors (Susser and Susser 1996a). The debates about high-risk versus population strategies of preventing disease illustrate well that sound knowledge is needed to inform interventions, and that it is knowledge about causal processes that facilitates choices between high-risk and population strategies. Discussing the weaknesses of measures of relative risk, Rose (1992) uses numerous examples of multiple causes and interactions among variables to show that 'simplistic approach(es) conceal gross inequalities of excess risk' (p. 41). Sound research can improve bodies of knowledge about how influences interact to cause disease, but population curves, statistical correlations and relative risk data cannot be simply transformed into assumptions about clinical disease in individuals. The cholesterol example illustrates that, contrary to the idea of saving resources and preventing unnecessary suffering, action based on limited or faulty knowledge wastes resources and can be dangerous.

It is also a myth that research on multiple causation is more time-consuming and costly than other types of research. If appropriate methods are used in a timely fashion, the way influences interact to affect outcomes can be mapped to provide information needed for effective interventions. There was actually evidence available in the research literature of other disciplines in the 1980s that could have provided insight for designing more effective and safer interventions to promote cardiovascular health (Dean 1996).

MEASUREMENT IN HEALTH PROMOTION RESEARCH

Measurement provides the foundation on which research investigations build. Health promotion research draws on both the social and the biological sciences. Research on disease relies heavily on biological measurement. When the focus of measurement shifted to health it became necessary to draw on social science approaches to measurement in order to study the multiple dimensions of health and variables related to health in data collected from samples of populations. Many of the most important research challenges in health promotion revolve around the shift in focus from disease to health. Identifying the forces that protect health and understanding how they operate depends on valid measurement of conceptual domains that can be complex and multifaceted. Health status measurements are necessary for identifying causal influences, examining how they operate, and evaluating the interventions developed from the knowledge they help to provide. This means that dealing with issues in the construction and validation of measures of health status is perhaps the most basic methodological challenge facing quantitative health promotion research.

During the era dominated by prevention research, health status was often measured in terms of specific diseases or of disease-specific or all-cause mortality. While these variables are seriously limited for measuring health and have well-documented problems related to data quality and measurement bias, mortality or diseases included in classifications generally accepted by health researchers provide measures that are relatively straightforward. The shift in focus from disease to health highlights difficulties faced in measuring multifaceted phenomena.

In recent times there has been a growing tendency to construct scaled variables from information collected in population surveys. Scales constructed from survey data are often composed of measures of multiple domains of health or behaviour that are summed into a composite variable. Since these scales are increasingly often being constructed and used in the field of health promotion, this discussion of measurement will take up methodological issues in scaling data.

WHAT ARE SCALED VARIABLES?

Briefly stated for our purposes, index scales are variables created from observations, generally in the form of answers to questions covering a common domain that are administered to respondents. The domains represent theoretical or conceptual areas. They may cover a conceptual state such as health or well-being, a psychosocial concept such as social support or a behavioural concept like lifestyle. Items representing the domain are summed or otherwise consolidated into variables that are considered to measure the domain. Index scales are then data reductions that, if executed correctly, become constructs that measure the theoretical domain.

WHY CONSTRUCT SCALES?

In measurement theory the construction of scales is based on the idea that they represent some type of underlying variable that cannot be measured directly such as intelligence, anxiety, coping or variables that are considered to measure personality types. In research on populations, scaled variables may also be constructed because it is believed that scores derived from data reductions can provide single or simple measures that can be used to monitor developments, compare groups or assign individuals relative values on variables of interest. Measures of health, functional ability, social support and socio-economic status are types of variables used in this manner in population health research. The ability of scales to achieve these goals depends on the extent to which they are valid measures of given theoretical domains. In performing data reductions to create scaled variables, numerical or ordered relational systems are developed to represent the theoretical/conceptual domains (Anderson *et al.* 1983). The procedures for performing a data reduction must obtain an accurate representation of the domain, so that the constructed variable can be used to investigate the theoretical domain.

WHAT IS NEEDED TO CONSTRUCT A VALID SCALE?

In quantitative measurement it is necessary to operationalise magnitudes. In data reductions the process of operationalising magnitudes is called variable construction. The proper execution of this process allows mathematical operations on the constructed variables to be interpreted (Andrich 1988). For data reductions to achieve valid measurement they must adequately represent the theoretically tenable conceptual domain and no other domain. This means that valid measures must be unidimensional. If it is believed that multiple dimensions are meaningful in a variable, at the very least it must be assured that they do not confound measurement or the results of the analysis of group data. Camilli and Shepard (1994), psychometricians working predominantly with Item Response Theory (IRT) methods, used the example that an item on an index used in educational testing might require two abilities, ability to reason and ability to work quickly. If this were the case, an item would not measure a single ability. Since IRT models are unidimensional, confounding and misinterpretations of the results are dangers to be considered. In such cases, it is necessary to know and understand the dimensions in relation to the purpose of the scale, and carefully to analyse – theoretically and logically – the cause of differential outcomes. This means that, when individual or group differences are obtained with a measurement scale, it must be assured that they are relevant to the construct being measured and not to multiple dimensions, biased items or artefacts of the validation methods. It is essential to recognise that no statistical procedure is accurate enough to be applied mechanically (Camilli and Shepard 1994). The results of using a technique must always be assessed in terms of the theory behind the conceptual domain, the limits of the statistical validation tool, and the intended use of the results of the measurement. In health promotion, the purpose of measurement generally shifts from psychometric assessments of educational abilities or clinical attributes of individuals to sociometric assessments of group data. The special measurement problems of working with data collected from population samples, such as the serious problems of confounding with multidimensional scales, are often ignored.

Since measurements are used to compare subjects on specific variables or to examine the relative importance of a variable compared to the influence of other variables on an outcome, a valid measure must be able to place individuals relative to each other on the domain of interest, assuring that no other domain is confounding the results. If the logic of the theory does not hold or the numerical system of assigning numbers does not represent the domain, then the mathematical procedures performed on the numbers will not answer questions about the empirical relationships in the domain, or worse, will answer them incorrectly (Anderson *et al.* 1983). Therefore, besides assuring that only the theoretical domain of interest is represented in the variable construction or validation, it must also be assured that the items used to tap the domain are not biased.

There are two major paradigms based on different theoretical models and statistical approaches used for constructing and validating scaled variables and testing for item bias: classical test theory and item response theory (Bohrnstedt 1983; Camilli and Shepard, 1994; Hambleton *et al.* 1991). Both traditions are concerned with the analysis of latent structures or underlying variables in theoretical domains.

The classical paradigm is based on a theory of true scores and unbiased measurement errors. The latent variable represented by the 'true score' and the measurement error sometimes called 'random noise' are considered independent. Additional assumptions developed so that this model can be operationalised are that the true score is a linear function of the latent variable and that both the latent variables and measurement errors are normally distributed. In this paradigm, problems in variable construction arise from violating the assumptions of the theory and by the introduction of non-random error. Construction and validation of scaled variables in this paradigm focuses heavily on obtaining reliable measures. Validity is often assessed in terms of criterion variables. The measure of the theoretical domain should predict other measures (criterion variables) that are considered to tap the same concept.[1]

In contrast, the item response theory (IRT) paradigm builds on a latent variable model in which the items are direct representations of the latent variable/theoretical domain in a given population. Measurement error is the difference between the value of an item parameter and the latent variable. Latent variables and measurement errors are not assumed to be independent

(Kreiner 1993). These more modern methods for developing and evaluating index scales have also been called 'total score categorization techniques' (Camilli and Shepard 1994). While having different statistical properties, they share a similar conceptual framework with earlier methods. Item Response Theory does not contain ideas about true scores that are linear manifestations of latent variables. Assuring construct validity and identifying item bias are fundamental. In this paradigm the focus of variable construction and validation is on obtaining items that adequately measure the domain and that are not biased. Test bias refers to systematic error in measurement outcomes for members of a specific group of people. Thus, 'bias is systematic in the sense that it creates a distortion in test results for members of a particular group' (Camilli and Shepard 1994).[2]

The ability of a measure to predict criterion variables is not considered adequate evidence of validity. It happens that such predictions may occur even when index variables represent domains other than the one the variable intends to measure. In the field of psychometrics, this has been well documented with examples of intelligence test scores, intended to represent the theoretical construct of intelligence, that were biased for cultural group differences or differences arising from economic or educational opportunities (Camilli and Shepard 1994).[3] An example in the field of health promotion is the body of research that predicted differences in mortality based on a measure of the theoretical construct of social support. Only later did it become recognised that the scaled measure used in the studies tapped domains other than social support that affect survival (Dean *et al.* 1994). (See discussion of this example below.)

Before a scale that predicts criterion variables can be accepted as a valid measure of the theoretical concept or latent variable it is supposed to measure, several conditions must hold (Rosenbaum 1989). The first condition is that higher values on the criterion variable must be associated with higher values on the scaled variable. Secondly, it must be determined that the scale measures the theoretical domain rather than systematically measuring something else. Finally, it must be assured that the scale predicts the criterion variable because the items included in the scale measure the theoretical domain and not because they represent something else. To illustrate these requirements one might examine a measure of health, perhaps a morbidity scale, that statistically predicts another measure of health, say a measure of functional ability. In order for this to support the validity of the morbidity scale, it must be assured that prediction occurs only because the scale measures a morbidity domain of health status and not because it taps another domain that is correlated with functional status, say age or socio-economic status. Similarly, *all* the items of the scaled variable must actually measure the domain of interest. For example, all the items of a behavioural risk scale must measure a tendency towards risky behaviour and not anything else, such as gender differences in alcohol consumption, exercise or eating behaviours (Dean and Salem 1998).

Methodological conditions for variable construction were developed so that social measurement can achieve the goal of interpretable comparisons. Fulfilling methodological requirements for the construction and validation of variables rules out possibilities that make comparisons ambiguous, tentative or false (Anderson *et al.* 1983; Andrich 1988). It has been shown that fundamental measurement is achieved when units of the measure have the same meaning over the range of the variable. The units must also provide constant or invariant comparisons. These conditions make summation possible. The data collected with the variable are then cumulative. This means that the probability of a particular response varies monotonically with the amount of the concept or characteristic. Monotonicity is required for data transformations to produce measurements (Andrich 1988).

The demand that the units of a measure have the same meaning over the range of the variable corresponds to the criteria of unidimensionality and to Rosenbaum's condition that an index scale measures the theoretical domain rather something else. When the units of the measure are constant or invariant over the range of the variable, they provide constant or invariant information about the concept or characteristic, irrespective of the group to which an individual belongs. The items of the measure are then free of bias.

IGNORING METHODOLOGICAL REQUIREMENTS FOR VALID MEASUREMENT HAS SERIOUS CONSEQUENCES

Recent assessments of knowledge used for population health initiatives direct attention to the consequences of ignoring methodological problems in health promotion research. The cholesterol example cited above is only one of numerous examples of problems arising from insufficient knowledge or misleading information. Inconsistencies and contradictions in risk factor research are widespread (Berkman 1984, 1986; Dean 1993; Dean *et al.* 1994; Rose 1985; Susser and Susser 1996a, 1996b; Taubes 1995). Since the valid measurement of variables is the foundation on which knowledge is built, weaknesses in measurement unavoidably lead to problems in the soundness of research results. Yet the validity of variable construction is often ignored or taken for granted by referencing validity claims made by researchers about measures validated in other samples. Norman Breslow, discussing problems in research on risk factors, points out that statistical confidence means considerably less than believed because systematic errors and biases that are not detected 'almost invariably overwhelm the statistical variation' (Taubes 1995, p. 168).

A few examples are illustrative. In 1988, it was claimed, in an article in *Science*, that evidence documenting the causal influence (the protective effects) of the social network on health approximated the evidence available on smoking at the time of the widely cited US Surgeon General's report on smoking and health in 1964 (House *et al.* 1988). The evidence cited in the article was produced in prospective studies of mortality using a composite measure of social network. While mortality had been consistently predicted in research using the composite measure of social network, there were serious inconsistencies in the predictions. The findings with regard to cardiovascular disease were especially confusing and contradictory. Numerous explanations were given for the contradictions in this body of research (Berkman 1984, 1986; House *et al.* 1988), but none of the explanations considered the possibility that methodological problems in the construction of the measure of social network might be responsible.

The scale used in the studies is a composite of subscales and items. The scale covers multiple dimensions: number of relatives, number of close friends, frequency of various kinds of social contact, membership in community groups, church attendance and marital status. The components of the scale represent not only multiple dimensions of social network activity and support, but also other conceptual domains. Serious bias has been found for both the subscales and individual items in the index (Dean *et al.* 1994). The bias detected in the scale is particularly strong with respect to the employment status, income and gender of the respondents.

The different dimensions of the scale represent variables other than support obtained in social networks that affect health. For example, items in the scale represent not only potential support, but also economic resources and opportunities. Because domains are confounded in the scale, it is not possible to get sound and consistent results when the scale is used as a measure of network support. In spite of the strong claims made for this body of research in the 1988 article, little work to understand the importance of various types of social support for health and well-being has occurred since that time. Rather, this subject has been relatively neglected in recent years. This is unfortunate, because the functioning of social networks, while poorly understood, clearly exerts influence on health and well-being (Cassel 1976; Cohen and Syme 1985). Understanding the nature of the influences under varying health and social conditions would be extremely useful for health-promotion interventions.

The social support example illustrates that the population groups that are known to be at greater risk for numerous health problems may contribute disproportionately to the measurement error and bias that, as pointed out by Breslow, can overwhelm statistical variation (Taubes 1995). This means that research purporting to measure one conceptual domain may in fact measure others. Thus a measure can represent educational or economic resources when it is intended only as a measure of psychosocial support. Another example is relevant to consider in this regard. Well-documented statistical relationships between some habits of daily living and variables measuring health or functional status have generated interest in the construction of behavioural risk scales. The idea behind combining behaviours in risk scales is to measure a latent dimension of risk-taking in order to study determinants of risk behaviour. Alternatively, a goal may be to measure the health outcomes of risky behaviour. In either case, to be valid, a risk index must measure risk behaviour without being confounded by other conceptual domains.

There is evidence that cautions against summing risk behaviours into additive scales. Using risk indexes constructed from behaviours correlated with health outcomes could produce misleading results. Work to construct and validate a behavioural risk index found that the most widely studied risk behaviours do not represent sufficiently similar types of phenomena to form additive scales (Dean and Salem 1998). The commonly studied risk behaviours were found to represent different dimensions of behaviour. Item bias, especially with regard to gender and education, was also a serious problem detected in attempting to construct a behavioural risk scale with the commonly studied behaviours. The findings suggested that the behaviours have quite distinct meanings and consequences for different subgroups of the population.

WHAT ARE THE IMPLICATIONS FOR MEASURES OF HEALTH STATUS?

These methodological aspects of measurement apply equally, perhaps even more fundamentally, to health status measurement. Measures of health status are used to identify the determinants of health and to evaluate the outcomes of interventions. Clearly, measures that suffer from systematic errors or bias will produce misleading results. The tendency to construct multidimensional scales can seriously compound the problems. The determinants of different dimensions of health and function may vary considerably. The importance of specific causal influences are not likely to be the same for physical, psychological and social dimensions of health.

The issues are basically the same as those taken up long ago by social scientists working on measures of socio-economic status. Methodological problems faced in constructing variables to measure these complex phenomena were widely debated. A basic measurement issue was whether socio-economic status could be considered unidimensional. Multiple dimensions of social stratification were identified (Caplow 1954; Hatt, 1950; Haug 1977). Hodge (1970), noting that different indicators of SES are associated with well-being, cautioned that any attempt to combine educational attainment, occupational pursuit, family income or occupational origins into composite variables of socio-economic status would prove unsatisfactory because the component parts of a composite SES variable would have different consequences for a given study variable.

Composite health scales often include domains of symptom experience, functional status, perceived health status and medically diagnosed conditions. There is evidence that each of these domains is subject to various types of measurement bias. There is evidence that symptom scales may themselves be multidimensional, with the same variables, such as age or gender, affecting the dimensions differently (Dean and Edwardson 1996; Kreiner 1993). Thus, not only is it likely that the determinants of separate domains represented in composite measures of health status differ considerably, but causal influences may operate in opposite directions from domain to domain. Thus the results of summing the domains would be confounded and could be seriously misleading. Measurements of health status must meet the same demands for valid measurement as any other variable.

SUMMARY

Attempts to pit methodologically sound research to improve knowledge against evaluation studies of health promotion interventions create a false dichotomy. It is a myth that research investigations to achieve meaningful and sound variable construction and to understand causal processes are more time-consuming and costly than evaluation research. Action which is based on research that is not methodologically sound wastes resources and can be dangerous. Attention to methodological issues in measurement can help to remove the systematic errors and bias that often overwhelm statistical variation in causal research. Myths about scientifically sound research are perpetuated by traditions of relying on knowledge generated in other disciplines and by extremely limited educational opportunities for learning about the range of available methods and about the rapid advances in options for quantitative analysis of population health data.

REFERENCES

Andersen, E., 1973. 'A Goodness of Fit Test for the Rasch Model', *Psychometrika*, 38: pp. 123–9.

Anderson, A., Basilevsky, A., and Hum, D., 1983. 'Measurement: Theory and Techniques', in P. Rossi, J. Wright and A. Anderson, eds., *Handbook of Survey Research*. London: Acadmeic Press, pp. 231–81.

Andrich, D., 1988. *Rasch Models of Measurement: Quantitative Applications in the Social Sciences*. Newbury Park: Sage.

Berkman, L., 1986. 'Social Networks, Support, and Health: Taking the Next Step Forward', *American Journal of Epidemiology*, 123: pp. 559–62.

Berkman, L., 1984. 'Assessing the Physical Health Effects of Social Networks and Social Support', *Annuals of Research in Public Health*, 5: pp. 413–32.

Bohrnstedt, G., 1983. 'Measurement', in P. Rossi, J. Wright and A. Anderson, eds., Handbook of Survey Research. London: Academic Press, pp. 70–115.

Camilli, G., and Shepard, L., 1994. *Methods for Identifying Biased Test Items*. Thousand Oaks: Sage.

Caplow, T., 1954. *Sociology of Work*. Minneapolis: University of Minnesota Press.

Cassel, J., 1976. 'The Contribution of the Social Environment to Host Resistance', *American Journal of Epidemiology*, 104: pp. 107–23.

Cohen, A., and Syme, L., 1985. *Social Support and Health*. New York: Academic Press.

Conference Report on Low Cholesterol: Mortality Associations, 1992. *Circulation*, 86: pp. 1046–60.

Davey-Smith, G., Song, F., and Sheldon, T., 1993. 'Cholesterol Lowering and Mortality: The Importance of Considering Initial Level of Risk', *British Medical Journal*, 306: pp. 1367–73.

Dean, K., 1993. 'Integrating Theory and Methods in Population Health Research', in K. Dean, ed., *Population Health Research: Linking Theory and Methods*. London: Sage.

Dean, K., 1996. 'Using Theory to Guide Policy Relevant Health Promotion Research', *Health Promotion International*, 11: pp. 19–26.

Dean, K., and Edwardson, S., 1996. 'Additive Scoring of Reported Symptoms: Validity and Item Bias Problems in Morbidity Scales', *European Journal of Public Health*, 6: pp. 275–81.

Dean, K., and Salem, N., 1998. 'Detecting Measurement Confounding in Epidemiological Research: Construct Validity in Scaling Risk Behaviors', *Journal of Epidemiology and Community Health*, 52: pp. 195–9.

Dean, K., Holst, E., Kreiner, S., Schoenborn, C., and Wilson, R., 1994. 'Measurement Issues in Research on Social Support and Health', *Journal of Epidemiology and Community Health*, 48: pp. 201–6.

Lancet (editorial), 1994. 'Population Health Looking Upstream', *Lancet*, 343: pp. 329–30.

Hambleton, R., Swaminathan, H., and Rogers, H., 1991. *Fundamentals of Item Response Theory*. London: Sage.

Hatt, P., 1950. 'Occupation and Social Stratification', *American Journal of Sociology*, 55: pp. 438–43.

Haug, M., 1977. 'Measurement in Social Stratification', *Annual Review of Sociology*, 3: pp. 51–77.

Hodge, R., 1970. 'Social Integration, Psychological Wellbeing and their SES Correlates', in E. Laumann, ed., *Social Stratification: Research and Theory for the 1970s*. Indianapolis: Bobbs-Merrill.

Holme, I., 1990. 'An Analysis of Randomized Trials Evaluating the Effect of Cholesterol Reduction on Total Mortality and Coronary Heart Disease Incidence', *Circulation*, 82: pp. 1916–24.

Holst, C., 1995. *Item Response Theory*. Copenhagen: The Danish National Institute for Educational Research.

House, J., Landis, K., and Umberson, D., 1988. 'Social relationships and health', *Science*, 241: pp. 540–5.

Hulley, S., Walsh, J., and Newman, T., 1992. 'Health Policy on Blood Cholesterol: Time to Change Directions', *Circulation*, 86: pp. 1026–9.

Kreiner, S., 1994. 'Validation of Index Scales for Analysis of Survey Data: The Symptom Index', in K. Dean, ed., *Population Health Research: Linking Theory and Methods*. London: Sage.

Kreiner, S., 1987. 'Analysis of Multidimensional Contingency Tables by Exact Conditional Tests: Techniques and strategies', *Scandinavian Journal of Statistics*, 14, 2: pp. 97–112.

Muldoon, M., Manuck, S., and Matthews, K., 1990. 'Lowering Cholesterol Concentrations and Mortality: A Quantitative Review of Primary Prevention Trials', *British Medical Journal*, 301: pp. 309–14.

Pearce, N., 1990. 'White Swans, Black Ravens and Lame Ducks: Necessary and Sufficient Causes in Epidemiology', *Epidemiology*, 1: pp. 47–50.

Pearce, N., 1996. 'Traditional Epidemiology, Modern Epidemiology, and Public Health', *American Journal of Public Health*, 86: pp. 678–83.

Robertson, L., 1998. 'Causal Webs, Preventive Brooms and Housekeepers'. *Social Science and Medicine*, 46: pp. 53–8.

Rose, G., 1985. 'Sick Individuals and Sick Populations', *International Journal of Epidemiology*, 14: pp. 34–8.

Rose, G., 1992. *The Strategy of Preventive Medicine*. Oxford: Oxford University Press.

Rosenbaum, P., 1989. 'Criterion-Related Construct Validity', *Psychometrika*, 54: pp. 625–34.

Rosenbaum, P., 1984. 'Testing the Conditional Independence and Monotonicity Assumption of Item Response Theory', *Psychometrika*, 49: pp. 425–35.

Selltiz, C., Wrightsman, L., and Cook, S., 1976. *Research Methods in Social Relations*. New York: Holt, Rinehart and Winston.

Strandberg, T., Salomaa, V., Naukkarinen, V., Vanhanen, H., Sarna, S., and Miettinen, T., 1991. 'Long Term Mortality after 5-year Multifactional Primary Prevention of Cardiovascular Diseases in Middle-aged Men', *Journal of the American Medical Association*, 266: pp. 1225–9.

Study group of the European Atherosclerosis Society, 1987. 'Strategies for the Prevention of Coronary Heart Disease: A Policy Statement of the European Atherosclerosis Society', *European Heart Journal*, 8: pp. 77–88.

Susser, M., and Susser, E., 1996a. 'Choosing a Future for Epidemiology: I. Eras and Paradigms', *American Journal of Public Health*, 86: pp. 668–72.

Susser, M., and Susser, E., 1996b. 'Choosing a Future for Epidemiology: II. From Black Box to Chinese Boxes and Eco-Epidemiology', *American Journal of Public Health*, 86: pp. 674–7.

Taubes, G., 1995. 'Epidemiology Faces Its Limits', *Science*, 269: pp. 164–9.

Tjur, T., 1982. 'A Connection between Rasch's Item Analysis Model and a Multiplicative Poisson Model', *Scandinavian Journal of Statistics*, 9, 1: pp. 23–30.

World Health Organisation, 1992. *The Crisis of Public Health: Reflections for the Debate*. Washington: WHO and American Health Organisation, Scientific Publication No. 540.

NOTES

1   Camilli and Shepard (1994), Kreiner (1994) and Hambleton et al. (1992) present overviews of methods based on Classical Test Theory and inadequacies that have been documented when these methods are used for validating scaled variables. The methods used to develop and validate index scales to measure variables in population data are based on methods first used for psychological testing. In early psychological testing, no demands other than the initial theoretical logic were required to verify a measurement tool. It was later recognised that just as other scientific theories had to be tested, inferences based on measurement scales had to be tested and evaluated as well. In the 1985 Standards for Educational and Psychological Testing, more stringent demands for construct validity requirements for all measurement tests were adopted. It was recognised that neither content validity nor predictive correlations are sufficient (Camilli and Shepard 1994). The psychometric demands adopted for construct validity must be considered minimum standards for sociometric measurement which also involves technical issues related to constructing variables that will be used in multivariate analyses of population data.

2   While it is beyond the scope of this chapter to take up in any detail the technical issues and debates within the field, it should be mentioned that there are different IRT models for testing the construct validity of measurement scales. A central debate focuses on the appropriateness of choosing among 1-parameter, 2-parameter and 3-parameter IRT models. For example, one body of opinion cautions against using only the 1-parameter model because it focuses on how well the items test the construct domain but does not test for differences in item discrimination, as does the 2-parameter model, or for possible guessing, as does the 3-parameter model (Camilli and Shepard 1994). A second body of opinion points to limits in the theoretical foundations for the 2-parameter and 3-parameter models and to problems identified in empirical work. For example, it is concluded that with the 2-parameter model subjects cannot be compared in a fashion that is specifically objective in a probabilistic sense (Holst 1995). Researchers

working with the 1-parameter model use a range of procedures to test the fit of the model and extend the validation to different types of deviations from the model. These include tests for item homogeneity (Anderson 1973), local and conditional independence of items (Rosenbaum 1984; Tjur 1982) and item bias (Kreiner 1987).

3   Early researchers discussed observed social class differences on tests of ability in terms of genetic or environmental differences in ability, much as debates about many subjects in the area of health occur today. Only after years of such debates did the focus shift to the possibility that measured differences on IQ tests might be due to the content of test items rather than accurately reflecting important underlying differences in ability (Camilli and Shepard 1994).

NINE

Methodologies and Evaluation in Public Health and Health Promotion

KLIM McPHERSON

INTRODUCTION

It is self-evident that public health policy, health promotion strategies and medicine are best if based on hard evidence of attributable effect. However, this simple assertion is fraught with problems about the nature of evidence and the methodologies used for deriving hard evidence (McPherson 1994; Sackett and Wennberg 1997). In the interdisciplinary collaboration that is essential to the full understanding of most of the questions in these areas, the struggle to obtain answers can sometimes polarise to absurd positions. One may be asked to believe that Evidence Based Medicine, for example, is merely an illegitimate expansion of a positivist discourse, one upheld in order to consolidate a professional hegemony over health promotion. In the middle of all this the randomised controlled trial (RCT) receives the brunt of much ridiculous polarisation as the 'gold standard' for hard evidence for a therapeutic or behavioural effect on outcome.

RCTs are a brilliant device for controlling unknown (and known) selection criteria, which might lead to confounding between treatment or intervention choices and their effect (Kleijnen et al. 1997). Hence observational (non-randomised) comparisons are interpreted with appropriate caution and cannot lightly represent the basis for strong evidence for such effects, since treatment *choices* themselves can depend so much on prognosis. Thus, discerning the difference between a real therapeutic effect or a confounding by selection effect is impossible, unless one can identify or exclude all differences in outcome that could be a result of differential aggregate prognosis.

In this chapter I want to use just this kind of argument about RCTs in the context of the problems of evaluating public health or health promotion interventions, as well as clinical interventions. I shall argue that, just as observational studies are in general uninterpretable unless very strict conditions are met (Britton et al. 1999), so RCTs which are not blinded (i.e.

in which the allocation to treatment is not hidden from the subject) are also uninterpretable unless other conditions are met. Of course there are many large RCTs evaluating new treatments in cancer or heart disease which are of necessity unblind and hence cannot, by the arguments to follow, be properly interpreted. The basic reason for this is that if preferences for treatment affect their effectiveness then unblind trials will incorporate such preference effects under certain conditions – which will be taken to be evidence of effectiveness unaltered by preference.

Thus, such trials or meta-analyses are widely believed to provide strong evidence in favour of a particular effect of treatments which are commonly used and simply biological/physiological/pharmacological in mechanism. The circumstances in which randomised trials cannot be blinded are very common, and of course the more the participation of subject or carer is required specifically for a treatment the less possible genuine blinding becomes. In particular interventions like surgery, or methods of encouraging behaviour change, blinding is often near enough to impossible.

The nature of the general methodological problem is that some kinds of health-related interventions are amenable to excellent methodological devices, like double-blind RCTs, to discern their specific effects, and other kinds of intervention are less amenable (McKee *et al.* 1998). Whether these interventions are amenable or not carries no necessary implication about their utility, their acceptability or their potency. Moreover, of course, there may be a variety of other brilliant devices which may be developed by different groups of people to solve different problems. These may be less familiar, and comply with different criteria of rigour or of evidence, to other groups working in health.

DIFFERENT KINDS OF INTERVENTION

Treatments expected to have consistent biological or physiological effects on specified groups of (possibly ill) people can have these effects disentangled from all other exogenous or endogenous effects on the relevant biological processes by random allocation. The disentangling is thus essentially averaging over the whole complexity of whatever these other effects actually are, which are made to be evenly balanced (in probability) by randomisation. The implied model is that the biological effect will occur almost in whatever circumstances the intervention is proffered. In effect the pragmatic question of whether the treatment works in such a consistent and aggregated way dominates the legitimate quest for hard evidence, in circumstances where such a question is obviously the most important one to address.

When we say that the treatment 'works' we mostly mean something like, people on the treatment do (say) 20% better on average overall, measured in some way, than those not on the treatment. Clearly this is an average statement of an effect, and among individuals the attributable benefit, if we could measure it, might of course be different. In particular, among certain *kinds* of individuals it might well be different in ways which might affect outcome, and these aspects can be measured. But concentrating on the main effect subordinates these possible complexities of *interaction and effect-modification*[1] to second-order questions, on the implied assumption that they are either relatively unimportant or too difficult to investigate or both. But this is usually merely an assumption.

Given the need for hard evidence this is often a wise assumption to make, since detecting important interaction and effect-modification in any biological treatment or intervention process with another influence, which is subject to variation, is relatively insensitive. Anyway, uncovering consistent main effects without investigating interaction or effect-modification is a necessary first step to understanding. Moreover, obtaining reliable evidence about these latter is just very difficult and generally an order of magnitude more expensive to do, with comparable precision and reliability, than testing for the main effect.

Many interventions, however, are expected to work by just this sort of complicated mechanism. That is to say that the existence of a particular interaction between a straight biological process and intrinsic features of people or communities and behavioural or psychological states of individuals must be commonplace. However, in clinical medicine such effect-modifiers will probably be rare, while in health promotion they can be expected to be much more common.

Thus, reducing the risk of lung cancer in populations could be achieved by developing an antidote to the harmful carcinogenic effects of tobacco which people who smoke could eat every day. This would be a biological/ medical intervention in which such a treatment would not be expected to work for absolutely everybody and whose biological properties would provide benefit only among those for whom the initial insult, tobacco, was present. Life-long non-smokers would accrue no benefit, presumably. On the other hand, to give people nicotine chewing-gum would be expected to work by having a different kind of effect. Basically, some would be assisted by the gum to quit tobacco forever, while others would not. Quite possibly some would smoke as much or more as a consequence of the intervention.

The important evaluative agenda to discover whether either 'worked' would be different from the detection of an aggregate effect among smokers in the first case, with the possibility of an *interaction* by amount smoked, to a possibly crucial *effect-modification* effect in the second. The effect-modification effect would be as dominant in that latter agenda as the *main* effect. The antidote, if it worked and had few side-effects, would probably be taken by most. Many might smoke more as a consequence and, depending on how it functioned, this might therefore attenuate its aggregate attributable effect. Many of the smokers would never get lung cancer anyway, of course, and for them the antidote would be ineffective, although it might well take the credit. Just as in the use of nicotine chewing-gum, the assessment of effect might be strongly affected by the population among whom, and the time when, the intervention was provided.

In these examples a double-blind trial is possible where placebo gum or antidote is offered to one group and active gum or antidote to another (although the two gums are in fact easily distinguishable to an addict!). Thus, a blind RCT would in principle detect the main physiological effect among the groups randomised. But possibly the dominant mode of action would be via a crucial and consistent interaction between physiology, attitude and character, for example. These would be deliberately missed in a blind trial, even if it were feasible to ensure blindness, and often this is impossible. The methodology for reliably detecting such things is much more complex and difficult than in the case of biological main effects, and it is naive to assume that every important effect of health interventions can be as easily tested as can straightforward aggregate biological effects. It follows, therefore, that it is naive to assume that, since the evidence for such effects may not be strong, they are therefore fanciful. This is important.

PATIENT (OR PERSON) PREFERENCES

One particular kind of interaction of interest here, and whose detection is highly subject to these intrinsic problems of methodology, is that between an organic and a possible psychological or even social effect of a medical therapy. A simple and typical example of this might be the therapeutic effect of patient (or consumer, possibly client) preferences (Antonovsky 1992); there are many other related descriptions, including of course the well-known placebo effect (Kleijnen *et al.* 1994, pp. 1347–9), with which this phenomenon is clearly related.

In clinical medicine, treatments work because of pharmacological or physiological effects on biological mechanisms. Thus, drugs which kill rapidly dividing cells or compounds which have (anti)-hormonal effects can be expected to go to the root of a particular pathological process – which will be common to all who suffer from it. In public health and health promotion, relevant interventions tend to be less specific. Thus an intervention designed to enable people to improve their health, by for example lifestyle change, does not have the same kind of simple (in principle) underpinning and theoretical justification. This is because the processes of making the change interact with the health consequences of that change, not to speak of the complex determinants of the behaviour in the first place.

The health effects may well have a simple biological underpinning, but the roots of the behavioural change processes are much less likely to do so.

The true complexities of these behavioural changes must include social and structural group-specific influences – which are actually often dominant determinants of action and belief. People never do, or believe, important things ignoring their own overwhelming context (Weber 1958). Thinking in public health has tended to ignore the true dialectic that exists between people's actual chances and their real possibility of making choices, because biological processes are assumed not to be subject to such influences. This is palpably not an entirely individual business, because both the realities and the possibilities are determined by status and context, themselves in turn variously real and perceived and volatile.

The so-called placebo effect of modern medicine is quite as complicated, and accordingly poorly understood with respect to both where and how it works (Chaput de Saintonge and Herxheimer 1994). But it may well be subject to similar influences of style and preference. That is to say that the nature of the interaction discussed here between treatment efficacy and the patient's hope and expectation is similarly likely to be subject to changing context and clearly may have strong components which have absolutely nothing to do with intrinsic need.

If such interaction or effect-modifying effects exist for medical treatments or health interventions, our capacity to detect them reliably at all is always compromised by a serious possibility of confounding by selection. People who tend to prefer something may well be different in some other consistent ways, plausibly related to prognosis, from those who do not. But, obviously, one can never randomise between enthusiasts for a treatment and those who hate the whole idea of it, in order to average over these other possible differences. Unless one knows that preference is unrelated to prognosis, randomisation will unfortunately be essential to discern any intrinsic preference effect (Silverman and Altman 1966). In addition, where people have strong preferences the whole possibility of randomising is difficult anyway (Lilford 1995).

Hence an essential, but neglected, part of the evidence-based agenda for medical or health promotion treatments is to disentangle the therapeutic effect of a health-enhancing intervention from any possible benefit of preferences themselves (McPherson 1996). Unfortunately, randomised trials, whose main purpose is to reliably detect aggregate biological effects, start by having to find a way of overcoming or circumventing unmeasured preference effects, otherwise they cannot detect therapeutic effects reliably. This is why double blinding is important.

EVIDENCE FOR SUCH EFFECTS

In health promotion it is axiomatic that changes which will bring benefit occur mostly among those most willing and able to change, since empowering people is basic to effective health promotion (WHO 1985). Thus some preferences are often a necessary condition for any intervention to work at all, basically. Certainly in aggregate the effect of intervention will to a large measure be determined by the popularity and acceptability of the measure, compared with alternatives, among the putative beneficiaries.

Irrefutable evidence for significant psychological preference effects among medical treatments on health outcome are, however, sparse. This may be because they are both difficult to detect reliably and because the dominant agenda has, perforce, to subordinate them to possibilities to be controlled, but not measured. Certainly, strong evidence for such effects can only come indirectly from classical randomised trials.

A well-known example, the Coronary Drug Project (The Coronary Drug Project Team 1980), provides a strong hint. Treatment for the secondary prevention of CHD among middle-aged men was observed to be dramatically more effective at delaying death when a *placebo* was 'properly' taken, than when not. If drug compliance here is a measure of some enthusiasm for the treatment, and non-compliance a measure of little enthusiasm, then individual preferences may seem to have an important effect on outcome which is not strictly or directly pharmacological. Adjusting for 40 potential confounding variables, most of which were physiological measurements, when comparing adherers with non-adherers made little difference to the comparison. In circumstances where confounding is a possible explanation for an effect, adjustment which changes the risk estimates strengthens that as an explanation. In this example, adjustment for a large number of variables changes the risk estimates hardly at all and hence the explanation of a preference effect (as opposed to confounding) is easily the most plausible. Since the drug was a placebo the therapeutic effect, by definition, was zero, but the adjusted difference in the five-year mortality among men between adherers and non-adherers was 26% and 16% and highly significant.

Although this example compares adherence to treatment it is not plausibly adherence itself that is responsible for a lower mortality, since the drug (placebo) was designed to be inactive, whether taken or not. It remains possible that adherence predicts compliance to other incidental aspects of care, but it is difficult to imagine what might have such a large effect. This example provides quite strong evidence that there might be an important effect of belief in treatment and in consequent lower mortality, which could be large.

If there is, we need firstly to understand the consequences and secondly to set about understanding where such effects might be important. There is a great deal of indirect evidence for such effects, none of which is absolute, and an equally fascinating debate exists on the possible biological pathways for such psychogenic effects (Cassileth *et al.* 1985; Levy *et al.* 1991; Phillips *et al.* 1993; Redd, *et al.* 1991).

In so far as individual enthusiasms or preferences for certain interventions can affect the effectiveness of those interventions, so randomised comparisons may estimate these true effects in a misleading way, or not at all, as we shall see. They may also, in the absence of good understanding about such effects, estimate the straightforward aggregated organic effect in a misleading way.

In health promotion a well-discussed theory discusses stages of change in which a progression is imagined among people, from no inclination whatever to alter behaviour (precontemplation) to being entirely prepared to change behaviour (contemplation or preparation). Thus the proportion in the latter category may strongly predict the apparent effectiveness of interventions – quite apart from their intrinsic merits in aggregate. In a randomised comparison, however, the proportions will be statistically similar, but different interventions might have a very different ability to persuade some categories of people to contemplate changing behaviour than others. Thus the net RCT outcome will be affected by the proportion prepared to change behaviour as well as the differential effectiveness of the two treatments among different categories of preparedness, in so far as these are remotely understood.

This will necessarily give rise to confusion about the true mechanisms involved, when one has no idea *a priori* for which categories such treatments work and what proportion of any population exhibits such categories anyway. It might also give rise to systematic and important confusion about the nature and extent of such effects. What are the possible effects of strictly adhering to randomised comparisons as the gold standard in order to estimate the true effectiveness of treatments, when such a strategy clearly must ignore patient choices and preferences in order to identify an average therapeutic effect? How large a bias can be induced by such a strategy, and how much confusion (McPherson *et al.* 1997)? For simplicity we shall ignore the effect of selection and generalisation associated with people with strong preference being selectively excluded from trials (MacIntyre 1991). We assume that, whatever individual preferences exist, patients are persuaded of the formal state of uncertainty described as equipoise (Lilford 1995).

A SIMPLE ADDITIVE MODEL

Imagine two treatments designated as A and B. Assume that 'biologically', or strictly organically as it were, treatment A affects (i.e. works on) a proportion P of eligible people, and treatment B a higher proportion $P + x$.

This might be the cure rate or simply the proportion of people affected positively by the intervention, in the absence of any effect of preferences. Assume also that having a preference for A bestows an extra average advantage for treatment A of an amount y to $P + y$ for any of the reasons alluded to above. Similarly, a preference for B bestows a similar additive affect y to $P + x + y$ for treatment B. Conversely, of those who prefer A, only $P + x - y$ will be affected if given treatment B, and of those who prefer B, $P - y$ will benefit if given A. Of the people who are indifferent to the treatments, P benefit on A and $P + x$ on B. These are postulated average effects of that group of patients for whom these treatments would be appropriate. B is better than A by $100x\%$ among people without any preference and having a preference adds another $100y\%$ to the benefit, while preferring the other treatment subtracts $100y\%$. These effects are summarised below.

Postulated treatment effects if:	indifferent	prefer A	prefer B
on treatment A	P	$P + y$	$P - y$
on treatment B	$P + x$	$P + x - y$	$P + x + y$

Figure 1.

Invoking a simple additive model in this way illustrates immediately why randomising among people who believe in treatments may be problematic. Usually nobody knows whether the 'y' interaction exists and how large it might be, among whom. If the proportion of the eligible population who prefer treatment A is alpha, and if beta prefer B and gamma are indifferent, then we shall require that (alpha + beta + gamma) = 1. More complicated models could, of course, be imagined, in which the effects of preference were graded, multiplicative or asymmetric, but since the effects of preference itself on outcome is so poorly understood, perforce the simplest possible model is to be preferred.

It can easily be shown that, in a large, well-conducted randomised comparison, on the above assumptions, the estimate of the effect of treatment B over treatment A (by subtracting the mean effect among those randomised to B from that among those given A) will be $x + 2y$ (beta – alpha). This will be different from x by an amount equal to $2y$ (beta – alpha) and hence such an RCT will only estimate x correctly either if y is zero or if beta = alpha. This of course ignores sampling error and hence represents the estimated treatment effect of an infinite number of meta-analyses, with coincident confidence limits. So long as y is non-zero (i.e. preferences have some effect on outcome), if more people prefer treatment B than treatment A, such a trial will overestimate the 'biological' effect; if otherwise, it will be underestimated. If the preferences are evenly distributed then there is no bias, in the sense that the trial will on average estimate x correctly. But the question is, by how much can there be this kind of 'bias', under reasonable assumptions on y and on beta – alpha? And what might this do to our understanding of evidence-based medicine and health promotion? Randomised trials are important precisely because they estimate effects without any biases associated with unknown patient selection problems.

Firstly we have to postulate the size and sign of the difference in the proportions preferring the two treatments. The sign does not matter, since the algebra is symmetrical and indeed preferences for old treatments against new ones (treatment B is the new treatment here, representing some improvement) may well go either way, but clearly will depend on their nature. It is not difficult to imagine strong reasons for either circumstance, but for the present argument the size of the difference alone is important. Thus if 5% prefer treatment B and 30% treatment A, the difference is 25%, i.e. (beta – alpha) = – 0.25

Secondly we have to assume a coherent effect of patient preference on outcome in circumstances where such things are nearly impossible to measure reliably. In this set up, if the average 'biological' effect of B over A (i.e. x) is 10% (it does not matter what the effect of A alone is, but imagine it to be 50%, say) and if the preference advantage (i.e. y) is 5%, then the treatment effects look like this:

Postulated effects of treatment if:	indifferent	prefer A	prefer B
on treatment A	50%	55%	45%
on treatment B	60%	55%	65%

Figure 2.

If these values for the extent of any preference effect, with the given organic effect, are ever appropriate then simple substitution will indicate that a fair RCT will be 25% 'out'.

(i.e., in this case) 2 y (beta – alpha) is 25% of x

That is, x (the 'treatment' effect) will be 'unbiasedly' (because it is an RCT) estimated as 3/4 x. If, on the other hand, 30% prefer B and 5% A, then the unbiased RCT estimate will be 11/4 x. Either way these results are both wrong, in the sense in which they would be understood by a conventional interpretation of such a trial, ignorant (as we must usually be) of the size of the effect of patient preferences, since these estimated differences will be taken as attributable to the treatment alone and hence generalisable. They will be different depending somewhat on the distribution of effective preferences, not on the organic effect of the treatment alone.

Clearly, if the difference in the proportions who prefer A or B rises to 50% then the size of the 'bias' from a randomised comparison itself rises to

50%, for these hypothetical values of x = 10% and y = 5%. If, however, y is only 1% then the 'biases' in the results of RCTs will be reduced to 5% for a 25% difference in proportions with contrasting preferences, and 10% for a 50% difference. However, if y is 10% (i.e. the role of preference is more profound than the intrinsic treatment effect) then the trials will be respectively 50 and 100% 'out', on average (i.e. the treatment effect will be estimated as $11/2$ x or $2*x$). This is clearly non-trivial, if such large differences in the prevalence of such important (i.e. potent) preferences are plausible.

The Coronary Drug Project observed around a 26% 5-year mortality among non-adherers and 16% among adherers to placebo in the placebo arm of a double blind clinical trial of drug prophylaxis. A value for y of around 5% (2 y = 10% = 26 – 16) would therefore be reasonable in this case. In this trial 67% took more than 80% of the prescribed dose and 32% took less than this, a difference of 35%; and they all knew that there was an even chance that they were taking a placebo. We might assume that a 25% difference in the proportion of men suffering a heart attack who adhere (to what they may have believed to be an active treatment), compared to those who do not, is a more reasonable estimate of the difference in the proportions who prefer 'effective' drug treatment to those that do not. If so, then on average trials of such interventions will overestimate the absent therapeutic pharmacological role of such drugs by 2.5% or more.

IMPLICATIONS

We might consider trials of a supposedly active new treatment, which may have enormous biological plausibility, but which in fact has no (aggregate) organic therapeutic effect, being compared with a placebo in an unblind trial. It may be that in these circumstances the true difference in the prevalence of preferences is much larger: possibly 90% preferring the new 'active' treatment, maybe 5% preferring the placebo and 5% being indifferent. The idea of preferring a placebo for its therapeutic benefit at all does sound slightly fanciful, however. If this is plausible, 'beta – alpha' becomes 0.85 and hence the 'bias' would be 8.5% in absolute terms. In other words, if the natural history is such that 50% 'survive' anyway, such a trial would suggest that the new treatment improved this to 58.5%. What might this say about cancer and cardiovascular treatments, and much else besides, which have been evaluated in many large unblind trials with highly significant estimated benefits of around 10%?

These simple calculations indicate that the supposed benefits, reliably estimated from many trials, may be wrongly attributed to straightforward organic responses; at least in part and possibly systematically. The placebo effect may indeed be profound. Double blind randomised comparison was designed to distinguish it from organic mechanisms. However, it cannot do so in many common circumstances where blinding is impossible (or deemed to be unnecessary) and where preferences are important. But randomised trials themselves, by their very nature and objective, have to try to control the potential of preferences to affect outcome. Hence the nature and extent, and indeed the mechanisms, by which such things might work will remain difficult to disentangle, unless we can understand all the possible consequences.

CONCLUSION

Rothman (1996) enjoins us to avoid placebo mania by randomising between successive new treatments rather than comparing every new treatment to placebo. In this circumstance the average net treatment effect ('x' above) is minimised, since the new treatment on average is likely to be less different from the old than from nothing. The implication of this on the dynamics of understanding about effectiveness are interesting to speculate about. People prefer treatments because they conform more or less with their own understanding of the nature of (disease and behavioural) processes being addressed. Something which is thought to be useful may be more useful because of that belief; the first assumption made, but not proven, throughout this article. That belief is likely to be reinforced by an overestimate of the true 'biological' effect in the absence of any coherent understanding of the extent of any effect of individual preferences.

Patients with a chronic disease for which the current treatment is known not to be a panacea, although it might be importantly better than nothing, will usually be advised by enthusiastic doctors concerned and eager to get their patients better. If a new treatment is on offer it will only be proposed if it confers some important theoretical benefit in the eyes of the adviser. Although Chalmers (1997) demonstrates that new treatments are just as likely to be worse, as better, than their predecessors, such a finding is unlikely to be widely absorbed either by enthusiastic clinicians or by their patients who want to recover. For precisely similar reasons people buy lottery tickets in their millions, against all the odds. We might again assume that in general new treatments have much more enthusiastic support than old treatments (that are clearly not panaceas), for example with chronic diseases such as cancer and heart disease that are not always amenable to treatment.

Clearly, believing in a treatment does not necessarily enhance its effectiveness at all, but it might, and if it does we would in general be unlikely to know. On these two assumptions – that belief does affect effectiveness and that people faced with poor therapeutic prospects are likely to believe in an untried treatment more than the conventional one – then organically ineffective treatments are, on average, likely to gain in apparent effectiveness as 'unbiased' evidence accumulates from RCTs and more people prefer them. If so, it is important that this process does not simply and systematically accrue more and more expensive (and possibly nasty) placebos, unless we are sure there is no other way to enhance the effect of interventions (because they will be enhanced by whatever mechanism) more cheaply and less harmfully. Presumably there is likely to be a limit to this process, when the organic state of the illness simply does not allow any further opportunity for important interaction with the psychology or preference of the patient or subject. But discerning that plateau requires us to begin to discern any effect of this interaction at all reliably.

So long as the preference component of effect ($2y$ above) is smaller than the so-called biological component, giving people treatments they do not prefer may well nonetheless confer some important advantage. However, whenever the preference component is as large or larger, then trials can badly misrepresent the true effect, both in aggregate elsewhere and among particular groups, and hence favouring one treatment, because of its apparent effect, may cause some to suffer a net disadvantage.

Many things follow from this analysis and it behoves us to understand the nature of the phenomenon better. We need to know where preferences are important and where they are not, and what the implications of this are on our understanding of the results of randomised comparisons. For example, interventions designed to affect behaviour as the main outcome might well be much more susceptible to important preference effects than those with organic outcomes such as death. Thus health promotion placebos might well more easily be consolidated into health care, unless for them most people prefer the old intervention. In which case new interventions may look like placebos, when they may be highly effective only among those who like the idea.

In general, health promotion interventions work because there are systematic effect-modifications in the nature of the intervention. They generally involve at least two components of mechanism, firstly a change which alters the physiological milieu and a consequent change in health status in the longer term. Randomised trials which assess outcome by measuring the effect on the former will measure the complicated interaction of desire and belief on behaviour and the consequent effect on cholesterol, cotinine, FEV levels or whatever. The simple model used here to illustrate the role of RCTs may only go some way to enhancing our understanding of these phenomena. The real complexities may well be much more profound. But, for sure, the interpretation of such a clinical trial, by the existence of a significant effect or not, is likely to be far too simple. What must happen is a trial which is likely to give important insight into the nature and extent of interaction and effect-modification. These mechanisms are simply not straightforward biological phenomena – which can realistically be expected to have overriding aggregate effects.

Even such biological effects are often subject to too simplistic inter-pretation in the absence of knowledge about patient preferences. When they are not blinded then the interpretation is problematic unless patient preference effects are known to be absent, just as the interpretation of non-randomised studies is problematic unless confounding by prognosis is known to be absent. In the first, measuring these effects reliably is extremely difficult and, in the second, having exhaustive information on the determinants of prognosis is just as hard.

WHAT TO DO NEXT

Clearly, comparing the outcome among patients who choose their treatments cannot be a reliable source of information on preference effects when the treatments differ too. On the other hand, depending on the extent of preference effects, choosing treatments might be optimal (McKee and Sasi 1995; Wennberg 1990). Comparing them among patients on the same treatments both might exclude those with strong alternative preferences and also allow legitimate but subtle questions of the effect of compliance with the active treatment.

The obvious progression is to mount randomised trials from which the size of preference effects can be reliably measured. Gerta Rucker (1989) has postulated a two-stage design where randomisation takes place between two groups: one a random allocation between treatments and the other treatment choices among those with a preference and randomisation of those without. Thus the two arms compare, on the one hand, no choices, with, on the other, patient preferences where they exist. The problem here is a practical one of interpretation since, while discerning the existence of organic main effects over complex biological mechanisms is relatively straightforward, such interactions as $2y$ are difficult to discern.

In this case comparison between the two randomised groups provides an estimate of a complex combined function of the main organic effects, x, and any preference effect, $2y$. The organic effect itself will have to be estimated from the randomised arm, but with an unknown preference component, as above, based on imprecise estimates of the proportions alpha and beta from the preference arm. Thence a preference effect might just be estimable from comparison of the results from the two arms. The algebra, which is laborious but simple (and available from the authors), convinces one again that estimating these effects reliably is just difficult. The estimate depends on the reliability of other estimates in the formula which dis-aggregates the effects. Thus, only large effects of preference with large differences in these proportions (beta – alpha) can be reliably detectable, even with very large trials. Such trials will provide a better estimate of y when the aggregated treatment effect (x above) is precisely known, but clearly randomising large numbers of people to a treatment, which is known to be sub-optimal by an amount x in aggregate, is unethical.

Whilst perhaps easier to put into practice and ethically sound, the trial design described by Brewin and Bradley (1989) will produce results for which a preference effect cannot be disentangled from possible confounding arising from systematic differences between patients with strong treatment preferences and those without, putting the inference back to observational studies.

Large trials usually require a formidable biological or clinical justification to obtain enthusiastic support, where the 'biomedical model of disease is so pervasive that we often fail to see it as such, but view it as a reality' (Phillips *et al*. 1993, pp. 1142–5). Thus, invoking alternative mechanisms which sound slightly fanciful themselves and for which there is not much evidence is unlikely to be enough on its own. It therefore remains to be seen whether sufficient evidence to justify such trials in any area can be derived from what we now already know and can agree upon. If it cannot, the much larger question will be whether it can ever be derived from what we can ever know and agree upon, however hard we try. Perhaps this positivist discourse has not so much to recommend it after all. For we certainly do need to know eventually! How much of modern medicine or health promotion is 'merely' a placebo is, after all, quite an important question. The possibility that the postulated mechanism may itself be transitory gives some urgency to the question, but serves also to seriously complicate matters.

REFERENCES

Antonovsky, A., 1992. 'Can Attitudes Contribute to Health? Advances', *The Journal of Mind-Body Health*, 8, 4: pp. 33–48.
Brewin, C.R., and Bradley, C., 1989. 'Patient Preferences and Randomised Clinical Trials', *British Medical Journal*, 299: pp. 313–15.
Britton, A.R., McKee, M., Black, N., McPherson, K., Sanderson, C., and Bain, C., 1999, full text in preparation. 'Choosing between Randomised and Non-Randomised Studies: A Systematic Review of Internal and External Validity'. London: Sage.
Cassileth, B.R., Lusk, E.J., Miller, D.S., Brown, L.L., and Miller, C., 1985. 'Psychosocial Correlates of Survival in Advanced Malignant Disease', *New England Journal of Medicine*, 312, 24: pp. 1551–5.

Chalmers, I., 1997. 'What Is the Prior Probability of a Proposed New Treatment Being Superior to Established Treatments?', *British Medical Journal*, 311: pp. 74–5.

Chaput de Saintonge, D.M., and Herxheimer, A., 1994. 'Harnessing Placebo Effects in Health Care', *Lancet*, 344: pp. 995–8.

Kleijnen, J., Gotzsche, P., Kunz, R.A., Oxman, A., and Chalmers, I., 1997. 'So What's so Special about Randomisation?', chapter 4 in *Non Random Reflections on Health Services Research*, BMJ Books. The Nuffield Provincial Hospitals Trust.

Kleijnen, J., de Craen, A.J.M., Everdingen, J.V., and Krol, L., 1994. 'Placebo Effect in Double-Blind Clinical Trials: A Review of Interactions with Medications', *Lancet*, 344: pp. 1347–9.

Levy, S.M., Herberman, R.B., Lee, J., Whiteside, T., Beadle, M., Heiden, L., and Simons, A., 1991. 'Persistently Low Natural Killer Cell Activity, Age, and Environmental Stress as Predictors of Infectious Morbidity', *National Immunity Cell Growth Regulation*, 10: pp. 289–307.

Lilford, R.J., 1995. 'Equipoise and the Ethics of Randomisation', *Journal of the Royal Society of Medicine*, 88: pp. 552–9.

MacIntyre, I.M.C., 1991. 'Tribulations for Clinical trials: Poor Recruitment Is Hampering Research', *British Medical Journal*, 30: pp. 1099–100.

McKee, M., and Sasi, F., 1995. 'Gambling with the Nation's Health: The Social Impact of the National Lottery', *British Medical Journal*, 311: p. 521.

McKee, M., Britton, A., Black, N., *et al.*, 1998. 'Choosing between Randomised and Non Randomised Studies', in N. Balck, J. Brazier, R. Fitzpatrick, and B. Reeves, eds., *Health Services Research Methods*. British Medical Journal Books.

McPherson, K., 1994. 'The Best and the Enemy of the Good: Randomised Controlled Trials, Uncertainty, and Assessing the Role of Patient Preference in Medical Decision Making'. The Cochrane Lecture, *Journal of Epidemiology Community Health*, 48: pp. 6–15.

McPherson, K., 1996. 'Patients' Preferences and Randomised Trials', *Lancet*, 347: p. 1119.

McPherson, K., Britton, A.R., Wennberg, J., 1997. 'Are Randomised Controlled Trials Controlled? Patient Preferences and Unblind Trials', *Journal of the Royal Society of Medicine*, 90: pp. 652–6.

Phillips, D.P., Ruth, T.E., Wagner, L.M., 1993. 'Psychology and Survival', *Lancet*, 342: pp. 1142–5.

Phillips, D.P., Ruth, T.E., and Wagner, L.M., 1993. 'Psychology and Survival', *Lancet*, 342: pp. 1142–55.

Redd, W.H., Silverfarb, P.M., Anderson, B.L., Andrykowski, M.S., Bovbjerg, D.H., *et al.*, 1991. 'Physiologic and Psychobehavioral Research in Oncology', *Cancer*, 67: pp. 813–22.

Rothman, K.J., 1996. 'Placebo Mania', *British Medical Journal*, 313: pp. 3–4.

Rucker, G., 1989. 'A Two-Stage Trial Design for Testing Treatments, Self-Selection and Treatment Preference Effects'. *Statistics in Medicine* 8: pp. 477–85.

Sackett, D.L., and Wennberg, J.E., 1997. 'Choosing the Best Research Design for Each Question', *British Medical Journal*, 315: pp. 1636–7.

Sheppard, B.H., Hartwick, J., and Warshaw, P.R., 1988. 'The Theory of Reasoned Action: A Meta Analysis of Past Research with Recommendations for Modifications and Future Research', *J. Cons. Res.*, 15: pp. 325–39.

Silverman, W.A., and Altman, D.G., 1966. 'Patient Preferences and Randomised Trials', *Lancet*, 347: pp. 171–4.

The Coronary Drug Project Team, 1980. 'Influence of Adherence to Treatment and Response of Cholesterol on Mortality in the Coronary Drug Project', *New England Journal of Medicine*, 303: pp. 1038–41.

Weber, M., 1958. *From Max Weber: Essays in Sociology*. Trans. and ed. by H.H. Gerth and C. Wright Mills. New York: Oxford University Press.

Wennberg, J.E., 1990. 'What Is Outcomes Research?', in Institute of Medicine, ed., *Medical Innovation at the Crossroads. Vol. 1, Modern Methods of Clinical Investigation*. Washington: National Academy Press.

WHO, 1985. *Targets for Health for All, 1991–1993*. Health for all series, No. 1. Copenhagen: WHO Regional Office for Europe.

NOTES

1   For simplicity I assume no interaction or effect modification if the odds ratio for a particular outcome of attributable effect among treated compared to not treated groups is constant over all kinds of people. Clearly, for treating disease this will only sensibly include diseased people. *Interaction* I take to mean a different degree of potency (measured by the odds ratio already defined) according to measured aspects of need, while *effect-modification* refers to different potencies according to other characteristics which may be entirely orthogonal to need. These definitions have an element of arbitrariness about them, which is inevitable. I do not wish to be at all prescriptive here – only to clarify meaning.

PART TWO

Health Promotion:
Contexts and Settings

TEN

Understanding Health:
Biomedicine and Local Knowledge
in Northern Uganda

TIM ALLEN

This chapter is about how different perceptions of health and affliction relate to choice of therapies and to public policy. It begins by making some general points about concepts and then focuses in particular on the Madi of north-west Uganda. The changing, interactive, pluralistic conceptions of causality and healing which have characterised the population's response to sometimes extreme circumstances are contrasted with the narrow parameters of the biomedical approach, as it is articulated by expatriates working for an international medical non-governmental organisation (NGO). These different understandings of health are often combined with a disturbing lack of communication. A result is that well-meaning medical aid workers can be turned into not very effective immunisation commandos, who have minimal contact with their target populations except at the end of a needle. The predicaments which arise here are by no means confined to the African setting in which I observed them; as an extreme but by no means exceptional case, they bring into stark relief a number of problems which beset health-related therapy and policy in general.

PERCEPTIONS OF HEALTH AND AFFLICTION

A fundamental problem that arises when trying to understand perceptions of health is that the word 'health' itself is ambiguous. In its broadest sense it means something like 'being well', and its connotations might include having a happy family life and enjoying a reasonable level of material affluence. The definition formally adopted by the World Health Organisation (WHO) is only slightly more specific: 'a state of complete physical, mental, and social well-being'. This suggests a kind of ideal, which perhaps most people never expect to attain. It is also something rather different from the actual objectives of most public health programmes. Indeed, in practice it is rare for health to be assessed in relation to this definition even by the WHO itself. Usually, what are referred to as 'health statistics' are mortality rates and morbidity rates. In other words, when health is measured, assessments are made in relation to its apparent absence, or in relation to the prevalence of certain kinds of affliction. People understood to be health professionals are usually trained in biomedicine, and are thereby equipped not to directly promote health, but to combat a very specific conception of ill-health.

Biomedicine is a powerful kind of knowledge. It recognises the existence of microbiological phenomena and explains symptoms of ill-health in terms of ideas about germs and/or malfunctions in a patient's body. It is associated with a sophisticated technology, clinical investigation, and a fairly rigid hierarchy of skilled therapists. Considerable emphasis is given to the curing and control of diseases, which are afflictions that can be scientifically veri-fied as failures in normal physiological activities. Biomedicine is sometimes referred to as modern, scientific, conventional or cosmopolitan medicine. The term 'Western medicine' is also commonly used, both because biomed-icine is so dominant in Western countries and because it was in the West that this approach first gained acceptance as an integrated set of theories and practices. However, 'Western Medicine' seems a rather misleading term, given the fact that biomedicine is now established as the basis of formal health-care services run under ministry of health auspices throughout the world. Moreover, the importance of biomedicine in Western countries does not preclude the existence of other forms of healing.

There is no doubt that biomedicine exerts considerable influence on popular as well as professional understandings of ill-health. Nevertheless, broader conceptions remain prevalent. Even those who accept the accuracy of biomedical interpretations will recognise that other kinds of ill-health exist. In Western countries, biomedical therapies are widely available and biomedical practitioners are accorded a high social status, yet non-biomedical therapies are still widely used either in preference or in combination. Acupuncture, homeopathy, aromatherapy and a host of other 'alternative' techniques are popular. Psychosomatic disorders are recognised as common, and so are forms of illness which psychoanalysts link with the unconscious. Many individuals will seek remedies for spiritual afflictions in religious organisations and will use prayer as a form of healing. Some Roman Catholics make pilgrimages to the miraculous shrine at Lourdes in France if their condition is serious. It is probably true to say that everyone feels unwell on occasion as a consequence of interpersonal problems, depression, a sense of inadequacy or inner conflict.

It is also important to note that popular views of diseases are by no means restricted to narrow, scientific categorisations. In the West, cancer and AIDS are often imbued with ideas about probity, and sufferers may be viewed as morally unclean. As Susan Sontag has argued, diseases can function as a 'symbolic metaphor' for social values. Contact with an afflicted person 'feels like a trespass; worse, like the violation of a taboo' (Sontag 1979, p. 6). So diseases may have meanings beyond their existence as clinically observed bodily malfunctions. However, in other instances they may be experienced as less significant than they appear in biomedical terms, because people who are diseased may consider themselves to be healthy. A person who is infected with HIV may be unaware of it, and may feel perfectly well. In Britain certain potentially fatal diseases are commonly thought of as an almost inevitable part of daily life. Influenza, blood–pressure problems and asthma may fall into this category.

In response to these kinds of confusion and the prevalence of non-biomedical therapies, anthropologists tend to draw an analytical distinction between disease and illness. They use the term 'disease' in a specifically biomedical sense to refer to objective phenomena of which an infected individual may or may not be aware, and use the term 'illness' to refer to subjective perceptions of ill-health. Thus the social stigma associated with AIDS may be viewed as relating to AIDS as an illness, rather than as a disease. It is also possible to be diseased without being ill, just as it is possible to be ill without being diseased. The distinction may be questioned on the grounds that it assumes the biomedical definition of disease is culture-free, and that the way diseases are conceptualised by biomedical practitioners is in reality always the same. Critics point out that, while there may be 'objective' aspects of biomedicine, its diagnostic procedures are influenced by local norms. Clinical practice and biomedical taxonomies vary. Nevertheless, the distinction remains useful, especially in parts of the world in which biomedicine is less culturally hegemonic.

Although biomedicine has become the basis for most formal public health care programmes throughout the world, this is a relatively recent development. The conceptualisation of illness in the form of individuality and the objectification of the body in a clinical setting – what Michel Foucault called the 'the anatomo–clinical gaze' (1973) – only emerged in the late eighteenth century. It did not achieve its current status in Western countries until the breakthroughs in medical science and increased access to formal education in the course of the past hundred years or so. Elsewhere it is often a legacy of European colonialism, and is linked to the formation of new states and the activities of international organisations like the WHO after the Second World War. Especially for the mass of the population in economically poor countries, it remains a kind of knowledge and range of therapies associated with the relatively affluent.

In much of Africa, formal health-care facilities and formal scientific education are still not readily available to the majority. Partly for this reason, clinical objectification of the human body is unlikely to be the only starting point for understanding symptoms which might be ascribed by a biomedical professional to disease, and bodily malfunctions may be less readily separated from other forms of affliction. It is common to find people who accept as 'normal' symptoms which might be linked to bilharzia or malaria or intestinal worms. Sometimes they may even think of the absence of such symptoms as an indication of illness. On the other hand it is very common for individuals to think of themselves as unwell without any biomedical cause. More so than in the West, illness, and indeed affliction generally, may be seen as expressing social values, and in more tangible terms than is suggested by Sontag's notion of 'social metaphor'. Ideas about interpersonal causality are crucial here, not only for understanding why combinations of therapies are adopted to heal an individual, but also to comprehend how mutuality is negotiated and moral probity asserted within a community.

While it would be misleading to suggest that there is something homogeneous which might be termed 'African aetiologies', implicitly or explicitly, discussions of affliction causality in Africa draw from Evans-Pritchard's famous book on the Azande, first published in 1937. Usually, summaries of *Witchcraft, Oracles and Magic among the Azande* emphasise its analysis of the logic that underpins witchcraft accusation, the crux of which is that the Azande are concerned primarily with the why, not the how, of sickness and misfortune. Those parts of the book are highlighted in which the Azande are described as caught in a 'web of belief', where 'every strand depends upon every other strand' and cannot be escaped from because it is the 'texture' of thought itself (Evans-Pritchard 1937, p. 194). The secondary elaborations, which deflect the attention of the Azande from the contradictions that seem so obvious to an outsider, are then outlined. It is this 'closed-system' model that Winch (1972) and Horton (1967) ascribe to Evans-Pritchard in their influential discussions of rationality and scientific thinking.

However, as Max Gluckman and others have pointed out, even in terms of this 'closed-system' model of African causality, incorporation of new ideas is not necessarily problematic. For example, if a child dies of typhus, an educated relative might well continue to maintain that witchcraft was the cause, reasoning that: 'I know that it was a louse from a person ill with typhus who gave my child typhus, and that he died of typhus, but why did the louse go to my child and not to the other children with whom he was playing?' (Gluckman 1944, p. 65; 1955, p. 85).

Janzen (1981, p. 188–89) takes the argument further. He maintains that Evans-Pritchard's book did not show that witchcraft and empirical causes were in any sense mutually exclusive but that among the Azande during the mid-colonial era it was witchcraft that gave social events their moral value. Furthermore, Janzen emphasises the lengthy sections of *Witchcraft, Oracles and Magic* that deal with 'natural' causation, a term used for an assortment of aetiologies, including lack of common sense, broken taboos and the remote work of God.

Other anthropological studies have taken up this issue of medical pluralism to great effect. It has been shown that, although events may be discussed in certain circumstances as if they take place within a 'closed' system, this does not mean that thinking is closed or static in practice. Research on African therapeutic systems has confirmed a vigorous and long-standing pluralism, which incorporates aspects of biomedical treatments with numerous other practices (e.g. Buxton 1973; Comaroff and Comaroff 1993; Feierman 1979; Janzen 1978; Ngubane 1977; Whyte 1997).

Anthropological studies have also highlighted another important point, one that is oddly overlooked by biomedically-trained professionals and indeed by many health researchers. The word 'health' is complicated in English. As we have seen, it is not a precise concept, and in practice it is usually evoked in a roundabout way with reference to its absence. It may be that it is possible to express most of its vague resonances in other international languages, but this is hardly likely to be the case for languages spoken by a few thousand people, most of whom are not literate and live in poverty.

It is a salutary experience to translate health education manuals into an African language, and then have them translated back into English, or to discuss the full connotations and associations of the concepts used. The local terms chosen for 'health' vary hugely in meaning between groups. Amongst groups I have worked with in east Africa, back-translations of 'health' range from 'having a strong body', to 'having no worries'. Amongst the Madi of north-east Uganda, the local word used is 'cwe', which basically suggests something which is 'good'.

Moreover, it may be impossible to adequately translate the word 'illness', let alone 'disease'. In Madi both are translated as 'laza', but this term can also refer to almost any kind of suffering, misfortune or pain. This does not necessarily imply that people who do not speak English (or French, Arabic or Swahili) in Uganda cannot understand what a disease is, or how it might be cured with a clinically-formulated, manufactured medicine. There have been several attempts by governments to control particular diseases since the time of British rule. Amongst the Madi it is recognised that certain diseases exist, including sleeping sickness and malaria, and that they can potentially be cured by biomedicine (or by a local substitute for biomedicine). Nevertheless, different languages reflect different philosophies of the person, and different perceptions of what it means to be well.

THE MADI AND SOCIAL UPHEAVAL

Most of the Ugandan Madis live in Moyo District – a territory located in the far north of the country on the border with Sudan, and divided by the White Nile. The word 'Madi' itself is an ethnic label introduced in colonial times. It is probably derived from a local word for 'a person' (ma 'di). The Madi language is closely related to that of the neighbouring Lugbara, and the Madi way of life is also comparable in many respects (Baxter and Butt 1953, p. 104). The two groups were deliberately separated and classified differently by British officials, largely for administrative reasons, during the first decade of the present century. There is also a great deal of overlap in customs with other groups in the region, such as the Acholi to the east. The Acholi language is very different from that of the Madi and Lugbara, but numerous words and concepts are shared and many people are multilingual.

To some extent the complex interrelation between languages and customs is a consequence of social upheavals since the mid-nineteenth century, which have prompted large-scale population movements and interaction between social groups. The area which has become Moyo District was devastated in the 1860s by slave and ivory traders operating from Khartoum and later was occupied by Turco-Egyptian forces. In the early part of the present century, when the land to the west of the Nile was under Belgian control, white hunters moved around at will with armed retinues. Under British rule, what was then the sub-district was seen as something of a hardship posting, prone to famine (1927, 1942), locust infestation (1930, 1938) and disease (meningitis, sleeping sickness, malaria, bilharzia).

In the later colonial period, until the upheavals of the 1970s, the mainstay of the local economy was cotton, supplemented by the sale of cattle and, in riverine locations, dried fish. In addition, most families had at least one male member who travelled to the south to work on plantations, in factories, or in the armed forces. These factors, combined with seventy-five years of Roman Catholic missionary activity and relatively high rural education levels for such a 'remote' place, mean that it makes little sense to attempt an under-standing of the Madi as if they were a homogeneous and discrete group, exist-ing in their own static, tradition-bound world. By the late 1960s, the district, as it had officially become at independence, could be viewed as a labour reserve, populated by a commoditised peasantry who had to pay their taxes.

During recent years, the Madi have been caught up in the tragedy that has engulfed northern Uganda as a whole. At the turn of the 1980s, the Madi and the Lugbara were seen as having been sympathetic to Idi Amin, and following the Tanzanian invasion and return to power of Milton Obote atrocities were perpetrated against civilians. North-west Uganda became the scene of protracted guerrilla warfare, and perhaps a quarter of a million people fled across international borders – the bulk going to Sudan, where they became the recipients of relief and development aid. A large number self-settled. Others, including the majority of the Madi, were herded into official camps.

By 1984, the refugees tended to be self-sufficient in food production and a few became relatively well off, compared to the host population. A handful also played a role in the complicated and increasingly bitter divisions in the politics of the southern region, which partly led to the return to war in Sudan. This made the refugee camps an obvious target for the Sudan People's Liberation Army. In April–May of 1986, the guerrillas drew upon local resentment of the Ugandans, fuelled by the aid that had been channelled in the refugees' direction, and attacked the camps to the east of the Nile where many of the Madi were settled, killing several people. Neither the Sudanese authorities nor the aid agencies were in a position to offer protection, so the refugees returned home as fast as possible. They left crops in the fields and, in a matter of three months, thousands had crossed back into Uganda.

Meanwhile, Yoweri Museveni's National Resistance Army had seized power in Kampala at the beginning of 1986 and established a National Resistance Movement government. Although there was still fighting going on in parts of the country, including Acholi-land, Moyo District was fairly stable. However, the returnees found themselves in a devastated environment. Marketing and transport facilities had collapsed. School buildings had been demolished, and government health-care services hardly existed outside Moyo town, where the hospital was in a poor state of repair. Two NGOs had been working in the district for some time under the auspices of the Office of the United Nations High Commissioner for Refugees (UNHCR) – namely, Lutheran World Federation and Médecins sans Frontières (MSF). However, coverage of the emergency in international media ensured that funding was increased, and several other agencies became operational, either in Moyo District or Arua District to the west, where further influxes of returnees were anticipated.

Such was the context in which I undertook fieldwork for about twenty months between 1987 and 1991. I established myself at Laropi, a small trading centre and location of the Nile ferry. Almost everyone had returned during the preceding months, having fled from the East Bank camps in Sudan. My initial research interest was in small-scale agriculture in the context of crisis, but I was concerned with all aspects of resettlement.

As time passed, I became increasingly drawn into thinking about health issues. This was essentially for two reasons. First, relative well-being, or the ever-possible occurrence of severe misfortune, was of immense concern for the people among whom I was living. I knew of no family that did not have at least one member who became seriously ill during the time of my stay and none that failed to incur the adverse consequences attendant on the death of a close relative. Second, during the course of my research, I developed close personal contacts with several of the expatriates working with the medical NGO teams in nearby towns. When I became ill myself, I consulted them and rarely would a week go by without my paying one of them a visit. The compounds acted as a refuge for me when what could be a grim situation in

Laropi became too much. I came to view their activities from two angles. On the one hand, as an expatriate myself, I inevitably observed things from the expatriate medics' point of view and could sympathise with their frustrations. On the other, I gradually learned to see their activities from the village recipients' point of view of aid-agency intervention. As my understanding of what was happening around me in Laropi deepened, the dichotomy between these perspectives became ever more acute.

AFFLICTION, ILLNESS AND CHANGE

In this section and the next one I try to make it clear how Madis themselves think about suffering. Using the distinction between disease and illness, I indicate ways in which the subjective experience of ill-health relates not only to the physical and psychological problems of individuals, but also to wider concerns. I then go on to discuss the view from within an aid-agency compound.

Given the chaos of recent years, I begin with some observations about how people dealt with affliction in the past. A danger of doing this is that an ideal of what things were once like ends up being contrasted with the confusion of the present. It would be hard to avoid this if the Madi were treated as a discrete cultural unit, because very little research had been carried out amongst them before my own, and there would be little to go on except the oral testimonies of living elders, many of whom might tend to view the past as a 'golden era'. However, this has not been the case for neighbouring groups. Information about the Lugbara in particular is extensive, due to the very high-quality ethnographic publications of John Middleton, based on fieldwork in the 1950s, and to doctoral research by Virginia Barnes-Dean in the 1970s. What material that is available on the Madi, mainly reports by colonial officers, suggests that much of what they say applied to the Madi as well.

At the time Middleton carried out his fieldwork, the Lugbara, particularly the male elders, believed that 'azo' (a term for misfortune/affliction and illness which is equivalent with the Madi word laza) should be explained in terms of an ideally unchanging socio-moral order (Middleton 1960, p. 252; 1963, p. 261). The Lugbara lived in small, exogamous, patrilineal/patrilocal groups, each headed by an elder. The lineage was the primary sphere of direct social relations, and neighbours, who were also kin, were the core of the moral community. Within the community there was intense competition among male elders for seniority, which eventually led to lineage fission. Competition between elders and the control they exercised or sought to exercise over their families was expressed through a cult of the dead (Middleton 1960; 1965, pp. 73–86). Deceased ancestors, usually males, were believed capable of sending 'azo' to people whom they considered harmful to the well-being of their lineage. Virtually anyone who felt wronged could invoke ancestral ghosts to inflict 'azo' on their behalf, but a senior male was expected to do so. It was part of his work, to 'cleanse' the lineage home. In addition, ancestors sent 'azo' without invocation if they felt the living were neglecting them. Thus, azo showed the living when ancestors were displeased.

Therapy proceeded in the following manner (Middleton 1963, pp. 261–71; 1965, pp. 75–83, 89–92; 1967, pp. 57–67; 1969, pp. 220–31). The ritual guardian of the afflicted person consulted male-operated, God-empowered oracles to discover the identity of the ghost concerned as well as the nature of the sacrifice to be made when the patient recovered. If recovery did not occur, it was said that 'God refuses', indicating that it was futile to do more, because God had decided to take that person away in death. Ultimately, death was always thought of as God's will.

However, sometimes when a patient failed to recover it was thought that the oracles had made a mistake or that they did not know the particular 'azo'. The oracles were either consulted again or alternative explanations for sickness were taken up. These alternatives reflected a recognition among the Lugbara that social order was not as stable as it ought to be. Quite apart from the upheavals of the early colonial period, when the Yakan cult rebellion occurred, there had been commoditisation by the 1950s as a consequence of short-term male labour migration to the south and the introduction of cash cropping. In addition, the authority of the elders was being directly challenged by the protégés of the government and the missions. Middleton describes various aetiologies that could not be known by oracles: certain illnesses caused by God through wind spirits, afflictions with those 'self-evident' causes, and witchcraft and sorcery.

'Azo' associated with wind spirits were epidemic diseases like cerebrospinal meningitis, while those with 'self-evident' causes included venereal diseases. There probably was some connection between these beliefs and limited exposure to biomedicine via dispensaries and government control programmes for particular diseases, notably sleeping sickness and yaws. Significantly, treatment was given by an 'ojo' (diviner) and administered to effect a cure for the specific symptoms in the patient's body (i.e. for these illnesses no interpersonal explanation was sought).

'Ojo' were almost invariably women who, at puberty, had been 'seized' by the much-feared aspect of God, which dwelt in the bush and near streams. They were diviners and often also local healers. As a healer, an 'ojo' would remove objects from the bodies of patients, attend births, and presumably (I do not recall Middleton mentioning this anywhere) administer herbal remedies. Her central role, however, was in mediating that which was 'outside' ('amve') the social and moral order. She could identify what caused those illnesses not sent by ancestors, for she 'knew the words' of the feared aspect of God and those of witches and sorcerers.

The Lugbara believed that 'onzi' (evil/amorality) was in the world because of ambition and envy. In particular, there were certain people who could cause 'azo' and death in mysterious ways. These were people with 'ole', a term that encompassed both notions of witchcraft and sorcery. Middleton follows the old anthropological convention of distinguishing between witches and sorcerers on the grounds that the former have an inherent power that, possibly unintentionally, can harm others, whereas the latter use technical means, termed 'enyanya' (poison/magic), in full deliberation.

Witchcraft was associated only with men. The accused was usually an elder who was losing authority, a person with physical disabilities, or someone marginal in the lineage. When a diviner indicated that witchcraft was the cause of the affliction, an attempt might be made to cool the envy of the witch, perhaps by inviting him to a meal. There were stories that night witches, those that danced outside their victims' homes in the dark, were speared, but Middleton found no case of a man who was ever actually put to death owing to witchcraft. While bad, witchcraft could be comprehended in that it occurred as a result of normal masculine ambitions within a lineage.

In contrast, sorcery was a heinous crime. If it occurred between agnatic kin, it amounted to fratricide, for 'enyanya' killed victims, something that ghost invocation and witchcraft rarely did. Sorcery also cut across spheres of ritual authority in a manner that threatened the very fabric of moral interaction. Accusations often occurred where obligations of kinship and neighbourhood were ambiguous. Sorcerers in these cases tended to be men from the outside, such as returning labour migrants or clients living within the home. If an 'ojo' revealed that such a person was involved, he might be beaten and have to flee the area.

Sorcery, in addition, was believed to have been practised by both sexes, and punishment for females could be more violent. The female sorcerer acted because of sexual jealousy. She poisoned co-wives and their children, who were, of course, children of her husband's patrilineage (unlike herself). If caught, she might be put to death by her husband's agnates by cutting off her limbs, burning or spearing, the latter a practice that seems to have been quite common in the 1920s and 1930s (Middleton 1963, pp. 266, 274). Middleton argues that this violence towards women and the driving away of strangers were responses to rapid social change. The concentration of the population, from cash cropping (which placed wives in direct competition with their husbands over land), markets, administrative convenience and the improvement in government services, together with such factors as labour migration, had greatly exaggerated the normal tensions of social life. In Lugbara terms, they had become out of hand.

Underpinning what Middleton writes about witchcraft and sorcery is the notion that women, like the dangerous forces that, as ojo, they might know, could be thought of as 'outside' and onzi (evil/amoral) themselves (Middleton 1960, pp. 248–50). A woman was never truly 'of the home', because she left that of her father at marriage and became part of her husband's lineage only through her children. It was therefore predictable that, when ritual or other institutionalised vengeance became untenable, women would end up as scapegoats. More positively, the spiritual powers and symbolic attributes vested in women might become legitimising avenues of traumatic change (Barnes-Dean 1986, p. 339; Casale 1982, pp. 385, 395; Middleton 1969, p. 230).

This latter issue has been taken up by Barnes-Dean (1986). In 1973, she found that azo was diagnosed either as 'enyanya', now including some practices that Middleton would have termed witchcraft, or as 'other illness'. Ancestor invocation seemed to have stopped. 'Azo' understood as 'other illness' had impersonal aetiologies and could be contracted by Europeans. Local remedies were known for many of them, but it was recognised that cures were also possible at mission or government hospitals. 'Azo' from enyanya, on the other hand, could only be contracted by Africans and could not be cured by biomedicine.

Local treatments for both enyanya and some 'other illnesses' were administered by 'ojo'. They cured a range of specifically named ailments, from headaches and itchy skin to the effects of poisons. Several of these treatments involved making small cuts on the patient's body and rubbing in the concocted remedy. Interestingly, treatment for venereal diseases involved drinking a liquid containing certain pounded leaves in combination with going to the hospital for an injection. Barnes-Dean maintains that the work of 'ojo' as herbalists was linked to the perception of women as 'outside' and of the bush, from where herbal remedies were collected. But, whereas in the 1950s it was this dangerous aspect of women that enabled ojo to mediate the evil forces that impinged upon the sphere of moral action, they had become the healers of 'true Lugbara sickness', now understood exclusively as 'enyanya'. The former medical system had 'in a sense been turned inside out by culture contact' (Barnes-Dean 1986, p. 344).

The therapies Barnes-Dean describes had arisen out of processes occurring in the context of, and largely as a consequence of, the emergence of a relatively stable, colonial then postcolonial state superstructure. The preceding two decades had been marked by increased provision of biomedical facilities and the promotion of empirical causality in schools, churches and government offices. The broadening of a general category of impersonal affliction was an obvious consequence of this. It is probable, furthermore, that the emphasis on 'enyanya' as the only viable aetiology had rather less to do with the cognitive inversion she posits than with an increased recourse to local-level courts. Records were kept in English, and, although it was usually impossible to make accusations of 'witchcraft', enyanya could be introduced into proceedings because it was translated as 'poison'. Court records indicate that this was common.

Since the 1970s, political turmoil and mass migration have forced most Lugbaras and Madis into a semi-subsistence economy for prolonged periods. Acute competition for scarce resources and extreme misfortune have become commonplace. With the drastic deterioration of government services, mechanisms for airing disputes and ensuring social accountability are chronically weak. Conceptions of affliction causality have become much more vigorously pluralistic than is suggested by Barnes-Dean, and can be grounds for heated argument. Occasionally, when therapy fails, there is appalling interpersonal violence. During the 1980s some Lugbaras and Madis (as well as Acholis and other groups of the region) became involved in witch-cleansing and in witch-killing, both in the refugee settlements in Sudan and following their return to Uganda (Allen 1991a, pp. 158–9; 1991b; 1992; 1994; 1996, pp. 252–8; 1997; Behrend 1991; 1995; 1998; Harrell-Bond 1986, pp. 309–29). In the following section I discuss the variety of aetiologies and therapies prevalent among the Madi at the time of my fieldwork.

HEALING AMONG THE MADI

A Madi informant might reply to the question 'What causes illness?' with a proverb: 'awo otu kwe ku', which might be translated literally as 'crying does not climb a tree'. It suggests a rejection of coincidental or impersonal causation in favour of an interpersonal explanation. But the very existence of such a saying suggests that debate over the issue is not a recent phenomenon.It may be countered with another expression, 'laza Rubanga dri'i' (affliction [is] given by God), or with a remark such as 'we are just born to suffer'. There are, in addition, Madi words for a range of specific ailments, which similarly suggest that spiritual or moral aetiologies of suffering have not been the only possible interpretations. As among the Lugbara, these labels for particular sets of symptoms can often be linked to disease eradication or control programmes during the colonial era (e.g. 'mongoto', sleeping sickness; 'loboto', yaws; 'njuku', syphilis/gonorrhoea). There are also certain general terms, like 'jue' (boils or swelling), that are used to refer to many illnesses, with the implication that an interpersonal explanation is not being sought, at least not at that point, by the person using the term.

Nowadays, an afflicted person's relatives may be deeply divided over diagnosis. It is common for factions to pursue alternative therapeutic pathways at the same time or to explain sickness with reference to causalities within causalities (in much the same kind of way as in the example given above by Max Gluckman). The broad division between interpersonal and impersonal aetiologies, which Barnes-Dean observed among the Lugbara in the early 1970s, is the primary focus of debate, and healers tend to specialise in one or another area. Some idea of the present situation may be given by looking at the current range of healers available to the population of Laropi and at the sorts of affliction they deal with.

Turning first to the healing of interpersonal aetiologies, we may begin with elders, who seem to have been the moral arbitrators of the past, much as they were among the Lugbara at the time of Middleton's fieldwork in the 1950s. In exile, the people of Laropi had often lived among non-kin in refugee settlements. In 1986, they had little option but to return to live in their ancestral lands, something that a number of them had not been doing before they left, since they had been working in other parts of Uganda. Old people, not necessarily those who are elders in terms of inherited lineage authority, tried to use this enforced recongregation to assert themselves in the fraught process of establishing a degree of community cohesion. They did this by drawing upon old beliefs, of which younger people profess ignorance. They argued that harvests were poor because ceremonies should be performed to placate the ancestors and to cleanse the land of the blood spilled upon it. Similarly, laza, especially when the afflicted person was a former soldier, was linked to past antisocial behaviour, now being punished by outraged patrilineal ghosts. Stories were told of individual men dying or becoming deranged with remorse in the vicinity of shrines. In these cases, however, elders were less involved in therapy than in explaining misfortune with reference to a morality they sought to promote. Oracles were not consulted, but the affliction showed justice being done.

In all the time I lived in Laropi, I never encountered an instance where a promise to perform a sacrifice at a shrine by elders was the only therapy adopted. Occasionally, it was combined with a biomedical cure. Thus, in the case of a boy with sleeping sickness, his aged step-grandmother insisted on a commitment to 'feed' the ancestors before she would agree to his father taking him for treatment at Moyo Hospital. More often, elders are called upon to play a role only when a specialised healer divines that ancestral ghosts are involved. These specialists are often called 'witch doctors', the English word having been incorporated into the vernacular, and include a 'traditional' 'ojo', a Zande refugee living in Moyo town, and new kinds of spirit mediums, sometimes also referred to as ojo, but more usually called 'ajwaka'.

If we use the term 'ojo', as Middleton and Barnes-Dean do for the Lugbara in the 1950s and 1970s, to refer only to those healers who were possessed by God as an adolescent and who act as diviner/herbalists, they were now rare. Their work as midwives and herbalists had been taken over by semi-professionalised traditional birth attendants (TBAs) and 'daktaris' (local doctors), and their work as diviners by 'ajwaka'. I met only one elderly woman who claimed to be an 'ojo' in the old sense. She dismissed her local competitors as fraudulent but respected the conscientious, trained midwife employed at the government health centre situated close to her home and was in fact registered as a TBA herself.

The Zande healer living in Moyo town, four hours' walk from Laropi, also operated as both diviner and herbalist. He had a high reputation, and charged high prices. Consulting him was an option only for the few who could afford to pay. In one case I know of, a former soldier became seriously ill. He was twice treated at Moyo Hospital but each time sent back to Laropi uncured. After other local healers had been consulted, the Zande healer was approached as a last resort. He explained that the patient had looted a house and that the owner had paid a witch doctor to ensorcell him in revenge. He offered to cure him, which he could do because the looted property had not been brought to the home. The family had to sell two bulls to meet the demanded fee, although in the end the money was not paid because the man died before it was handed over.

At the time of my fieldwork, it was normally the 'ajwaka' that dealt with laza when an interpersonal cause is suspected. Unlike 'ojo', 'ajwaka' were women permanently possessed by named, usually non-kin, spirits. One in Laropi was possessed by five spirits, including that of a murdered bishop. 'Ajwaka' did not treat 'laza' from ancestors or the retributions of the wronged deceased. These cases were referred to elders. But they could be efficacious in the treatment of 'inyinya' (the Madi equivalent of 'enyanya') and possession by wild spirits, particularly a kind of wild spirit usually referred to as 'jok' (an Acholi word for spirit/ghost). Both 'inyinya' and jok-possession were so common that many think of them as daily hazards.

Since the people of Laropi did not live together in exile, even closely related neighbours might be strangers to each other. However, the attempted reassertion of the moral and economic values associated with patrilineal relations meant that those not of the patrilineage were more suspect of having ole, the motive for inyinya, than others. Those who fell into this category included Muslim Lugbara from Aringa County, who operated as traders; migrants, like the Zande healer in Moyo town; men who were living with their wives' families (and are therefore not of the patrilineage); and married women who had not produced children or for whom bride-wealth had not been paid. When inquiry was made into knowledge of 'inyinya', a frequent response was that the Muslims use it. But when it came to direct accusation, most instances involved recently married women for whom virtually no bride-wealth payments had been made.

Talk of 'inyinya' came up at most funerals, being initiated by maternal uncles of the deceased who use it as a lever in negotiations for compensation. Efforts were made by the men of the patrilineage to quash it, and angry scenes were common. Occasionally the suggestion was taken up within the patrilineage, and a woman thought of as 'angwe' (the Madi equivalent of the Lugbara word 'amve' [outside]) was blamed. In a neighbouring home to my own (on a day I was visiting Moyo town), a man whose son had died accused the daughter (by a former husband) of his father's second wife. The girl and her mother were tortured horrifically and eventually beaten to death.

Violence towards women is not new in north-west Uganda. Apart from Middleton's references to it, Rowley writes of the Madi 'addiction to the use of various kinds of poison' and gives an instance of an old woman being severely beaten to extract a confession (Rowley 1940, p. 282). It is hard to establish if accusation was now more common than in the past, but it was certainly widespread. Moreover, ideas about 'inyinya' had been influenced by the promotion of empirical causality, the introduction of biomedicine, the teaching of biology in schools, and experiences in exile. As 'poison', it readily allowed a scientific explanation to coexist with an interpersonal one, and even the compound of the Médecins sans Frontières team in Moyo town was not exempt. A driver was convinced that one of the new female cooks had 'poisoned' him, and a long meeting involving the French administrator was necessary to sort the problem out. Unlike the situation described by Barnes-Dean, 'inyinya' was not now thought of as an aetiology specific to local people. Harrell-Bond (1986, pp. 309–12) provided shocking examples of violence linked to 'poisoning' among Ugandan refugees in Sudanese camps; and when I had a severe hangover after drinking locally distilled liquor, it was speculated that I too had succumbed.

'Ajwaka' were not consulted over allegations at funerals but could divine if inyinya was causing laza. When it was, they refused to reveal the name of the sorcerer but would make vague hints and offer advice about what to do. They did not, as a rule, administer herbal remedies to a patient (this was done by a daktari), but they could find 'poison' put on a path or buried in a field that might afflict an entire neighbourhood, and received considerable rewards for doing so. They were also paid well for successfully dealing with 'jok' possession, again a phenomenon closely associated with women.

The terms 'jok' and 'ajwaka' were recent imports from the neighbouring Acholi to the east. In Madiland, 'jok' referred specifically to one or more named spirits that seized a victim, almost always a woman, and caused her to do peculiar things like sleep in a tree or dance wildly in the bush. Her male relatives would take her to see an 'ajwaka', who would arrange a ceremony at which she would go into a trance-like state and dance wildly with the patient and other women who came along for the occasion. Young men played drums, and quantities of strong alcoholic drinks would be consumed. It could be very exciting. The spirits of the 'ajwaka' would speak through her and call upon the spirits possessing the patient to reveal themselves and explain what they wanted. When they did so, in strange high-pitched voices, sometimes a grievance concerning the home was revealed. In one case, a woman turned out to be possessed by her dead father, who, through her, castigated her brothers as drunkards. The ceremony was relatively expensive, and often further ones had to be organised, particularly if a 'jok' 'loved' its medium and decided to stay permanently. If this was so, the woman might be initiated as an 'ajwaka' herself.

It is tempting to see many cases of 'jok' possession as a form of female expression or even resistance, rather than as illness. It highlights the weakened control men had over women as a consequence of the refugee experience and the chronic instability of marriage. It also confirmed to men the irrational nature of women. Several times I heard men complain that 'jok' dancing had become an epidemic simply because women enjoyed it. Men could be possessed themselves but, it seems, less benignly. This was so in the case of an ex-seminarian who attempted to murder his mother. He had formerly gone to Kampala for psychiatric treatment, which failed, and was taken to see an 'ajwaka'. After three days of exorcism ceremonies, his therapy-managing group was instructed to tell his elders to ensure the success of the cure by performing a sacrifice at the lineage shrine.

We may now turn our attention to those healers specialising in curing ailments with impersonal or God-given aetiologies. Therapy for these afflictions was of two kinds: local or herbal remedies, and biomedicine. Local remedies was usually administered by 'daktari' (who were normally men), or, in the case of pregnant women, by TBAs (who were women). Daktaris and TBAs were individuals who had responded to the half-hearted attempts to professionalise traditional healers since the late 1970s. TBAs were again being registered at the time of my fieldwork, and the trained midwife at the health centre was supposed to improve their skills. The basic problem she faced was that the concept of a 'traditional birth attendant', in the sense of a woman who specialises in antenatal care and child delivery, was a fiction. Severe suffering in childbirth could be interpreted as symptomatic of unrevealed wickedness, and the few women who gave birth at the health centre were thought to have done so because they had something to hide. The calling of 'ojo' to attend births in the past was to discover the reason for the difficult delivery, to find out if the woman had committed adultery, or to determine if she had 'inyinya'. In the late 1980s, TBAs generally denied being 'ojo', but in this respect they did sometimes fulfil a comparable role, particularly in cases of 'illegal' pregnancy; that is, when the impregnator was not known and therefore could not be fined by the woman's patrilineage. However, the modern TBA mainly prided herself on herbal remedies, which, like those of the 'daktari', were revealed by God in dreams.

The best-known 'daktari' in Laropi equated himself with district medical staff and saw himself as working in conjunction with a small village dispensary. Patients were referred to him by the medical staff working there, and he referred other cases to them. He told me that he had worked in Moyo Hospital in the 1970s. I was unable to confirm this, but I met numerous people, including highly educated people, who regarded him as very competent. However, in spite of his high reputation, he seemed to earn very little from his clinic, and he complained to me that the government ought to pay him a salary. He also vehemently rejected any association between his practice and the work of 'witch doctors'.

Although he did not practice any form of divination, his medicine (like that of TBAs) was in fact quite similar to remedies used by the old, 'traditional' 'ojo' living near the health centre and to cures that, according to Barnes-Dean (1986), were used by Lugbara 'ojo' in 1973. His medicines were derived from dried leaves and roots, which he collected himself. Among other ailments, he treated various body pains, boils, topical ulcers, worm and intestinal problems, hernia, measles, throat infection, and infertility. He also had different sorts of purges to cause vomiting or bowel movements, as well as potions to alleviate these symptoms. Purges were used in cases of 'inyinya' where the victim had swallowed the poison, and he would sometimes assist if 'inyinya' had been inflicted externally by touching or by leaving it on a path. It is was not his role, however, to locate a culprit. He treated 'inyinya' simply as another sickness. Most medicines were drunk, but others were rubbed into scores of tiny cuts made with a razor blade on the skin of the patient in the manner Barnes-Dean describes. It is possible that several of these cures could be assessed to be biomedically effective. Others, like the cutting out of the lower canine teeth of small children to cure diarrhoea, surely were not.

Part of the appeal of the 'daktari' was that the availability of manufactured biomedicines was very limited. They were mostly brought into Moyo District either as supplies from the Ministry of Health store in Entebbe or as part of the medical aid programmes administered by international NGOs, theoretically under Ministry of Health auspices. Unfortunately, district medical staff were so poorly paid that the only way that they could make ends meet was to find additional sources of income. The midwife at Laropi Health Centre made a living by selling a special sort of beer on Sundays. Others charged for services that were supposed to be free, and, one way or another, large quantities of manufactured drugs ended up on the open market. There was a never-ending demand for aspirin, chloroquine, and antibiotics, all of which were generally available in the small shops of the Laropi market, tucked behind piles of matches, soap and batteries.

In certain situations, an afflicted person would seek assistance from trained medical staff at an early stage. This was always the case with severe lesions or a broken bone. In instances where aetiology was more open to debate, there tended to be dissent between therapy managers over when, or if, a biomedical remedy should be sought. A few equated the use of biomedicine with being progressive and adopted it invariably as a first resort. This amounted to a public rejection of belief in 'inyinya', which could be dangerous if the patient's health deteriorated. Others would talk of hospitals as places where people go to die in the hands of strangers (as indeed they often did). However, in mild cases, usually with symptoms of bacterial infection, headache or fever, which did not require therapy managers, a visit to the health centre was unproblematic and common. Patients would not generally go there for diagnosis but rather to try to obtain drugs free of charge, and if they were informed that supplies had run out or that they were not really needed, there was the alternative of purchasing them for treatment at home. Home treatments included the external use of tetracycline powder, derived from tablets, the consumption of large quantities of chloroquine for 'malaria' (a term used to refer to a wide range of symptoms), and the widespread abuse of penicillin injections, administered with reused disposable syringes.

A fundamental problem associated with biomedicine was perceived as one of access. The popularity of 'daktari' and recourse to home treatments reflected this. People would say things to me like, 'In your country, you do not grow old quickly because you have plenty of medicine.' If drugs were readily available, it was suspected that many cases of 'laza' with impersonal aetiologies could be cured. It was, after all, well known that the white expatriates had their own private supplies with which they regularly dosed themselves; so why did they not simply bring more and give them out?

Médecins sans Frontières (MSF) cars came to Laropi every other day when I was living there, but on many occasions people expressed confusion to me about what the French expatriates were doing in the district. It seemed peculiar that they were so eager to inoculate children, which made them feel ill, but were reluctant to provide injections for adults. Rumours even circulated at one point that they were making a lot of money from experiments done on patients in Moyo Hospital. Personal relationships with them were, as a rule, impossible, because they stayed only briefly on visits outside of Moyo town, lived in an enclosure, were often not fluent in English, and were on short-term contracts. By and large, they are thought of not as real people at all but as a resource like the UNHCR, from which things ought to be forthcoming on a regular basis.

THE VIEW IN THE COMPOUND

The number of French expatriates in the MSF team based in Moyo town varied. It was usually around ten, including two administrators, two doctors, a laboratory technician, a pharmacist, a midwife and three nurses. They were engaged on contracts of six months to a year. All of them were young and often they had not been employed abroad before, but they were altruistic, paid low salaries, and were usually prepared to work very hard. The organisation had been operational in the district since 1984, mainly with UNHCR funding, providing emergency medical facilities for returnees and assisting the Ministry of Health in rehabilitating district health-care services. Expatriates collaborated with government health staff, and, in addition, the team directly employed many local people in a range of non-medical occupations (cooks, drivers, masons, carpenters, etc.). Expatriates worked on all wards of Moyo Hospital, with the exception of the surgery wards, and the team was involved in the reconstruction of static health centres and dispensaries, such as those in Laropi, as well as in the provision of medicines, in-service training of medical staff, child vaccination and sleeping sickness control.

That MSF's efforts cured individuals of debilitating diseases and saved lives cannot be questioned. Nevertheless, virtually all the expatriates working on the programme often expressed frustration. The attitude they encountered in the population was oppressively mendicant. They found themselves dehumanised and often forced to act as mere conduits for relief items. A great deal of time ended up being spent on attempts to police an effective distribution of drugs, an impossible task given the pressure on local staff to sell them to make ends meet.

Short-term contracts and the structure in which they worked made it difficult for the team to understand much of what was going on around them. They remained ignorant about the ways in which affliction was locally understood, and they were usually even unaware of whether there were Madi words for the diseases they treated. They were also very disturbed when they encountered the adverse results of some local therapics, or were confronted by attitudes which seemed very different from their own. Sometimes they would be presented with a baby with an horrific abscess caused by an injection given at home; or by infected cuts covering the body of someone treated by a 'daktari' using a razor blade; or a complete lack of interest in the suffering of non-kin in the hospital; or outright hostility towards a woman with labour complications.

The tendency was to respond by retreating into compound life, a 'rational', moral sphere that was emphatically French. One-half of the main living room had been turned into a copy of a Mediterranean bar. Sadly, by the time they left, some of them had developed strongly negative attitudes towards the people they had come to assist. Others felt angry at having been placed in such a position by the organisation that employed them. The institutional solution in both cases was the same, to bring out a fresh face.

It is striking that the views of departing personnel seem to have been largely ignored by MSF (and by other medical NGOs working in northern Uganda). There appeared to be no structured facility for accumulating

insights to formulate effective policy judgements, and decisions were commonly made by people with little knowledge of the area, and were mainly made
on a hand-to-mouth basis. Paucity of independent finance required MSF to
operate as an implementing agency for large donors (mainly UNHCR and
the EU), and this meant that, in practice, projects were determined more by
the availability of funds than by anything else. For this reason, MSF was
drawn into the medical screening of those returning refugees transported on
UNHCR's vehicles, a time-consuming and largely pointless exercise because
it could not involve much more than asking hundreds of people if they had
a headache or itchy skin. The overall emphasis was on the rehabilitation of
clinic buildings, and on distribution of drugs and inoculations. Such efforts
elicited approval from funders, because they seemed to produce tangible
outcomes, and also from Ugandan politicians, for they represented visible
and thereby politically expedient development strategies.

It could be countered that there were also funders and factions within the
Ugandan government who might have been enthusiastic about adopting a
comprehensive primary health-care approach. It would have accorded closely
with the National Resistance Movement's commitment to encouraging
popular participation, something which many donors were keen to support. To
the argument that this might have been a more effective way of promoting the
long-term improvement of health in the district than continued, excessive
emphasis on technological biomedical intervention, MSF administrators
based in Kampala and Paris replied that the organisation was not really
concerned with long-term objectives. MSF was not a development agency
but a relief programme, operating temporarily in a crisis.

In this respect, the organisation was similar to German Emergency
Doctors, and Swiss Disaster Relief, both of which also worked in north-west
Uganda for a period. But, as these agencies discovered, a dilemma arose
when it was time to leave. The services that expatriates administered were
in acute danger of deteriorating drastically, because the hard-pressed
Ministry of Health was just not in a position to run institutions at the same
level. Furthermore, it was becoming increasingly apparent that the
continued pumping of drugs into the area without adequate control over
prescription might be seriously counterproductive. The continued reuse of
syringes in Uganda, with its high incidence of HIV and hepatitis, was
fraught with obvious dangers.

In reality, the distinction made between relief and development by
medical NGOs did not make much sense. Northern Uganda had been in a
state of crisis for a long time and has remained so. MSF had been operational
in Moyo District for several years. The people living in Laropi watched
expatriates in relief programme vehicles pass by their homes day after day,
and from their perspective there was not much difference between one
agency and another. Aid had become a permanent feature of the landscape,

and talk of leaving was not taken seriously. When Swiss Disaster Relief pulled out of East Moyo County, the Swiss MSF replaced them, and the French MSF based in Moyo town was still operating in the late 1990s.

Continued attachment to the notion of relief, however, has the advantage of enabling an organisation to side-step the complex issues raised by development and to ignore critiques of top-down, technological intervention. No serious assessment of the effects of the programme seems to have been required. In the late 1980s, MSF undertook some nutritional surveys based on anthropometric measuring of children. The data were used to show that people were not starving, despite the fact that most of the food relief that was expected to be distributed in the district (by UNHCR and the World Food Programme) failed to arrive. In fact the results of the surveys were inconclusive, because sample sizes were very small, and because no mortality-rate data was collected (a slight decline in incidence of acute malnutrition might have indicated an overall improvement in nutritional status, or it might have been a result of a rise in mortality, and increased consumption by surviving children). It is reasonable to assert that, throughout the time I lived in Laropi, MSF and the other aid agencies working in the area had no clear idea of how local people were surviving or, indeed, whether they were not.

MSF did collaborate on a primary health-care project but of the selective variety espoused by UNICEF (UN Children's Fund) since 1983, which moved away from the principles established at the 1978 Alma-Ata Conference and concentrated on GOBI (Growth-monitoring, Oral-rehydration, Breast-feeding and Immunisation) (UNICEF 1983; Wisner 1988). As elsewhere, this amounted to rounding up children for inoculation and distributing pre-packaged rehydration salts (revealingly, one of the first UNICEF operations taking this approach, which was run in Burkina Faso, was called Operation Commando).

Some commentators have suggested that the attempt to subvert the primary health-care ideal was partly because of fears that it might take on political overtones (Lang 1988; Werner 1988). This is possibly credible with respect to the major donors, but one would expect NGOs to have had a degree of autonomy, or at least to attempt to assert one. Moreover, in other sectors of the development business, NGOs had become uncomfortable about purely technological approaches, even in crisis situations. Particularly in the realm of agriculture, the value of grassroots schemes, which drew upon indigenous knowledge, had become the orthodox rhetoric and sometimes also a reality. Robert Chambers' book *Rural Development: Putting the Last First* (1983) had become very influential, and NGO staff working in the agricultural sector in Moyo District would sometimes try to implement its suggestions. Yet medical NGOs persisted, unrepentantly, to operate in the apparent belief that technological inputs alone were unproblematic. Why was this so? Why did so many medical NGOs embrace the UNICEF agenda of the 1980s so enthusiastically? Why was it that, after years of working among the Madi, there were no pamphlets or posters in the vernacular to explain biomedical approaches to disease? Why were efforts not made to involve schools, scouts, church groups and local councils in grassroots health-care projects?

One answer, perhaps, is not to do with political ideology or financial constraints, but with the hegemony of biomedicine in international ideas about healing and the power of the biomedical establishment. Reflexivity in scientific agricultural knowledge, when faced with indigenous expertise, is one thing. Reflexivity in scientific medical knowledge is quite another, for biomedical knowledge relates to the way people conceive of themselves as persons, and is a body of information that is considered to be universally and objectively true.

For those whose world view is informed by biomedicine (including most senior Ugandan health professionals) 'medical thought is fully engaged in the philosophical status of man'. It was in medicine that the conception of the individual as both the subject and the object of knowledge first began to emerge, giving it a pivotal position in relation to the human sciences and directing 'our gaze into a world of constant visibility' (Foucault 1973, p. 198, x). To paraphrase Evans-Pritchard again, medical knowledge is a web of belief that cannot be escaped from because it is not an external structure but part of the texture of thought itself (1937). The awe in which doctors are held, the hierarchical organisation of the profession, and the rejection of emotion in the restraint of clinical discourse all act as secondary elaborations. Confronted by a strange world beyond the compound, rife with weird cures, manufactured drugs and clinical techniques, can become, even more than they are in the West, physical emanations of Foucault's 'anatomo-clinical gaze'. They are efficacious commodities that are more than tools. They are symbols, even fetishes, confirming that science describes actuality.

CONCLUSION: CLOSED MINDS, OPEN SYSTEMS

An article that appeared in *The Lancet* at the time I was living in Uganda argued that efforts to improve health in the poor world have tended to ignore the importance of behaviour (Meegan and McCormick, 1988, pp. 152–3). 'Ideas which are common in the rich world,' the authors state, 'have as a rule no place in the mental vocabulary of the rural population in Africa.' Germ theory is considered absurd, for the 'frame of reference does not accommodate scientific knowledge.' Moreover, 'traditional cultures have beliefs about aetiology and treatment of disease just as strong as we do' and these 'cannot be displaced by an alternative and alien system simply by extolling the latter's virtues'. In fact, 'integration of the two systems is impossible and probably undesirable. The best outcome is to add something which may remain an alternative rather than a preferred course of action.' According to the authors, the way forward is fluency in the local language as a base for understanding, for only in this way will trust be built up, which may prompt people to make 'an act of faith' and adopt better health-care practices.

The essay by Meegan and McCormick is a critique of current modes of technological intervention, centred on methods of biomedical evangelism. The authors present a view of African cultures as closed systems that, though ultimately mistaken, are logical in terms of themselves, resilient, and worthy of respect (1988). This is like a caricature of Evans-Pritchard's analysis of Azande causality, akin to those of Winch (1972) and Horton (1967). The proposed solution, furthermore, is a form of anthropological fieldwork that would enable biomedical knowledge to be transferred without trauma.

Two months after the publication of Meegan and McCormick's article, a rejoinder appeared that rightly pointed out that the authors 'display a woefully low expectation of the intelligence of traditional peoples' (O'Dempsey 1988, p. 686). Meegan and McCormick's view, however, is a prevalent one; indeed, many would regard it as a sympathetic perspective and see the proposed way forward as ideal, if impractical. It relates to a perception of African cultures that accords with Western ideas of what they should be like, ideas that are all too often loaded into the well-worn categories of 'traditional' and 'community' that retain widespread currency in aid-agency parlance. For expatriates working for medical NGOs in Moyo District, it is a view confirmed by experience, for, even when the 'truth' of the biomedical world is revealed through a microscope, this does not necessarily affect behaviour. By and large, expatriate medics see themselves as working at a tangent to the world beyond the compound, which most are prepared to believe is rational in terms of itself but which is clearly incomprehensible during a brief stay. I recall the surprise and irritation of one of the French doctors when a 'daktari' came to see him in the compound and asked for fresh, clean razor blades for his practice. For the doctor, it was extraordinary to imagine a connection between their professions. For the 'daktari', the connection was obvious.

Rather than enclosed by the Madi world, the expatriates were actors within it in a manner that their transitory conception of intervention masks. They were part of a long-term encounter that in its new form had lasted since the early 1980s but that has roots a century old. There is a closed system in Moyo, but it is not that of Madi culture; it is that of biomedicine. It is a body of knowledge that Westerners adapt and accommodate in the course of normal social interaction, but it lies at the core of their cultural identity, of the way in which they conceive of themselves. As has been noted, psychoanalysis, acupuncture, homeopathy and other non-biomedical therapies have established niches in the West, but the very manner of their espousal tends to reflect the polarisation of objectivity and morality, the hegemony of the biomedical, the post-mortem as the absolute, ultimate, arbitrator of sickness causality. They are all viewed as 'alternative' medicines. Confronted with the feared or the incomprehensible in a non-Western setting, reductionism sets in, and mediation occurs by recourse to the technological.

In the Madi medical system (if 'system' is the right word), diagnostic and therapeutic pluralism is fundamental. So are incorporation and adaptation. Impersonal aetiology is a possibility. But, frequently, biomedical and local herbal cures are combined and may be embraced by overlapping, sometimes competing, interpersonal explanations. The concept of disease as a distinct phenomenon is recognised, and biological knowledge is often considerably more than my own (for example), because former school students pore over textbooks all their lives. But use of biomedicine does not exclude non-biomedical ontological premises. Laza may not be distinguished from other aspects of personal suffering, and therapy can act as the medium through which social accountability is sought, partially established, and re-established in continually trying, intermittently awful situations.

This contribution has not been directly concerned with outlining prescriptions for better health-care programmes. Rather, I have tried to understand the dynamics of a social situation. I have examined ways of thinking about affliction and healing and some of the reasons for the miscommunication between Western expatriate medics and the population they have been sent to assist. But it is clear that this miscommunication has practical consequences. It adversely affects the manner in which expatriates relate to the recipients of their aid on a personal level, and it gears programmes towards a top-down approach. While it may save some lives in the short term, it both is unsustainable and encourages a dangerous abuse of drugs.

My own sympathy for a more broadly-based form of primary health-care is obvious. From this point of view, the shift that occurred in UNICEF's position during the 1990s towards a holistic, rights-based approach may prove to be a positive development. MSF too has begun to move away from a rigid emergency orientation, no doubt partly due to the changed funding climate, but also because the organisation has been forced to confront the counter-productive consequences of some of its programmes. However, the discussion presented here has not suggested a setting aside of policies premised on biomedical interpretations of affliction. It is not my intention to encourage the adoption of public health services delivered by profession-alised local therapists applying their own 'indigenous knowledge'. As Robert Chambers has pointed out, there are reasons why local understandings of crop production may be more like scientific understandings than are local understandings of the human body. Farmers everywhere apply the technique of trial and error in order to obtain desired crop characteristics, but parents will not be willing to experiment in the same way with their children. Often 'the coping mechanisms for the awfulness of the illness and death of those who are close are social and spiritual, and so linked with social and spiritual rather than physical explanation' (Chambers 1983, p. 97). The difficulties of working closely with so-called traditional healers are underlined by the activities of TBAs and 'daktaris' in Moyo District. It cannot be assumed that all therapists are engaged in the enterprise of alleviating the effects of bodily malfunctions, or that they have mechanisms for doing so. In many cases, it may be better to involve other individuals in grassroots medical schemes than local therapy specialists. Given the continuing lack of resources for formal education and public health facilities in most impoverished countries, and also the acute limitations of intermittent selective intervention, facilitating access to biomedical information should be a priority, while actively (and sensitively) propagating a biomedical interpretation of illness.

My basic plea, however, is that medical aid workers concentrate as much on understanding what is going on around them as on administering cures. It is important to be able to locate vulnerable groups (such as those who might be accused of 'inyinya'), rather than to treat communities as homogeneous entities, and it is crucial to have an awareness of what local healing means in order effectively to offer a biomedical alternative when appropriate. Moreover, a sympathy to social context and appreciation of other ways of thinking is invaluable for the aid workers themselves. The introversion of compound life, and the implicit conception of the surrounding population as an amorphous target, involves a paring away of humanity that is as damaging to the doers of development as it is condescending or even degrading to the recipients.

ACKNOWLEDGEMENTS

This chapter is a revised and expanded version of a chapter called 'Closed Minds, Open Systems', which was originally published in a book edited by David Brokensha in honour of Paul Baxter (Allen 1989). I am grateful to Melissa Parker, Georgia Kaufmann, James Appe, Ken Wilson, Barbara Harrell-Bond, Graham Clark, Teddy Brett, Wendy James, and Terence Ranger for comments on earlier drafts. Research in Uganda was financed by the University of Manchester and the Uganda office of the European Community.

REFERENCES

Allen, T., 1989. 'Closed Minds, Open Systems', in D. Brokensha, ed., *A River of Blessings*. New York: Syracuse University.

Allen, T., 1991a. 'The Quest for Therapy in Moyo District', in H. Bernt Hansen and M. Twaddle, eds., *Changing Uganda*. London: James Currey.

Allen, T., 1991b. 'Understanding Alice: Uganda's Holy Spirit Movement in Context'. *Africa*, 61, 3: pp. 370–99.

Allen, T., 1992. 'Upheaval, Affliction and Health: A Ugandan Case Study', in H. Bernstein, B. Crow and H. Johnson, eds., *Rural Livelihoods: Crises and Responses*. Oxford: Oxford University Press.

Allen, T., 1994. 'Ethnicity and Tribalism on the Sudan–Uganda border', in K. Fukui and J. Markakis, eds., *Ethnicity and Conflict in the Horn of Africa*. London: James Currey.

Allen, T., 1996. 'A Flight from Refuge', in T. Allen, ed., *In Search of Cool Ground: War, Flight and Homecoming in Northeast Africa*. London: James Currey.

Allen, T., 1997. 'The Violence of Healing', *Sociologus*, 47, 2: pp. 101–28.

Barnes-Dean, V.L., 1986. 'Lugbara Illness Beliefs and Social Change', *Africa*, 56, 3: pp. 334–51.

Baxter, P.T.W., and Butt, A., 1953. *The Azande and Related Peoples*. London: International African Institute.

Behrend, H., 1991. 'Is Alice Lakwena a Witch?', in H. Bernt Hansen and M. Twaddle, eds., *Changing Uganda*. London: James Currey.

Behrend, H., 1995. 'The Holy Spirit Movement and the Forces of Nature in the North of Uganda', in H. Bernt Hansen and M. Twaddle, eds., *Religion and Politics in East Africa*. London: James Currey.

Behrend, H., 1998. 'The Holy Spirit Movement: New World: Discourse and Development in the North of Uganda', in H. Bernt Hansen and M. Twaddle, eds., *Developing Uganda*. Oxford: James Currey.

Buxton, J., 1973. *Religion and Healing in Mandari*. London: Oxford University Press.

Casale, M., 1982. 'Women, Power, and Change in Lugbara (Uganda) Cosmology: A Reinterpretation', *Anthropos*, 77: pp. 385–96.

Chambers, R., 1983. *Rural Development: Putting the Last First*. London: Longman.

Comaroff, J., and Comaroff, J., eds., 1993. *Modernity and Its Discontents: Ritual and Power in Postcolonial Africa*. Chicago: University of Chicago Press.

Evans-Pritchard, E.E., 1937. *Witchcraft, Oracles and Magic among the Azande*. London: Oxford University Press.

Feierman, S., 1979, 'Change in African Therapeutic Systems', *Social Science and Medicine*, 13b: pp. 277–84.

Foucault, M., 1973. *The Birth of the Clinic*. London: Tavistock Publications.

Gluckman, M., 1944. 'The Logic of African Science and Witchcraft: An Appreciation of Evans-Pritchard's Witchcraft, Oracles and Magic among the Azande', *Rhodes Livingstone Journal* (June).

Gluckman, M., 1955. *Custom and Conflict in Africa*. Oxford: Basil Blackwell.

Harrell-Bond, B.E., 1986. *Imposing Aid: Emergency Assistance to Refugees*. Oxford: Oxford University Press.

Horton, R., 1967. 'African Traditional Thought and Western Science', *Africa*, 37, 1: pp. 50–71; 2: pp. 15–87.

James, W., 1988. *The Listening Ebony*. Oxford: Oxford University Press.

Janzen, J.M., 1978. *The Quest for Therapy: Medical Pluralism in Lower Zaire*. Berkeley: University of California Press.

Janzen, J.M., 1981. 'The Need for a Taxonomy of Health in African Therapeutics', *Social Science and Medicine*, 15B: pp. 185–94.

Lang, R., 1988. Selective versus Comprehensive Primary Health Care. Unpublished manuscript, Health Unit, Oxfam House, Oxford.

Meegan, M., and McCormick, J., 1988. 'Prevention of Disease in the Poor World', *Lancet*, July 16: pp. 152–3.

Middleton, J., 1960. *Lugbara Religion: Ritual and Authority among an East African People*. London: Oxford University Press.

Middleton, J., 1963. 'Witchcraft and Sorcery in Lugbara', in J. Middleton and E.H. Winters, eds., *Witchcraft and Sorcery in East Africa*. London: Routledge and Kegan Paul.

Middleton, J., 1965. *The Lugbara*. London: Holt, Rinehart and Wilson.

Middleton, J., 1967. 'The Concept of 'Bewitching' in Lugbara', in J. Middleton, ed., *Magic, Witchcraft and Curing*. New York: Natural History Press.

Middleton, J., 1969. 'Spirit Possession among the Lugbara', in J. Beattie and J. Middleton, eds., *Spirit Mediumship and Society in Africa*. London: Routledge and Kegan Paul.

Ngubane, H., 1977. *Body and Mind in Zulu Medicine*. London: Academic Press.

O'Dempsey, T.J.D., 1988. 'Health Education and Traditional Cultures', *Lancet*, 17 September: pp. 686.

Rowley, J.V., 1940. 'Notes on the Madi of Equatoria Province', *Sudan Notes and Records*, 23, 2: pp. 279–94.

Sontag, S., 1979. *Illness as Metaphor*. London: Allen Lane.

UNICEF, 1983 and annual. *The State of the World's Children*. Geneva: UNICEF.

Werner, D., 1988. *Empowerment and Health*. Unpublished manuscript, Hesperian Foundation, Palo Alto, California.

Whyte, S.R., 1997. Questioning Misfortune: *The Pragmatics of Uncertainty in Eastern Uganda*. Cambridge: Cambridge University Press.

Williams, F.R.J., 1949. 'The Pagan Religion of the Madi', *Uganda Journal*, 13: pp. 202–12.

Winch, P., 1972. *Ethics and Action*. London: Routledge and Kegan Paul.

Wisner, B., 1988. 'Gobi versus PHC? Some Dangers of Selective Primary Health Care', *Social Science and Medicine*, 26, 9: pp. 963–9.

ELEVEN

Reproductive Health or Population Control?

FRANK FUREDI

The question of global population is a public health issue about which it has conspicuously often been assumed – especially by the popular media – both that social issues are fundamental to populations' health, and that people's health can be improved by an obvious step: by limiting population. Scarcity and famine, it used at any rate to be thought, can be curtailed by limiting population. In this paper, I propose to deal with what at first appear to be more sophisticated and politically acute approaches to population questions. It is almost impossible to encounter any expert these days who professes to be an advocate of population control. Even terms like 'population problem' and 'population programmes' are going out of fashion and the vocabulary of ardent neo-Malthusians is continually peppered with terms like 'reproductive health', 'maternal health' and 'gender equity'. International conferences – Cairo (1994), The Hague (1999) – which are driven by the impulse of global fertility control self-consciously distance themselves from the language of demography. Examining some of the issues that arise in these settings, I shall show that attempting to alter other people's social attitudes and situations involves moral and practical pitfalls which appear to be unsuspected in much health-related literature. Altering aspects of other societies in the name of enhancing health (those societies' or our own) can only too easily cause a confounding of values which culminates merely in imposing our own preferred standards on other people. This does not mean that we should never make impacts on society in order to improve health, but it does entail that we must develop a stringently critical form of discourse for analysing the processes involved in doing so.

It is worth noting that the Programme of Action adopted at the International Conference on Population and Development in Cairo does not refer to any demographic factor as the main cause of any problem and does not even use the term 'population problem'. Instead of population, the Programme prefers to focus on the issues of gender equality, women's health, the empowerment of women and the elimination of violence against

174

women. In reality this was very much a conference about population, but its organisers took the view that demographic concerns could be most effectively sold through a different packaging. As one advocate of this consensus reported: 'The new thinking endorsed in Cairo is that population growth can be stabilised and development efforts enhanced by the advancement of women' (Ashford 1995, p. 2). This policy is seen to be the most effective route to the spread of family nucleation and the establishment of a regime of low fertility.

Since Cairo, advocates of population programmes have become even more sensitive about appearing to be motivated by eugenic and neo-Malthusian concerns. Many organisations, especially feminist-influenced NGOs, are reluctant to be associated with what they regard as a highly unpopular population agenda. In the run-up to the 1999 Hague conference, it was issues like sex education, maternal health, reproductive health, youth and violence against women which came to the fore. The importance of distancing from the Malthusian agenda has been continually stressed by health activists during the past four years. As one NGO declared:

> A significant shift in thinking is needed from the concept of population control programme imperative to that of reproductive health. The Family Reproductive Health Programme aims to promote equitable appropriate access to health and other life opportunities, which influence and affect people's reproduction. It is not motivated by demographic considerations, therefore it is important to establish that the Family Reproductive Health Programme is not a population control programme. (*Save the Children Ghana* 1996)

The anxiety arising from being associated with population control programmes is driven by a variety of motives. In some cases there is a genuine hostility to the coercive practices linked to the project of population control. Some feminist NGOs have drawn the conclusion that their own objective of gender equity could be usefully promoted through a pragmatic alliance with neo-Malthusians. Others have opportunistically decided that their work could be discredited through an exposure of their ties with the population lobby, whilst the main neo-Malthusian players have concluded that targeting women and discreetly downgrading demographic concerns is the way forward (Hodgson and Cotts Watkins 1997).

LOSS OF CONFIDENCE

As I argue elsewhere (Furedi 1997), the population control lobby has undergone a major crisis of confidence during the past two decades. There was a time when neo–Malthusians could confidently declare that poverty, underdevelopment and social tension in the societies of the South were the consequence of high rates of population growth. Statements which warned of 'population bombs' were disseminated and the term 'overpopulation' was routinely used to describe the continents of Africa, Asia and Latin America. But since the late seventies, economic arguments that served the cause of population control have been discredited. As a result neo–Malthusians are continually looking for new ways of justifying their cause.

Publications of the United Nations Population Fund (UNFPA) now treat the relationship between population growth and development as a side issue, and seek to mobilise support for population control programmes on other grounds. Even organisations and individuals who fervently promote programmes designed to curb population growth will now openly acknowledge that there is 'no evidence that population growth is the *cause* of poverty' (Ashford 1995, p. 31). To be sure, popular media representations of the issue still associate population growth with the problems of economic development, famines and food shortage. However, the more specialist studies, especially those based on empirical research, are far more circumspect. Today, professionals attached to the delivery of population programmes are far more likely to justify their action on the grounds that it will improve women's health or protect the environment than because it contributes to economic development.

The tension contained within the agenda of population control is expressed through a permanent search for effective arguments. Lack of confidence in the presentation of the case has shifted the focus to the packaging of population policies. Population policies are rarely marketed in explicitly demographic terms these days. The tendency is to integrate population policies into other, apparently more neutral, programmes such as health care, education and the empowerment of women. The words used to package population policies are chosen with care. So, often policies which are designed to reduce fertility are represented as giving women more choice. Donald Warwick has drawn attention to the cultivation of an inoffensive vocabulary used to market policies:

> Those who favour fertility control prefer the phrase family planning, which has overtones of rationality, self-direction, and human welfare, rather than birth control, which implies limits on free choice. (Warwick 1994, p. 190)

It is difficult to avoid the conclusion that the vocabulary associated with population issues is designed to mystify rather than clarify.

The linguistic acrobatics of the population lobby are symptomatic of an underlying defensiveness. In recent years the central theme of population policy has become the empowerment of women. An assessment of the Cairo Conference on Population noted, in passing, that during the proceedings 'no plenary speaker dared omit at least mentioning' the importance of empowerment of women. It added that 'agreement on the central role of women in development has become so non controversial that it was not even an issue at the IPCD' (Cohen and Richards 1994, pp. 274–5). An examination of most of the recent publications on the subject shows that the role of women and reproductive health have become a dominant justification for population programmes.

TARGETING WOMEN

Because of women's central role in reproduction, their attitude and behaviour has been of interest to those involved in population issues from the beginning of the eugenic tradition to today. Curiously, despite an appreciation of the way in which progress towards women's emancipation could impact upon fertility, the population lobby did not take this connection seriously until the late sixties. It was the rise of the women's liberation movement which alerted the population establishment to its potential importance. The women's liberation movement was dynamic and possessed considerable moral authority. At a time when the population lobby was on the defensive, the temptation to link up with the women's movement must have been strong. Those interested in population control saw the demand of the women's movement for access to contraception and abortion as lending credibility to their own agenda. The potential importance of the women's movement for the population lobby was spelled out in 1972 by the American political scientist Peter Bachrach:

> The interest of supporters of population control would be significantly served if they used their power to aid women's liberation groups to realise one of their goals – compelling the government to enforce its policy of providing for equal education and economic opportunities for women – for the anti-natalist sentiment that would be generated by such an enforcement would be profound. (Bachrach 1972)

The perception that the advance of the women's movement would help to create a climate in which anti-natalist ideas could enjoy legitimacy won significant support in the population field.

By the early seventies, many of the high-profile population controllers had jumped on the women's bandwagon. Increasingly they came to regard the export of women's issues to the Third World as an important component of indirect population programmes. The Ehrlichs were particularly enthusiastic about promoting population policies through the medium of women's rights. They outlined their approach:

> There are many possibilities in the sphere of family structure, sexual mores, and the status of women that can be explored. With some exceptions, women have traditionally been allowed to fulfil only the roles of wife and mother. Anything that can be done to diminish the emphasis upon these roles and provide women with equal opportunities in education, employment and other areas is likely to reduce the birth rate. Any measures that postpone marriage, especially for women, would also help to encourage the reduction in birth rates. (Ehrlich and Ehrlich 1970, p. 253)

Here was a bold platform designed to harness the dynamism of the women's liberation movement to the cause of population control. From this perspective, changes in the position of women could provide the answer that the population lobby had long been looking for in its search for a good argument.

The connection between the changing status of women and the reduction in family size has been enthusiastically embraced by most sections of the population lobby as an important theme in their campaign. The targeting of women is now routine in the various surveys and reports on population. The report of the International Commission on Peace and Food (1994) clearly expressed this sentiment: 'Concrete steps must be taken to generate greater educational, training and employment opportunities for the poor, and most especially for females – the best-known methods for eradicating poverty and bringing down the rate of population growth' (International Commission on Peace and Food 1994, p. 186). Since changing the position of women is apparently the 'best-known' method for bringing down the rate of population, it has been adopted as a policy by all the relevant agencies.

Many women writers and feminists have been disturbed by the way their concerns have been manipulated and co-opted by population activists. Bonnie Mass was one of the first women to warn against this manipulation of feminist rhetoric, arguing that imperialism had veiled 'its interest behind the mask of false feminism'. She pointed to how female-oriented propaganda had become a device for selling population control (Mass 1976, pp. 230–1). Amrit Wilson has warned against the 'cynical attempt' to use feminist rhetoric against women (Wilson 1994, p. 2202). Lakshmi Lingham commented that the incorporation of women's reproductive rights into the population agenda in practice meant that 'the rhetoric of the feminist movement' was being appropriated, though not its concerns. She wrote:

> At present women's status or health is being seen as a means to an end in the following way: improving women's status speeds fertility decline thus reducing considerably 'the overall negative impact' of population on environment and development. (Lingham 1994, p. 85)

Third World women's groups have also expressed suspicion about the manner in which reproductive rights have been co-opted into the international population agenda.

Many feminist writers are not so much hostile as ambivalent in their relationship to the population lobby. The contribution of Betsy Hartmann well illustrates this tendency. Her book *Reproductive Rights and Wrongs* (1987) provides a well-documented critique of the ideology and practices of the population lobby. Moreover Hartmann is sensitive to the instrumental way in which the issue of women is used by international agencies. She warned that feminists were in danger of being outflanked, noting that 'there is always the danger that these individuals' genuine commitment to women's welfare will be twisted and manipulated by others in the population establishment who want to appropriate feminist language and concepts in order to give population control a better image' (Hartmann 1987, p. 295). Despite these reservations, Hartmann did not reject population policies as such. She was prepared to give some initiatives the benefit of the doubt and called for an alliance with 'liberal family planners' against what she called the 'hard-line population camp' (p. 143).

Hartmann's call for an alliance of feminists and liberal family planners reflects a clear tendency within the international population establishment. Most feminists argue that redistribution, equity and improvement in the position of women should be the key element in any population policy. Many of them are aware of the instrumental way in which these issues are used. However, because they accept a common premise, namely that population growth is the problem, their criticism of the more traditional population lobby tends to have only a tactical character.

In practice, the tension between the priority of population control and that of improvement in the position of women remains unresolved. This is not merely due to a conflict of priorities. Whereas the precondition of the emancipation of women is far-reaching socio-economic change, population policies merely require organisation and effective targeting. Consequently, the commitment to change the position of women is treated as a long-term objective, while family programmes are seen as practicable in the here and now. For example, critics of India's Draft National Population Policy have pointed to the cynical way in which in practice the role of women is ignored:

> The report is virtually silent on the growing feminisation of poverty in India. Its reference to gender equity and to free and informed choice for women merely reflect the report's uncritical and deliberate assimilation of the vocabulary of women's groups and women activists. (Anon. 1994, p. 2471)

One reason why the tension between the two priorities remains unresolved is that, at the level of policy-making, anti-poverty measures have gone out of fashion. Since the eighties, international agencies have promoted structural adjustment programmes, whose effect has been the intensification of inequalities in developing societies. Many of the international agencies which have called for a greater integration of women into population policies have also promoted structural adjustment programmes. It is surprising that the contradiction between these two objectives has not been rigorously explored by the protagonists in the debate (see, for example, Sen *et al.* 1994, p. 4, who merely refer to the parallel evolution of women-oriented and structural adjustment policies as a 'paradox').

The interweaving of population and women's policy is confusing. This confusion is perpetuated by the tendency of contributors to the discussion to accept the presentation of family planning policies at face value. One of the questions regarding family planning programmes that is rarely posed is this: are they about improving the position of women or are they about controlling population? In their discussion of such policies, writers rarely distinguish between the public relations packaging, the fundamental aims and the means used to implement them. Consequently, even those critical of population policies seldom entertain the conclusion that they might have little to do with the stated goal of improving the position of women.

In most instances, policies oriented towards women's status and education are, in practice, motivated by demographic considerations. Critics who demand that such policies be less instrumentalist towards women miss the point of why such programmes exist, and why international agencies finance them in the first place. If, for example, the real objective was the improvement of female education, then this would be promoted independent of demographic considerations. But that would presuppose that education was the end rather than the means to realise another agenda. The insistence that family planning programmes increase their emphasis on women misses this point. Even when such programmes talk about nothing else but women, the issue of equality remains an expedient to be manipulated for demographic objectives. An illustration of this is Lily Hsia's editorial in a recent issue of the *Journal of Nurse-Midwifery*, entitled 'Stemming the Tide of the Global Population Explosion: The Key Role of Women'. Hsia celebrates the increasing importance attached to the role of women by family planners. However, an examination of her argument reveals that the position of women is peripheral to the discussion:

> In the past, family planning was considered to be the most effective means to stabilise and slow world population growth. Today, other initiatives such as quality reproductive health care, increased educational and economic opportunities for women, reduction in infant

and child mortality rates, and increased employment of women are considered important adjuncts to population decline. (Hsia 1995, p. 2)

It is in the capacity of 'adjuncts to population decline' that women's issues acquire relevance in demographic discourse. In the same vein, an article entitled 'Empowering Women: An Essential Objective', published in the *UN Chronicle*, goes straight to the point. Its opening sentence reads: 'the empowerment of women – a basic human rights objective – is key to achieving development and population goals' (September, 1994).

The emphasis of demography on women is heavily influenced by the objective of winning the propagandist war against the critics of population policy. That demographic narrative is shaped by the exigencies of public relations and propaganda has already been alluded to. The need publicly to distance population policy from traditional Western anti-natalist objectives became increasingly important in the seventies. During that period, demography self-consciously divested itself of the remnants of its past eugenic and racist vocabulary. Traditional welfare issues, health and the status of women were used to repackage population policies. An important component of this shift in vocabulary was the adoption of a more *indirect* approach to population control. The implications of this approach were clearly spelled out in an important American government document titled 'Implications of Worldwide Population Growth for U.S. Security and Overseas Interests' (all references here to this document, known as National Security Study Memorandum 2000, are taken from Information Project for Africa 1991, pp. 3–38).

The document argued that population policies designed for the Third World had to be presented as if they were motivated by altruism rather than national self-interest. To 'minimise charges of an imperialist motivation behind its support of population activities', it was suggested that programmes had to be presented as if they were about social reform. The document also suggested that terms like 'population control' and 'birth control' should be avoided by personnel implementing such programmes in the Third World. Like other reports, this one proposed that population programmes should be disguised as a service promoting health or some other public good. It noted:

> In the case of LDC countries uncommitted to population programs our efforts must be fine-tuned to their particular sensitivities and attitudes. In the main, we should avoid the language of 'birth control' in favour of 'family planning' or 'responsible parenthood', with the emphasis being placed on child spacing in the interests of the health of child and mother and the well-being of the family and community. Introduction and extension of primary health services are, in fact, the

principal ways of successfully introducing family planning into many of these countries.

The introduction of population control through the back door – under cover of concern about health, education and so on – was a central component of the strategy. A final component of this approach was the use of *intermediaries* for promoting population policies. The document advocated the use of non-governmental organisations and other agencies not directly linked with Washington as the appropriate vehicles for implementing population policies.

The propaganda techniques used by the population lobby today rely on the use of intermediary organisations. Such organisations – groups of women, reproductive health professionals, community groups – are sometimes set up with the explicit aim of creating a demand for population policies. According to Howard Wiarda, 'considerable pains have been taken to disguise' US government involvement in population programmes. He noted:

> Much of the funding has been channelled through third-party agencies to disguise the extent of United States involvement. Various fronts have been set up to make it appear, particularly in the early stages as though it is a private association that is supporting the program, not the United States government. Care has also been taken to find local doctors and concerned citizens in the countries affected so as to provide the appearance of local control, even though the funding and much of the direction may come from outside. (Wiarda 1987, pp. 61–2)

It is worth noting that the US government does not have a monopoly on the use of front organisations. Such front organisations, claiming to represent authentic local interests, are routinely deployed by both sides of the population debate.

The promotion of population policies through the rhetoric of health, particularly women's health, is one of the most important innovations of the propaganda techniques that emerged in the eighties. Programmes that were once labelled as policies of 'population control' and then called 'birth control', only to change to 'family planning', now go under the appellation of 'reproductive health'. The integration of population programmes into health services has become central to the marketing of fertility control. This medicalisation of population concern is seldom contested, because it appears to be entirely about the non-controversial subject of health.

The medicalisation of population control has been central to the approach adopted by Western governments over the past twenty years. For example, a report commissioned by the American government in 1981 advised that population activities 'should be integrated with maternal and health care delivery' because projects that focus too narrowly on family planning as a solution 'only increase suspicion in the host country' (cited in Simons 1995, p. 36). Since the early eighties, it has become customary unobtrusively to insert population measures into a broader health initiative. In that way, fertility control is presented as part of a long list of health measures. Invariably population control is promoted as a major contribution to women's health. With this redefinition of the objective of family planning, patients may be excused for failing to grasp that contraception is about reducing numbers of children.

In response to the demands of public relations, the term 'reproductive health' has been expanded to include virtually every women's condition, from menstruation to menopause. In this way, the underlying agenda of fertility control becomes inconspicuous to the designated target audience. Ironically, some radical critics advocate the expansion of the meaning of 'reproductive health', since they believe that it represents an important step in the direction of a more holistic, women-oriented approach. Gita Sen argues that there has been important progress because 'women's health activists have increasingly joined the population debate' (Sen 1994, p. 63). This optimistic interpretation can be countered by the view that women's health has become the latest in a long line of fashionable policies through which the population lobby seeks to influence fertility.

Reproductive health, like education, has become in practice another form of isolation exercise, aimed at reducing fertility. Reproductive health is above all about the indirect administration of contraception. Like education, the issue of health in general is isolated from wider issues of social development for the specific objective of influencing fertility. From the perspective of human well-being, the isolation of health is necessarily counter-productive, since it is so much bound up with every aspect of social life. This point is well made by Rosa Linda Valenzona in her criticism of the manipulation of the health issue by the 1993 Philippine Demographic Survey:

> The document concludes that the high risk infant, neonatal, child and maternal mortality is associated with pregnancies where mothers are too young, too old, or have already had several children. But a discussion of poverty is missing from the list of factors related to health. It would be difficult to deny that poverty, lack of access to safe water, poor housing, poor hygiene and unsanitary conditions all have a strong bearing on the health of the mother and child. (Valenzona 1994, p. 21)

Health programmes which fail to tackle the issue of poverty are either just ineffective or are promoting an agenda which has little to do with human well-being.

Many health activists would concur with Valenzona's criticism of the neglect of the crucial role of poverty. But in some cases the narrow emphasis on health, and specifically on birth control, is interpreted as just an isolated error. Ines Smyth's discussion of the Safe Motherhood campaign in Indonesia accepts that it gives 'too much importance to family planning as a strategy to reduce maternal mortality'. But she adds that there is 'insufficient evidence to suggest that there is a sinister explanation for the stress that Safe Motherhood initiatives give to family planning'. So how does she account for the emphasis of the campaign?

> However, it is common to consider reproductive health primarily from a demographic perspective and to link it to family planning. The cost-saving benefits of family planning over the more radical measures necessary to improve women's general and reproductive health are perhaps a more realistic explanation of this emphasis. (Smyth 1994, p. 25)

Smyth is loath to draw out the implications of her own words. If health is promoted from a 'demographic perspective' then the central objective is not the well-being of women but the reduction of population. Campaigns that are genuinely committed to reducing the rate of maternal mortality would be driven by a concern with maternal mortality and not by something else. This is not what motivates the Safe Motherhood campaign. The Safe Motherhood campaign uses the issue of maternal mortality to influence the fertility of Indonesian women. It is the failure of many health activists to demand the separation of health from what Smyth calls a demographic perspective that has allowed population programmes to masquerade as projects about reproductive rights.

The failure to demand the separation of health from demography or of education from demography or of poverty from demography is not accidental. Even the most critical voices are often trapped by their own consciousness of demography. Left-wing writers, feminists and health activists often accept the premise of the population lobby. Sometimes their criticism of narrow population policy is grounded in a shared perception of the fundamentals. The arguments of Sen, Germain and Chen for a radical and empowering policy are instructive in this respect: 'We argue that investing in people's health, empowerment, and human rights is not only worthy in its own right, but would probably be more conducive to population stabilisation than narrowly conceived policies of population control' (Sen *et al.* 1994, p. 11). To justify investment in health in terms of its contribution to the stabilisation of population is to elide the distinction between two very different concerns. Such arguments offer only a minimalist alternative to traditional population policies. To the 'narrowly conceived policies of population control' they counterpose a more widely conceived programme. A difference in scale but not of substance!

In the run-up to the Hague conference, maternal mortality has been identified as the key issue for reproductive health care. The figures –

580,000 deaths annually – for maternal mortality are truly horrific. But if maternal mortality is the fundamental concern, then the campaign should be oriented towards the building of maternal hospital services and ante-natal clinics, and not on simply preventing pregnancies in the first place.

COERCION BY ANOTHER NAME

Outwardly, promoters of reproductive health present their cause as the very antithesis of coercion. Many supporters of reproductive rights are genuinely hostile to population control programmes, and regard their approach as fundamentally different from the neo-Malthusian perspective. They uphold the inviolate right of women freely to determine their own fertility. They claim that a woman has an 'absolute right to bodily integrity and to decide herself on matters of sexuality and childbearing with no interference from her partner, family, health care professionals, religious groups, the state, or any other actor' (Reed *et al.* 1994, p. 100). Unfortunately, this admirable commitment to the inviolate right of each woman freely to determine her fertility is rarely pursued consistently. Experience has shown that the social and cultural values of reproductive health activists often lead precisely to disregarding the rights of women to make choices about their fertility.

As Hodgson and Cotts Watkins have observed, 'Internationally, the practice of many couples aborting female foetuses in order to give birth to more sons has made it difficult for any feminist to absolutely support the individual's reproductive autonomy. So although reproductive rights feminists theoretically are opposed to any form of coercion', they have worked hard to include in the Cairo Programme of Action a 'call for state intervention to stop such prenatal sex selection' (Hodgson and Cotts Watkins 1997, p. 507). But if reproductive coercion to accomplish a gender-equity goal is acceptable over this issue, it becomes unclear why it should be considered unethical in relation to other matters.

A selective approach towards the right of women to make decisions about their fertility is evident in the approach of reproductive health activists. In recent years, activists have become increasingly intolerant of what they consider to be unacceptable cultural obstacles to the realisation of their objectives. A recent publication jointly published by *The Guardian* and Marie Stopes International clearly reflects the authoritarian instincts of neo-Malthusianism. One of the authors, Yasmin Alibhai-Brown, condemns the lack of political will of the international community towards the implementation of 'maternal health rights' in societies that regard reproductive health issues as 'Western values'. She claims that these are human rights that are of universal significance and must therefore override all local objections. 'Donor agencies need to use human rights instruments more vigorously', writes Alibhai–Brown. She advocates breaking down local resistance through a policy of social engineering, which makes use of those aspects of culture that help the cause whilst destroying those which resist it. Her approach is straightforward: 'a better balance is needed between respecting cultural values which can be part of the solution and breaking down cultural values which are central to the problem' (Alibhai–Brown 1998). Cloaked in the language of human rights, this approach is driven by another right – the right of enlightened people to break down the cultures of societies of which they disapprove.

The moral authority assumed by those who claim the mantle of human rights allows many reproductive health activists to treat cultural obstacles as if they were a physical disease. From their target audience, they demand compliance rather than dialogue. This relationship is more comparable to that between parent and child than to one between equal partners. In this relationship, between those who know best and those who are ignorant of vital reproductive health issues, there is always the implication of coercion. Anyone familiar with the dynamic of interaction between an international agency and a small rural community will grasp the enormous pressure that will be exerted on the local people. The implication of this dynamic was clearly avoided by Tony Baldry, British Parliamentary Under-Secretary for Foreign and Commonwealth Affairs. When asked what constituted coercive population control, he replied:

> Population activities would be considered coercive if they sought to infringe the basic right of couples and individuals to decide freely and responsibly the number and spacing of their children. (Hansard 23 May 1995, col. 514)

Since population programmes are designed to reduce fertility, their aim is not to provide free choice but to influence people towards a particular outcome. A village where people 'freely' decided to increase their rate of fertility would not be considered a success by those in charge of a repro-ductive health project. The pressure is clearly in one direction – and the line between pressure and coercion is, in practice, blurred.

Most studies of fertility practices do not take the views of their subjects seriously. If their investigation reveals a general preference for large families, they have no hesitation in assuming responsibility for changing people's attitudes. Studies of 'unmet need' for contraception are quite open about the fact that their aim is to make people aware of this need, whether they like it or not. Family planning programmes contain an important focus on propaganda. Bongaarts and Bruce, two leading experts working with the Population Council, advocate not just providing family planning services, but also changing attitudes on the issue. They argue that 'an effective program is frequently one that goes far beyond the provision of family planning and contraceptive services by addressing social obstacles to use, such as fear of side effects and social or familial disapproval' (Bongaarts and Bruce 1995, p. 57). Bongaarts and Bruce are so convinced about their cause that they never pause to ask who gave them the right to tell others how to live, to undermine what they euphemistically refer to as the 'psychological and cultural barriers' to contraception in an African or Asian society.

For family planners, the cultural norms and values of target societies are obstacles that need to be overcome through a variety of techniques. Central importance is attached to encouraging women to adopt aspirations, lifestyles and identities which are at variance with the prevailing norms of their societies. 'To reduce unwanted sexual contact and pregnancy, we must assist girls to envision future identities apart from sexual, marital and mothering roles' argue Bongaarts and Bruce' (p. 72). The far-reaching implications of this perspective on social engineering in developing societies are rarely spelled out. This attempt to foster new aspirations and identities system-atically undermines the moral foundation of the target society. Whether societies have a capacity to absorb the effects of such changes is an issue that is simply evaded by the proponents of the new morality.

The issue at stake is not whether one approves of a particular idea or practice. There are many practices in *all* parts of the world which offend different groups of people. The real issue worth considering is, from where do a group of population professionals derive the authority to decide what is in the best interest of people in societies around the world? It seems that, for all their talk of rights, the one right which they clearly reject is the right of a people to decide how they should regulate their fertility. Their selective adherence to human rights indicates that they are not just the purveyors of reproductive health services.

REFERENCES

Alibhai-Brown, Y., 1998. 'Earth Mothers', in *Birth Matters*, a special supplement on reproductive health in the developing world. London: *The Guardian*.

Anonymous Note, 1994. 'Politics of Population and Development', *Economic and Political Weekly*, 17, September.

Ashford, L.S., 1995. 'New Perspectives on Population: Lessons from Cairo', *Population Bulletin*, 50, 1.

Ashford, L.S. 1995. 'New Perspectives on Population: Cairo', *Population Bulletin*, 50, 1.

Bachrach, P., 1972. 'The Scholar and Political Strategy: The Population Case', in R.L., Clinton, W.S., Flash, and R.K., Godwin, eds., *Political Science in population Studies*. Lexington, MA: Lexington Books.

Bongaarts, J., and Bruce, J., 1995. 'The Causes of Unmet Need for Contraception and the Social Context of Services', *Studies in Family Planning*, 26, 2.

Cohen, S.A., and Richards, C.L., 1994. 'The Cairo Consensus: Population, Development and Women', *Family Planning Perspectives*, 26, 6.

Ehrlich, P.R. and Ehrlich, A.H., 1970. *Population, Resources, Environment*. San Francisco: W.H. Freeman and Co.

Furedi, F., 1997. *Population and Development: A Critical Introduction*. London: Polity Press.

Hartmann, B., 1987. *Reproductive Rights and Wrongs: The Global Politics of Population Control and Contraception Choice*. New York: Harper Row.

Hodgson, D., and Cotts Watkins, S., 1997. 'Feminists and Neo-Malthusians: Past and Present Alliances', *Population and Development Review*, 23, 3.

Hsia, L., 1995. 'Stemming the Tide of the Global Population Explosion: The Key Role of Women', *Journal of Nurse-Midwifery*, 40, 1.

Information Project for Africa, 1991. *Population Control and National Security: A Review of U.S. National Security*. Washington DC: IPFA, pp. 3–38.

International Commission on Peace and Food, 1994. *Uncommon Opportunities: An Agenda for Peace and Equitable Development*. London: Zed Books.

Lingham, L., 1994. 'Women, Population and Development Question', *Economic and Political Weekly*, 15 January.

Mass, B., 1976. *Population Target: The Political Economy of Population Control in Latin America*. Brampton, Ontario: Charters Publishing Co.

Reed, B., Rao, S., and Zeldenstein, G., 1994. 'Honouring Human Rights in Population Policies: From Declaration to Action', in G. Sen, A. Germain and L. Chen, eds., *Population Policies Reconsidered: Health, Empowerment and Rights*. Boston: Harvard University Press.

Save the Children Ghana Appraisal Study Report, 1996. August.

Sen, G., 1994. 'Development, Population and the Environment: A Search for Balance', in G. Sen, A. Germain and L. Chen, eds., *Population Policies Reconsidered: Health, Empowerment and Rights*. Boston: Harvard University Press.

Sen, G., Germain, A., and Chen, L., 1994. 'Reconsidering Population Policies: Ethics, Development and Strategies for Change', in G. Sen, A. Germain and L. Chen, eds., *Population Policies Reconsidered: Health, Empowerment and Rights*. Boston: Harvard University Press.

Simons, H., 1995. 'Repackaging Population Control', *Covert Action*, 51, Winter.

Smyth, I., 1994. '"Safe Motherhood", Family Planning and Maternal Mortality: An Indonesian Case Study', in E. Sweetman, ed., *Population and Reproductive Rights*. Oxford: Oxfam.

Valenzona, R., 1994. 'The Road to Cairo', *Far Eastern Economic Review*, 25 August.

Warwick, D.P., 1994. 'The Politics of Research on Fertility Control', in J. Finkle, and C.A. McIntosh, eds., *The New Politics of Population*. New York: The Population Council.

Wiarda, H.J., 1987. 'Ethnocentrism and Third World Development', *Society*, September/October.

Wilson, A., 1994. 'New World Order and West's War on Population', *Economic and Political Weekly*, 20 August.

TWELVE

Concepts of Health and Illness among Older People in Ireland

ANNE MACFARLANE

INTRODUCTION

The importance of exploring the knowledge and attitudes which people hold about health and illness has shifted towards a more prominent position in academic research since the 1960s. Understanding the concepts of health and illness held by older people in order to inform health-promotion work with this group is but one relevant focus within studies of so-called lay representations of health. The importance of such work has been highlighted by the World Health Organisation (1989) with reference to the task of delaying the onset of age-related health problems, as well as maintaining functional abilities to improve the quality of life experienced by older people. This paper will outline the need for qualitative studies of health beliefs among older people. A review of studies that have explored older people's definitions of health will be presented with reference to some findings from a recent Irish national study of health beliefs among older people. The relevance of older people's concepts of health and well-being for the health-promotion movement will be critically examined with reference to gaps between empirical data and practice initiatives.

RESEARCHING LAY REPRESENTATIONS OF HEALTH

The dominance of the biomedical model of health within professional discourses of health has been considered by Curtis and Taket (1996) and, also, Sidell (1995) in relation to the formal sanctioning of, and support for, biomedicine health services. Biomedicine, representing a reductionist approach to health, is characterised by a focus on illness rather than health, such that health is defined as an absence of disease. The biological and mechanistic focus of biomedicine is, as Sidell (1995) argued, 'bleak' for older people in terms of the likely increase in illness and disability during old age. Certainly,

189

the risk of chronic illness increases with age, and health services research indicates an age-related gradient (Nolan 1991). However, not all older people have chronic conditions and old age itself is not an adequate explanation for ill health (Peto and Doll 1997). Moreover, we know that some older people who *do* experience ill-health provide positive ratings of their health. Blaxter and Paterson (1982), for instance, found that older participants in their Scottish study reported that their health status was good despite evidence of poor health experiences from medical records. This indicates that self-assessment of health and quality of life among older people is not always directly dependent on objective indices of health employed, and endorsed within, the biomedical model.

Social constructionists argue that utilisation of objective and, typically, quantitative indices of health will not provide a satisfactory account of health status because it does not capture the social nature of health and illness. From this perspective, qualitative and ethnographic methods are advocated in order to understand lay interpretative processes within the context of the lay knowledge, attitudes and behaviour (for instance by Morgan *et al.* 1985; Stainton-Rogers 1991). The next section reviews studies that have employed qualitative methods to explore the concepts and meanings of health held by older people.

A REVIEW OF OLDER PEOPLE'S HEALTH DEFINITIONS

Qualitative studies of lay definitions of health have revealed a number of recurring themes or concepts. Some notions of health focus on the presence or absence of symptoms while others emphasise a more positive concept of health with reference to feelings of psychological well-being, vitality or energy. Another consistent theme within recorded health definitions is a functional one. Functional definitions can refer to health as the ability to perform one's work or duties as well as being physically fit and active. An overview of these themes within studies of health definitions is shown in Table 1.

People's ideas about health are likely to incorporate a number of dimensions at once (for example Baumann 1961; McCluskey 1989), thus highlighting the multidimensional nature of lay definitions of health. It is also known that ideas about health are context-dependent. Differences have been recorded, for instance, between health and illness as generalised rather than personal concepts. Definitions of health have also been found to vary according to social class (Pill and Stott 1982) and gender (Blaxter 1990). Variations in health definitions also occur across age-groups. Functional definitions of health, as stated earlier, can refer to a performance-orientation or a fitness-orientation. McCluskey (1989) reported that notions of health

Author(s)	Symptoms	Function	Psychology	Reserve
Apple 1960	Ambiguity of symptoms	Interference with activities		
Baumann 1961	Absence of illness	Physically fit	Well-being	
Herzlich 1973	Health in a vacuum		Equilibrium	Reserve of health
Blaxter and Paterson 1982	Absence of disease	Functionally able Physically fit, energy	Psychologically fit	
Williams 1983	Absence of disease	Fit for work		Continuum of health and strength
Calnan 1987	Never ill	Get through the day Fit and active	Cope with stress	
McCluskey 1989	Symptom-free	Performance orientation	Feeling state	Asset/ reserve
Blaxter 1990	Absence of disease	Functionally able		
Pierret 1993	Health-illness	Health-tool		

Figure 1. Definitions of Health: recurring themes

as a fitness-orientation were more commonly cited by younger participants than older participants. Similarly, Blaxter and Paterson (1982) found that the younger generation of mothers in their study were more likely to consider physical fitness as a definition of health. Members of the older generation tended to perceive health as an ability to get through the day and keep working. Blaxter and Paterson (1982) concluded that, overall, the older women interviewed by them held 'negative' notions of health, for references to health as a feeling of well-being were largely lacking. Moreover, definitions of health as the absence of illness were also very common:

> The norms of what constituted good health, now, were conspicuously low. Good health was being able to work, being healthy enough for 'all practical purposes', not being admitted to hospital, having no 'big operations'. (Blaxter and Paterson 1982, p. 28)

Williams' (1983) in-depth analysis of older people's ideas about health and illness produced similar findings. Specifically, he found that health was defined along three main themes: health as being free from illness, health as the strength to resist illness and, finally, health as a capacity to function. Of these themes, health as the ability to perform one's daily work was of particular importance to participants. This finding was recorded as well by Pierret (1993). Following a study of health beliefs in urban and rural France she referred to tensions between having health and using health to work. Specifically, health was perceived as a form of wealth that made everything possible, especially work. Work, for older people, has typically been defined as activity in the home or garden rather than paid work (Blaxter and Paterson 1982; Williams 1983).

A particularly interesting point pertaining to functional concepts of health among older people is that the ability to be active has not only been defined as health but, also, as a means of maintaining health. Williams (1990) found that the ability to engage in daily tasks and jobs within the home or garden was perceived to be an effective means of preventing illness and generating health. Participants in Williams' study also reported that one should try to remain active even in the face of ill-health. Participants described their reluctance to withdraw from their daily tasks and duties even when they were unwell. A strong reason for this was fear of criticism from others, which operated as a form of social sanctioning against hypochondria. A small number of others explained that they had had to develop alternative ways of being active if a particular illness became too serious. These ideas reflect a basic determination to be active. Sidell has identified a finding common to both Blaxter and Paterson's (1982) study and Williams' (1983, 1990) work, as follows:

> there was a strong moral implication to having the strength to resist illness and disease and if not to resisting the disease then at least not giving in to the symptoms. (Sidell 1995, p. 29)

Sidell's own case-study analysis of states of health among older people (1986, 1991; Fennell *et al.* 1982, cited in Sidell 1995) revealed the same kind of beliefs regarding 'normal' daily living as a means of preventing, and minimising, experiences of ill-health. Attempts to understand the emphasis placed on activity by older people within their concepts of health have focused on the morally problematic nature of health and illness within lay ideologies. The influence of a work ethic as espoused in economic models of industrialisation and capitalism (Pierret 1993) as well as Christian traditions (Turner 1984) have been considered relevant to these ideologies. Also, Cornwell (1984) has argued that the importance placed on maintaining a positive attitude and outlook on life, which is related to people's sense of control over health, is relevant:

> one factor that it is assumed individuals can control (which) is their state of mind, or their approach to life in general as well as matters of

health and illness, and in doing so they establish the moral criteria according to which individuals can be judged 'good' or 'bad'. (Cornwell 1984, p. 133)

A national qualitative study of the health-related concepts of older people in Ireland was conducted recently by this author (MacFarlane 1998). Fifty-one older people, drawn from a representative Economic and Social Research Institute (ESRI) 1993 database of older people in Ireland aged sixty-five years and over, participated in an interview study. As part of the interview schedule, participants were asked to define health in their own words. Three broad conceptual categories were evident from their responses. Three-quarters of those interviewed defined health as a functional concept (performance orientation) and just over half provided definitions of health as the absence of illness (symptom-free orientation). A quarter of participants defined health in relation to feelings of well-being (feeling state orientation).

Definitions of health as the ability to perform were expressed in relation to an overall notion of health as the ability to get up each day, to go and do whatever one desired and, therefore, to be independent. The ability to get up in the morning was cited as a specific indicator of health. Both male and female participants from rural areas as well as city-dwellers mentioned this aspect of health:

What's health? Number one, to be able to get up in the morning.

. . . sure that I can get up every morning.

. . . anybody that's able to get up in the morning.

Details of the kind of tasks performed by participants each day were frequently provided. The nature of 'performance' was largely discussed in terms of work rather than leisure activities, with the exception of gardening, which was mentioned relatively frequently. Gender differences were apparent in the descriptions of daily work provided by those interviewed. References were made by female participants, for instance, to housework, such as chores including cleaning and shopping. Nora, from a large working-class suburb in Dublin, considered herself healthy, and lucky to be healthy, at the age of seventy years. The daily activities she referred to were housework and shopping:

> . . . I can do any jobs I want. It's very important. I'll be seventy next week so I am lucky. If you are able to do your housework and do your shopping it's good isn't it?

Similarly, Kathleen, who lived alone in a large town, explained that health meant she was able to:

> . . . do my chores and go to our Mass and do my little bit of shopping and come back and light my fire and so forth.

The normality of these daily activities is evident and was stressed by some participants. However, in some cases, there was a sense of frustration at the reduced range of tasks one could engage in. Kate, for instance, was widowed, living alone, and described herself as being fiercely independent. She explained that she had worked all her life in business. She talked about her capacity to work professionally as well as within the domestic domain during her younger years. While very determined to remain busy, Kate had osteoporosis, which limited her functional abilities. In the quotation shown below she acknowledges the impact of age on her activities. Essentially, while she can manage normal daily duties like housework and so forth, other kinds of job are not possible:

> I suppose at my age now, to be able to get out and do all your housework and things like that you always did. There is nothing as maddening as to see a job to be done and you can't do it. Ye young people don't realise this but when I was younger I could say 'Oh, I'll go and decorate this room,' and I'd strip the paper and start to do the ceiling and all sorts of things I couldn't even think of starting now.

Male participants cited 'jobbing around' or farmwork as examples of the work they undertook as part of their daily routines. Joe lived alone in a large, newly-built farmhouse which had been intended as a home for him and his wife. She died soon after they had moved into their new home and he explained the shock and sadness of this for him. Joe talked about his poor health in terms of having angina, as well as depression, and associated this with the death of this wife. However, at the same time, he considered his ability to work around his farm as a sign of good health and, moreover, as a means of maintaining health:

> Like you know as long as I can get around working or herding. I'd be knocking about. I keep a couple of cattle and that.

These kinds of activity were also mentioned by William, who lived with his wife on a small farm. His definition of health included the ability to get up each morning as well as being able to do certain farmwork:

> [Health means] up early in the morning anyway and eat a good breakfast, out working in the land. Working with the sheep or cattle, or training a dog. Training a dog was my hobby.

The benefits of good health, that is the ability to do one's work each day, were associated specifically with independence by some participants. As one woman explained, 'Health means independence.' Another emphasised that health meant being mobile so that she was not a burden on anyone else.

Another main conceptual theme noted in participants' reported health definitions relates to health as a symptom-free state. Some participants defined health very clearly as the absence of symptoms: 'if you are not sick or anything like that' or 'having no aches and pains'. Others defined their health in terms of low levels of contact with biomedical health services, thus reflecting a symptom-free theme whereby medical attention would not be required if one had no presenting symptoms. Conversely, other participants associated the presence of symptoms with a lack of health. Typically, details of specific illnesses were provided within these health definitions. Joe, mentioned above, said, 'I'm not healthy you know, I have angina.' Geraldine, who lived alone in a small old farmhouse adjacent to her son's newly-built home, also defined health in relation to presence of illness. She explained that she considered herself unhealthy since the birth of her children over thirty years previously:

> Well, it's so long since I have been healthy because I'll tell you why. I had two boys and they were very big. One was eight and a half and the other was eight and three quarters and I had a boy thirteen months after that and he was nine pounds' weight and the muscles in my tummy dropped do you understand. All the support went and I've had a bad tummy ever since to be honest with you.

Finally, it was also apparent that, for some participants, one could be healthy despite the presence of symptoms. Participants perceived themselves, or others, to be in good health *apart* from an illness such as arthritis or diabetes. As one woman stated, 'Sometimes I don't feel well with arthritis but otherwise the health is there.'

Definitions of health as a feeling state were provided also by some participants. These health definitions were sometimes expressed in relation to a general feeling of good form, or 'good order' within oneself. In other cases, specific feelings of happiness and well-being were cited as indicators of health. It was also interesting to note that health was sometimes defined in relation to enjoying life or having a 'zest' for life. The emphasis seemed to be on being *interested* in enjoying activities. One man explained that health was about 'a wanting to do things' and another considered health as having an interest in a variety of things or subjects, and he cited his interest in sport, books and outer space, among other things, as examples. These views were expressed by both male and female participants. Martin, from a small town in the West of Ireland, developed the notion of health as the ability to get up each morning in terms of having an interest and sense of happiness in connection with whatever one was doing:

> If you can get up and go out and you're looking forward to doing something. You pass your time that way, you take an interest and you're happy at it. And you feel healthy at it.

Mary lived with her husband in a new home in a Dublin suburb and was perhaps better off than she had been during her earlier life. She expressed similar ideas about health as a psychological state. She defined health in terms of feeling interested in going out and about as well as maintaining one's physical appearance, speaking of health as:

> the way you feel. You feel good and like getting out and going for a nice long walk instead of sitting in the house feeling sorry for yourself. It's feeling good in yourself and looking good. You know you put an effort into doing yourself up, dressing yourself up.

Overall, these data suggested that, if one were not healthy in terms of psychological well-being, this might impact on one's ability to perform activities and tasks; they reflect a link between definitions of health as a performance orientation and definitions of health as a feeling state orientation. Indeed, a matrix analysis of recorded health definitions revealed that multiple definitions of health were cited by approximately one-third of those interviewed. Strong inter-category associations were evident between health definitions both as the ability to perform and as health as a symptom-free state. This result is not really surprising, as a lack of physical health would clearly affect functional ability. One woman's account of her health definition was particularly striking in this regard as she explained the consequences of an accident in relation to her impaired health status and loss of independence. Joan was recently widowed and described the terrible impact of her husband's sudden death on her life and her sense of well-being. They had been married for forty-nine years and she talked about the depression and loneliness she had experienced following his death. Joan had also had a bad fall at the time; she had never really regained her physical health or capacities and this, she explained, compounded her difficulties. In this quotation, Joan talks about her fall and the impact it has had on her life and, particularly, her ability to be independent:

> Well, health now for me, I was a person who had perfect health and was active up until the time I had this bad fall. Where did I go wrong? What happened to me that now I can't even cook my dinner? I can't stay standing longer than about five minutes. If I go to Mass, if I go out, I have to take somebody with me. I always drove my own car, I always did my own thing. I reared eleven children and I reared neighbours' children. I looked after them when their parents would be out and I looked after my grandchildren up to two years ago . . . now I am completely confined.

Interestingly, while strong associations were noted between physical health and functional status and, also, between functional status and psychological well-being, associations between physical health and psychological well-being were not made by participants.

The extent to which these Irish data are consistent with previous research in this area will now be considered. Particular attention will be paid to the pertinence of health as a functional concept among older people across studies. Alternative interpretations of this finding will be considered in order to enhance our understanding of meanings of health for older people and, thus, improve both the delivery of care and the development of health–promotion programmes.

'DOING MY OWN THING'

The findings from the Irish interview study concur with previous research about concepts of health and illness held by older people in many regards. The conceptual categories recorded – performance orientation, symptom-free orientation and feeling state orientation – were consistent with McCluskey's (1989) analysis of health definitions, which, in turn, reflect the major themes recorded across studies of this kind (see Table 1).

The extent to which concepts of health are age-related is supported by the current findings. First, McCluskey (1989) had recorded definitions of health as a fitness orientation in his analysis, but this did not feature in the present analysis. As discussed earlier, notions of health as a state of physical fitness are more common among younger people (Blaxter and Paterson 1982; McCluskey 1989). Thus, as expected, there was no reference to health as a state of physical fitness in the present study. Secondly, the significance of health as a functional concept to older people as documented by Blaxter and Paterson (1982) and Williams (1983, 1990), among others, was clearly illustrated in the collected data. Indeed, the centrality of health as a functional concept for older people has been shown in this analysis from both quantitative and qualitative points of view. Performance-orientation definitions of health were those most commonly cited by participants. Rich descriptive accounts of how and why the ability to perform *was* health were provided by participants. Also, references to health as a functional concept were also evident *within* other recorded definitions of health; namely, health as a symptom-free orientation and as a feeling state orientation.

The emphasis placed on functional abilities within older people's concepts of health has been considered previously by Blaxter and Paterson (1982) as indicative of low norms and expectations about health. Indeed, an emphasis on daily functioning along with implicit and explicit reliance on physical health does reflect traditional biomedical notions of health and illness. However, it is argued here that interpreting functional concepts of health as solely negative underestimates the importance and significance of functional abilities to the lives of older people. It is not as if health was perceived as the ability to function for purely 'functional' reasons. The richness of qualitative analyses has revealed several distinct reasons why the ability to 'do one's own thing', to get up each morning and complete apparently basic tasks each day, constitutes health for older people.

The extent to which moral aspects of illness impact on older people has been discussed earlier in terms of the fear of criticism from others if one is not able to perform one's tasks or duties (Blaxter and Paterson 1982; Williams 1990). The influence of social and religious ideologies about work have been cited as explanatory factors (Pierret 1993; Turner 1984), supplemented by Cornwell's (1984) analysis of people's ideas about control over health. Sidell (1995) has argued that the tendency among older people to minimise health problems may be explained in the context of challenging ageist attitudes or denying negative stereotypes of older people. Drawing on Wenger's (1988) work and Thompson *et al.*'s (1990) study, Sidell (1995) argues that older people have internalised negative stereotypes of old age – being old means being ill; therefore, denying ill-health is to deny old age. The consequences of this, she suggests, are a pressure neither to complain too much about symptoms nor to utilise health-care services excessively – in other words, not to become a burden. Thus, the frequency and consistency with which older people cite functional health definitions relates to two main factors: beliefs surrounding moral ideologies about work and productivity and, also, a desire for independence and autonomy in the face of ageist stereotypes in society.

But it is also necessary to acknowledge the appeal of independence for older people for more individual reasons. Associations between health as a functional concept and health as a psychological concept were noted in the present analysis. Specifically, a sense of psychological wellness was discussed by older people in terms of having an interest in, and being able to enjoy, events and activities. These ideas seem to reflect a sense of *joie de vivre* and highlight notions of positive health among older people which has been overlooked in previous analyses.

There is, however, another dimension to functional concepts of health among older people that requires consideration. Williams' (1983) finding that activity was not only defined as health by older people but also was considered health-*generating* is also relevant here. This concurs with the analysis by Fahey and Murray (1994) of health behaviours among people aged sixty-five years and over in Ireland. Eighty per cent of participants reported engaging in activities such as housework, odd jobs, gardening and walking to maintain or improve their health. Radley's (1994) analysis of activity as a means of generating health emphasised that activity cannot be perceived only as an index of health but also as a medium through which health may be built up or sustained. It is argued here that it must also be recognised that activity constitutes a medium through which health could be *regained*. Overall, then, it is apparent that an older person, such as Joan who was quoted earlier, who was in good health and functionally able until an accident, experiences several consequences at both an individual and social level. This analysis is consistent with Nettleton's (1995) argument that beliefs about health and illness should be perceived as both individual and social.

IMPLICATIONS FOR HEALTH PROMOTION

At this point, it is worth assessing the relevance of contemporary health-promotion initiatives for older people, based on their recorded health and illness concepts in Ireland and elsewhere. Notwithstanding criticisms of Irish and British health practitioners' approach to older people as compared with the more pro-active approach of some German or North American practitioners (see Edmondson 1997), current official aims and objectives of health promotion for healthy ageing appear congruent with the recorded concepts of health and illness among older people. A recent WHO publication (1997), for instance, bears an apparently appropriate title, *Active Ageing*. The articles included in this publication reveal an impressive range of health-promotion programmes, including ideas for suitable exercise regimens for older people (Morris 1997), specialised training programmes for primary health-care workers (Michel 1997), strategies for creating inter-generational links and activities (de Souza 1997), as well as examples of lifestyle peer counselling programmes across Europe (Greengross 1997). Certainly, health-promotion initiatives during mid-life may delay the onset of ill-health and disability and are undeniably extremely worthwhile. Yet a feeling of concern emerges regarding the emphasis on 'growing old in *good* health' (Nakajima, 1997, p. 3), the benefits of exercise 'to *resist* old age' (Morris 1997, p. 6) and remaining '*fully* functioning, active and productive' (Amosun and Reddy 1997, p. 19 [emphases added]). In essence, the focus appears to be on successful ageing in terms of good physical health and functional ability only. This appears to reflect a functionalist activity theory of ageing (Havighurst 1963) which has been criticised for portraying an unrealistically idealised model of ageing that ignores the structural and biological realities of ageing experienced by many older people (Jones 1994). The helpfulness of supposedly anti-ageist images of 'super-oldies' has also been questioned by Sidell (1995). She argues that these images serve as oppressive role-models based on exceptional individual experiences and that they distract from the real experience of ageing for the majority, which does involve a decline in physical functioning. Focusing on successful ageing does not challenge negative societal attitudes towards older people as 'a burden'. Nor does such an emphasis meet the needs of older people who may be feeling distress at their loss of health and consequent loss of independence, together with fears about criticism for being dependent on a family member, neighbour or health-care worker.

Moreover, this focus seems to reflect narrow biomedical notions of health as the absence of disease, i.e. to assume that the goal of health promotion is to keep older people disease-free and able-bodied. It is precisely this notion of health that the disability movement has questioned and challenged with reference to social models of health and disability which highlight social and environmental barriers to health and well-being for disabled people (Morris 1993). The need for health-promotion interventions to consider those who fall below the disability threshold in order to ensure the best possible quality of life has been discussed by Kalache and Kickbusch (1997), though they do not include specific details of how this might be done. I should argue here that attention to the essence of the disability movement, which is based on equality for, and the rights of, those who are disabled to participate fully in society, would be beneficial to the promotion of health among older people. While community-care policies have aimed to enable older people, among others, to remain living in their own homes or, alternatively, a 'home' environment, this initiative has not succeeded in providing people who are disabled with the means to 'go about their daily lives' with the assistance they require (Morris 1993, p. ix). Key questions for health promotion then might be: How can older people be empowered to remain active even in the face of ill-health? What kind of structural supports should be in place within the home or residential environment to facilitate activity?

One possible route to empowerment for all older people is through the education of health workers. Hodgins and Kelleher (1998) described a distance-education training programme for training Irish care workers. In Ireland, it is estimated that there are approximately 100,000 informal carers as well as large numbers involved in paid care work. There are, for instance, 10,559 people employed with the home help service (Lundstrom and McKeown 1994). However, carers are typically educationally disadvantaged

(O'Connor and Ruddle 1988). The distance-education programme, rooted within health promotion theory and delivered using an adult education philosophy, recognises the opportunities for care workers to promote health and well-being. Feedback from students indicates that they have developed a heightened understanding of older people and their health needs, of the heterogeneity of older people and, also, of health as a holistic concept. Clearly, such educational initiatives could have a significant impact on the lives of older people. A carer could assist an older person who has diminished functional ability to remain autonomous and in control of household tasks, choices about clothing, preparation of food, among other things. However, it must be acknowledged that, invariably, care workers do not have much autonomous capacity to influence the ethos of care delivery in more 'formal' care settings. Edmondson (1997) has questioned the extent to which residential homes for older people are based on positive models of ageing. She highlighted a lack of opportunities for activity, either 'occupational therapy' or more routine daily tasks that we know are valued by older people, and suggested that much needs to be done to widen the scope for the introduction of 'independent living' rather than 'care' in many of these settings. Here again, it seems to me that ideas from the disability movement may be transferred in a positive way to the domain of health care for older people.

Another route to empowerment for older people is through the process of consultation. Consultation, part of a client-directed approach and widely considered to be a feature of 'good-quality' health promotion, focuses on enabling and facilitating people to identify their own interests and needs as well as possible choices and solutions (Ewles and Simnett 1989). Moreover, consultation between health professionals and clients acknowledges the valuable contribution of people's life knowledge and experience to the attainment of health and well-being. The scope for older people to contribute in this way is plainly obvious and yet often ignored in contemporary Western societies. The extent to which consultation with older people occurs already was described at a recent Irish health-promotion conference. The Midland Health Board, in conjunction with Age and Opportunity, the National Council on Ageing and Older People and the Office for Health Gain, organised a conference on 'lifelong learning' as the key to health and well-being in older age in November 1998. The value of lifelong learning for older people, and society at large, was described by Cooley (1998). Drawing on Tennyson's writings, he considered that the extent to which older people 'rest unburnished' or 'shine in use' depends on the extent to which our culture promotes the involvement or disinvolvement of older people. Details of the way in which the experience and wisdom of older people contributes across sectors were provided with reference to business enterprises, sophisticated communication technologies, as well as the development of assistive technology such as accessible public transport. The example of transport that is truly accessible to older people with mobility difficulties is very relevant here because such transport would, of course, have a positive effect on the ability of older people to participate in daily life and society. Thus, future health-promotion initiatives for older people should centralise the importance of functional capacity for older people and, moreover, encourage consultation with older people regarding the nature and development of both practical programmes and social policies. This should ensure the preservation of independence among older people which, as Kelleher (1993) has argued, is a constant aim of health-promotion work. The successful attainment of this goal will produce healthy benefits for older people now and for all of us as we get older.

ACKNOWLEDGEMENTS

The Irish research described in this paper was conducted under the supervision of Professor Cecily Kelleher, Department of Health Promotion, National University of Ireland, Galway (NUI, Galway). Funding was provided by NUI, Galway, for a postgraduate research fellowship for the author from 1992 to 1995 and by the Cardiovascular Disease and Health Promotion Research Group (CHIRP), Health Promotion Unit, Department of Health, Dublin. Thanks are due to members of the Department of Irish Folklore, NUI, Dublin, the National Council for the Elderly, Dublin, and the Economic and Social Research Institute, Dublin, for their collaboration and assistance with this work. Thanks are also due to Ann O'Kelly, Social Care Programme, Department of Health Promotion, NUI, Galway, for her comments on earlier drafts of this paper. Finally, most sincere thanks to all those who participated in the interview study for their time and generosity.

REFERENCES

Amosun, S.L., and Reddy, P., 1997. 'Healthy ageing in Africa', *World Health*, 50, 4: pp. 18–19.

Apple, D., 1960. 'How Laymen Define Illness', *Journal of Health and Human Behaviour*, 1: pp. 219–25.

Baumann, B., 1961. 'Diversities in Concepts of Health and Fitness', *Journal of Health and Human Behaviour*, 2: pp. 39–46.

Blaxter, M., 1990. *Health and Lifestyles*. London: Routledge.

Blaxter, M., and Paterson, E., 1982. *Mothers and Daughters: A Three-Generational Study of Health Attributes and Behaviour*. London: Heinmann.

Calnan, M., 1987. *Health and Illness: The Lay Perspective*. London: Tavistock.

Cooley, M., 1998. 'To Rest Unburnished. Not to Shine in Use? Enablement and the Promotion of Self Reliance.' Paper presented at the Midland Health Board

Conference, Carry on Learning: Lifelong Learning – the Key to Health and Well-Being in Older Age, Tullamore.

Cornwell, J., 1984. *Hard Earned Lives: Accounts of Health and Illness from East London*. London: Tavistock.

Curtis, S., and Taket, A., 1996. *Health and Societies: Changing Perspectives*. London: Wiley and Sons.

de Souza, E.M., 1997. 'A New Lease of Life', *World Health*, 50, 4: p. 26.

Edmondson, R., 1997. 'Older People and Life-Course Construction in Ireland', in A. Cleary and M.P. Treacy, eds., *The Sociology of Health and Illness in Ireland*. Dublin: University College Dublin Press.

Ewles, L., and Simnett, I., 1989. *Promoting Health: A Practical Guide to Health Education*. Chichester: Wiley and Sons.

Fahey, T., and Murray, P., 1994. *Health and Autonomy among Over-65s in Ireland*. Dublin: Economic and Social Research Institute.

Greengross, S., 1997. 'Ageing Well', *World Health*, 50, 4: pp. 22–3.

Havighurst, R.J., 1963. 'Successful Ageing', in R.H. Williams *et al.*, eds., *Processes of Ageing*, vol. 1. New York: Atherton.

Herzlich, C., 1973. *Health and Illness: A Social Psychological Analysis*, trans. D. Graham. London: Academic Press.

Hodgins, M., and Kelleher, C., 1998. *Promoting the Health of Older People through Health Education and Training for Carers*. Poster presentation at the Health Promotion Conference, Galway.

Jones, L.J., 1994. *The Social Context of Health and Health Work*. London: Macmillan.

Kalache, A., and Kickbusch, I., 1997. 'A Global Strategy for Healthy Ageing', *World Health*, 50, 4: p. 4.

Kelleher, C., 1993. *Measures to Promote Health and Autonomy for Older People: A Position Paper*. Dublin: National Council for the Elderly. Publication No. 26.

MacFarlane, A., 1998. *Medical Pluralism in Ireland: 1930s–1990s*. PhD. thesis, National University of Ireland, Galway.

McCluskey, D., 1989. *Health: People's Beliefs and Practices*. Health Promotion Unit, Department of Health. Dublin: Government Publications Office.

Lundstrom, F., and McKeown, K., 1994. *Home Help Services for Elderly People in Ireland*. Dublin: National Council for the Elderly. Series No. 36.

Michel, J.P., 1997. 'Primary Care for the Aged', *World Health*, 50, 4: pp. 12–13.

Morgan, M., Calnan, M., and Manning, N., 1985. *Sociological Approaches to Health and Medicine*. London: Croom Helm.

Morris, J.N., 1997. 'Resist Old Age: Exercise!', *World Health*, 50, 4: pp. 6–7.

Morris, J., 1993. *Independent Lives: Community Care and Disabled People*. London: Macmillan.

Nakajima, H., 1997. 'Towards a Healthy Old Age', *World Health*, 50, 4: p. 3.

Nettleton, S., 1995. *Sociology of Health and Illness*. Cambridge: Polity Press.

Nolan, B., 1991. *The Utilisation and Financing of Health Services in Ireland*. The Economic and Social Research Institute. General Research Series: Paper No. 155.

O'Connor, J., and Ruddle, H., 1988. *Caring for the Elderly*, Part I. Dublin: National Council for the Elderly.

Peto, R., and Doll, R., 1997. 'There Is no Such Thing as Ageing', *British Medical Journal*, 315: pp. 1030–2.

Pierret, J., 1993. 'Constructing Discourses about Health and Illness and Their Social Determinants', in A. Radley, ed., *Worlds of Illness: Biographical and Cultural Perspectives in Health and Disease*. London: Routledge.

Pill, R., and Stott, N., 1982. 'Concepts of Illness Causation and Responsibility: Some Preliminary Data from a Sample of Working Class Mothers', *Social Science and Medicine*, 16, 1: pp. 43–52.

Radley, A., 1994. *Making Sense of Illness: The Social Psychology of Health and Disease*. London: Sage.

Sidell, M., 1995. *Health in Old Age: Myth, Mystery and Management*. Buckingham: Open University Press.

Sidell, M., 1986. *Coping with Confusion: The Experience of Sixty Elderly People and Their Carers*. Unpublished PhD thesis, Norwich, University of East Anglia.

Sidell, M., 1991. *Gender Differences in the Health of Older People*. Research Report, Department of Health and Social Welfare. Milton Keynes: Open University.

Stainton-Rogers, W., 1991. *Explaining Health and Illness: An Exploration of Diversity*. Hemel Hempstead: Harvester Wheatsheaf.

Thompson, P., Itzin, C., and Abendstein, M., 1990. *I Don't Feel Old: The Experience of Later Life*. Oxford: Oxford University Press.

Turner, B.S., 1984. *The Body and Society*. Oxford: Blackwell.

Wenger, G.C., 1988. *Old People's Health and Experience of the Caring Services: Accounts from Rural Communities in North Wales*. Liverpool: Liverpool University Press.

WHO, 1989. *Health, Lifestyles and Services for the Elderly*. Copenhagen: World Health Organisation.

WHO, 1997, 'Active Ageing', *World Health*, 4.

Williams, R., 1983. 'Concepts of Health: An Analysis of Lay Logic', *Sociology*, 17, 2: pp. 185–205.

Williams, R., 1990. *The Protestant Legacy: Attitudes to Death and Illness among Older Aberdonians*. Oxford: Oxford University Press.

THIRTEEN

Untimely Meditations on Ageing, the Good Life and a Culture of Friendship

MARKUS H. WÖRNER

The significance for the health of a society of its philosophy, and the philosophical implications of practices accepted within it, can scarcely be shown more clearly than in the case of ageing. Present life expectancy at birth compared with life expectancy at birth immediately after the turn of the century shows a remarkable rise.[1] In contrast to previous generations this century, Europeans and other members of 'developed' countries appear at the turn of this millennium to be living two lives instead of one. They can now be reasonably assured of reaching an age of at least 75 years (Olshansky 1990, 1993). Perhaps some have come to regard reaching this age virtually as a natural right. But this has had profound consequences for our views about the point of life in general and health and well-being in particular — consequences which can be argued to have reached crisis point.

Most people in the West now regard it as a secure expectation that their individual lifespan will include old age. In contrast, during the first thirty years of this century the actual length of life which could be expected was generally regarded as insecure. Plague, famine and war, the classical causes of a widespread decrease of life-expectancy, together with infectious diseases and death at childbirth, no longer seem seriously to affect us in the West since the Second World War and Vietnam, even in spite of AIDS.

The fact that more and more people are now able to rely on growing older than the majority of the newborn of previous generations, as well as the almost undisputed confidence with which they predict reaching the age of 75, has frequently been accompanied by an unexpected phenomenon, noted especially in developed countries. Apart from a reported increase in adolescent suicides, the number of reported suicides among elderly people (those above the age of 65) in Germany, Switzerland, France or Sweden has grown steadily over the last thirty years, particularly in the age-group of those over 75.[2] Moreover, there is scant information available about elderly persons who attempt to commit suicide and fail, or about those who seriously consider it 'the best solution' or 'a relief for everyone concerned' without ever attempting it.[3]

Frequently, then, numbers of elderly people who can no longer be ignored feel at a loss when facing questions about what to do with everyday life and how to continue to make it worth living. On the international agenda of health promotion, it is well recognised that adding days (let alone years) to life is not enough if it does not also involve adding life to days. This has become a cliché. But innovative ideas as well as political guidelines for deliberation and action concerning a life well lived during a whole life-course are required for dealing adequately with the problem of ageing. These ideas need also to find public consensus, particularly in increasingly dissent-filled and complex pluralistic societies. Nonetheless, they are necessary to help convincingly to clarify whatever contributes to living a life of flourishing as a human being in old age. Such ideas of a good life, as well as guidelines and practices expressing them, form constitutive elements of any given culture. By 'culture' I mean here the interacting beliefs, practices, conventions and institutions shared by members of communities – especially those helping them to flourish as human beings (*cf.* Edmondson 1997 and in this volume). Just as there are many sub-cultures within a society, there will be many philosophies, formulated or otherwise; my argument here is that it can be helpful or indeed necessary to make conscious and develop some philosophies rather than others – philosophies which explore and endorse the good life in older age rather than undermining it.

Ancient traditions of ethics and anthropology in Western culture (and elsewhere) maintain almost unanimously that members of a society who do not know how to live well, either individually or collectively, also do not know how to age and thus how to die well. Conversely, if they do not know how to die well, they also do not know how to live well. Due to the lack or the educational neglect of such knowledge, an entire society may become increasingly alienated from a common awareness of what it means to excel as a human being, even despite having a highly sophisticated knowledge of what it means to excel as a craftsman, a businessman or an economist.

A human society – *qua* human – embodies a culture of those who know that they are mortals. 'Mortal' is the oldest definition of 'human being'. Other definitions, such as 'rational animal', 'political animal' or 'social animal', all presuppose this one, which first occurs in Homer's *Iliad* (24, 525f.). But although mortality is certainly not a new phenomenon, we still have our problems with it.

A GOOD LIFE AND THE ART OF DYING

We are not happy with the fact that we are rational mortals. The notion has morbid undertones. Being a rational mortal is like having a tendency to systemic breakdown programmed into our DNA code – which, many feel, should be altered in order to combat senescence. The capacity to age, on this view, is like having a stigma. But since nothing can be done about it as yet, in spite of recent attempts to delay the cellular ageing process, what seems left as a reason for hope in old age is the reconciliatory idea of post-mortem, eternal existence. This is generally expressed as a hope in a temporally unlimited and fulfilled life after death.

For centuries, the idea of eternal life after death offered consolation; it will probably continue to do so. Some of its critics say that it used to provide consolation especially for those with a relatively low and insecure life expectancy, for those whose life of pilgrimage through the valley of tears[4] was painful, burdensome or lonely. If life here on earth could not be lived well, then the very experience of deficiency, pain or suffering nourished the hope that life would finally flourish in Heaven (*cf.* Aries 1975). According to this view, one might be justified in being reasonably relaxed about the lack of opportunities of enjoying a life well lived 'here below'.

This idea of eternal life as an unlimited and perfect possession of the good life was nonetheless far from undramatic. There existed the possibility of an eternally failed life which could only be escaped by keeping religious faith until the very moment of death. Books on *Ars moriendi* taught the believer how this could be done successfully (Imhof 1991; Wagner 1989). Although the sting might have been taken out of death through faith, the sting in the process of dying remained the characteristic mark of the vale of tears.

This idea of a post-mortem good life is obviously not accepted by everyone. The longer and the more secure our lifetime 'here' has become, the less convincing becomes – so it seems – the notion of a life 'beyond'. And the consequences of the weakening of a religious conception of human lifetime are quite staggering. Human lifetime, previously believed to be eternal, now appears to have been shortened by an infinity, even though it may be an atemporal and not a sempiternal infinity. At the same time, life expectancy at birth has doubled. Although people seemingly live two lives' worth of years now, lifetime has become very short indeed if considered *sub specie aeterni*: relatively short, but safe.

As a result of this development, there now exists an opposing set of assumptions concerning lifetime and the good life. Their proponents claim to be unable to make sense of the question whether there can exist a good life *after* death if our life *between* birth and death is more or less a failure.

Human life, it is said, can only flourish 'here', because this is the only place and time for it. Considerations concerning a life well lived become exclusively focused on lifetime between birth and death. Since time for living becomes increasingly short, more and more must be packed into it if nothing is to be missed which might enrich life. This stressful demand for more becomes even more aggravating given the fact that living is not an experiment which can be repeated under different conditions. The sting of death, in this case, is final. It is of the utmost importance, therefore, to become free from the fear of death if anything like a good life is to be achieved. Clearly, there is an urgent need for a new *ars moriendi*.

BEYOND METAPHYSICS AND ANTI-METAPHYSICS

Theories of a life well lived are, then, trapped between the horns of a dilemma. Before asking which of these two diametrically opposed positions concerning the length, purpose and quality of a lifetime may be true, their common ground should be analysed.

First, both positions presuppose the idea of a desire for a good life as a possession and fruition of life which is as perfect as circumstances will possibly allow. No one who has ever had the presentiment of a better life will simply choose to survive, or to live a life of permanent crisis management. The desire for a perfect possession of life, be it a natural or an acquired desire, incorporates the characteristic features of eternity mentioned by the Roman philosopher Boethius: 'Eternity is the perfect possession of illimitable life, possessed presently in its entirety' (*Consolatio Philosophiae* V, pr. 6, 422.9–11; *cf.* Wörner 1989). Admittedly, this definition was meant to explain the notion of an absolutely perfect mode of existence, supposed to be true of divine life. It is nonetheless relevant for human everyday life under conditions of contingency. Humans seem to share the desire to improve their mode of existing. They wish to possess life to its fullness. Although they may not actually become happy, perhaps, they certainly wish to be happier than they are.

Secondly, both positions also presuppose affirmative or negative assumptions concerning post-mortem existence. Neither position can be falsified or verified in a lifetime between birth and death. Neither can be made inescapably convincing to a potentially global community containing pluralistic convictions, histories and cultures. Both positions are metaphysically biased.

Suspension between the horns of a dilemma has frequently stimulated both philosophical thought and a sense of wonder, provided that the dilemma itself was not suppressed by denials of its relevance, of its very existence. If we firmly believe one side to be true and the other to be false, the dilemma no longer arises. A common technique for suppressing the dilemma in this case is to pretend – individually or as an entire society – that life is going to continue for ever, particularly the life of youth. This involves the fight against ageing. It is part of this struggle (and is regarded by it as health-promoting) to ban death and graveyards from locations where everyday life takes place.

HEALTH PROMOTION AND THE ART OF LIVING

Let us now attempt to formulate what human beings already know about living their lives *before* making any metaphysical assumptions; this will mean analysing those features which both positions have in common, where we can find the most likely expression of this knowledge.

Presupposed in the first common feature, i.e. the desire for a possession of life which is as perfect as the circumstances can possibly allow, is the *regulative idea* of a 'successfully lived', a 'flourishing' or a 'good' life. This idea is closely linked with the notion of personal identity, for both positions would claim that a good life in which people cannot determine or live out their personal identity is a contradiction in itself.

Nonetheless, the idea of a good life alone does not help to clarify what it means *materialiter* to live successfully or to flourish as a human person. The ideal will remain merely a formal one if its content cannot be specified step by step, starting from states of affairs such that it would be contradictory to deny their status as constituent elements of a good life. Random lists of 'goods' supposed to refer to specific features of a good life should also be avoided, on the grounds that they are not equipped with sufficient reasons for maintaining that, in fact, they are part of a good life.

The concept of a 'good life' or a 'life lived successfully as a human person' refers to an activity involving living. This activity can be performed successfully or unsuccessfully. It is not performed successfully simply by nature (necessarily), or only by chance. Provided that it can be performed successfully, a certain 'know-how' or method of learning and exercising this activity appears to be required. Since it is the very activity of living whose success we are examining, the know-how in question is knowledge of *how to live*. In antiquity, this was regarded as constituting an 'art' (*techne, ars*), the *art of living* (*techne tou biou, ars vivendi*). As an art, it could be taught and learned. It had the function of leading the way to a good life for the individual as well as for the community. Theoretical discussions in philosophical ethics/politics had the practical aim of improving the quality of human living both at individual and at community level. Contemporary dictionaries of philosophy or books on ethics, however, now barely provide articles on *ars vivendi*. The 'art of living' appears to have become the domain of novels, magazines for good housekeeping or the advertising industry. Yet there is some indication that health promotion, too, feels the need to be concerned with this discussion. The well-known WHO definition of 'health' involves not only the ability to keep working or freedom from pain, but also a (subjective) feeling of well-being and the capacity for successful social integration; reaching these states is, of course, part of an art of living. The WHO position implies that a healthy person is someone in whom doctors can find no signs or symptoms of illness – and who feels happy. Although this optimum state of health is one which few members of a given society might actually attain for any length of time, its emphasis by the WHO helps to indicate the significance of an art of living for the promotion of health.

The Stoic philosopher Epictetus says of this ancient art: 'The subject-matter of a carpenter is wood; of a statuary, brass; and so of the art of living, the subject-matter is each person's own life' (*Moral Discourses* XV, par. 1). But there is an obvious difference between arts or technologies using wood or bronze and the art of living. Its material, our lives, does not comprise a means to an end which is different from the material itself, as wood or concrete blocks are for a house. Human life is simultaneously the subject, medium and object of its own formation. A successfully lived life is a work (of art) whose artisan it is itself. Treating one's own life and lifetime or those of others merely as material for planning (perhaps planning in terms of health promotion, social planning and management) can lead to a social technology of ageing, but not to an art of living. Here the possibility of a well-lived life for individuals or for entire political communities is *eo ipso* frustrated.

SENSIBILITY AND THE ART OF LIVING

The practice of the art of living is characterised by two features in particular. It is accompanied (a) by an aesthetic of existence and (b) by an individual form (*Gestalt*) of existing. By 'aesthetic of existence' I mean *the capacity for increased and deepening responsiveness through openness to new experiences*. Here I am following the terminology used by Schmid (1991) in his discussion of Foucault's theory of the art of living and its relation to the basis of ethics; hence, by an individual 'form of existence' I mean a lifestyle.

As far as an aesthetic of existence is concerned, at the very beginning of his *Metaphysics* (980a 1f.) Aristotle points out that human beings love their senses dearly, particularly the sense of seeing, and that this is a sign of their natural desire for knowledge. Conversely, research in suicidology has shown that a depressive or suicidal state of mind is frequently accompanied by a decline in the capacity to perceive (Neuringer 1976). Since sensation and perception are usually directed to the 'other' and never exclusively have the 'self' as their object, any cultivation of our senses as an integral part of the art of living presupposes circumspect attention to the particular: the particular situation, object, person or set of events. Circumspect attention is characteristically directed to situations which allow us to experience ourselves as feeling fully present (as opposed to living in dreams, memories or expectations which obstruct us from the experience of presence).

I should like to call this capacity for attention 'sensibility'. It nurtures an openness to what is unforeseen, new and special in any situation. *Sensibility is the condition of the possibility of knowledge of life (life-experience) and thus it forms the basis of our theoretical understanding (the Noetical), of practical understanding (the Ethical), and of an understanding of beauty (the Aesthetic) as the most fundamental forms of knowledge.* Individuals as well as communities can cultivate sensibility. The degree and mode in which he or she has cultivated sensibility is one of the indicators of a person's culture, and the same applies to the culture of a community.

In so far as enrichment of life-knowledge also implies cultivating a relish for living, cultivation of sensibility is its necessary condition. Reducing sensibility beneath the parameters set by our common biological fate is self-destructive. Clearly, training and cultivating sensibility cannot begin only at the age of maturity, nor can it be done without public support. It has to be cultivated from childhood. This is part of cultural education. Failure to cultivate it, or common neglect of it, sets the agenda for depression in old age, possibly for a whole population.

As far as individual lifestyle is concerned, cultivating sensibility (which must be trained and supported individually as well as at community and at state level if it is to be part of a *common* culture) has the effect of evolving a know-how based on attitude- and habit-formation to be found at individual, group and community level. This know-how provides different styles of the activity of living. Since the cultivation of sensibility presupposes openness to new experiences, however, no lifestyle constitutive of a good life can comprise a permanently fixed set of attitudes and habits which defy the possibility of change, preventing the transformation of the self in the interest of a better life and enhanced self-identity. Training in the capacity for openness to new modes of existence, of living and thinking, therefore also forms part of the art of living. 'Life-plans' which are intended to provide the basis for fulfilling activities in old age must take this into account, since they need to avoid any solidifying of patterns of thinking, feeling and behaving – which are, ultimately, repressive.

By 'art of living' I mean the totality of intellectual and practical skills, techniques, attitudes and habits which constitute a successfully lived life as a human person. These skills have traditionally been discussed in connection with lists of ethical and intellectual aspects of human excellence or ways of flourishing as a human being (virtues) and techniques of the self.

Authors as different as Aristotle, Epicure, Cicero, Seneca or Foucault maintain
that these skills, techniques and attitudes need to be learnt from early youth in
order to provide the basis for a good life in old age. It is neither necessary nor
impossible to put them into practice. They are contingent. In so far as they
constitute a good life, they are nonetheless its necessary conditions.

Learning virtues (for example, practical wisdom, or adequate emotional
and activity responses), techniques of the self (for example, self-monitoring
through critical self-reflection, writing diaries or talking to friends), taking
physical and mental exercise or learning skills of improving perception and
interaction (such as painting, acting or playing music) presupposes that the
learning person has *autonomously accepted* the validity of the idea of a life
lived successfully as a human person and is also prepared to apply it to his
or her own act of living. Autonomous acceptance and application of the idea
of the good life is a basic condition of the traditional 'Care for the Self
(Soul)' (Foucault 1981). Governmental social policies, community or family
activities ought to make us *inclined* to maintain an appetite for living and for
happiness; they ought not to plan to *make* us happy. We have to want to be
happy ourselves – because this is part of our autonomy, just as autonomy is
part of our happiness.

RELATING TO NATALITY AND MORTALITY

Skills, techniques of the self and habits which form an integral part of the
art of living have to be learned by taking into account basic characteristics
of their joint object. This object is living in finite time. Seneca's remark
about lifetime, repeated by Michel de Montaigne at the transition from late
Humanism to Modernity, provides the clue to an understanding of basic
characteristics of living. Seneca said, 'A man who has learned how to die has
unlearned how to be a slave' (*Epistolae morales ad Lucilium* XXVI;
Montaigne's version [*Essays*, 1991, p. 96] was 'To philosophise is to learn
how to die'). Seneca's brief remark, as well as Montaigne's comments on it,
highlight two basic and interrelated conditions of the good life.

The first condition is to *unlearn how to be a slave*. Taken in its positive
sense, this means self-determination, autonomy, freedom. This is the moral,
political and historical programme of the Enlightenment, whose critical
heirs we are. To *unlearn* how to be a slave means quitting the state of
immaturity imposed by ourselves on ourselves.

Any unlearning of this kind is the negative aspect of learning to live well.
Its positive aspect is the process of self-constitution via emancipation from
internal or external varieties of unjustifiable or intolerable domination. This
process is guided by the idea of becoming, and the desire to become *masters
of our own lives*, to possess our lives and not to be possessed.

This desire has its roots in a basic mode of experiencing existence, on account of which persons may experience their lives as processes of finding themselves, of renewing themselves, even of being reborn. This is frequently connected with moods and feelings of delight and exultation, lightness and ease. Following Hannah Arendt (1960), I should like to call this basic mode of experiencing existence 'natality'. Unlearning to be a slave means learning to appreciate natality.

The second condition of the good life is *to learn how to die*. Mention of this condition indicates that Montaigne was not a philosopher of modernity: he was post-modern. 'Learning how to die' does not refer to the intellectual, moral and political emancipation from intellectual, moral and political institutions and powers; it refers to the emancipation from a power which dominates both the dominator and the dominated. This is the emancipation from death and from its precursor, from dying. Death and dying seem initially to be the very contradiction of living and, *a fortiori*, of any chance of living well. Nonetheless, the contradiction to life appears to be a necessary element of life itself.

Learning how to die, in this case, is to learn to deal with a basic mode of experiencing human existence which is the opposite of natality. This is the experience of living in terms of something which is a burden, loss, failure or 'illness unto death' (Kierkegaard). The basic moods or feelings connected with this apparently unavoidable trait of life-experience are those of depression, dejection, resignation. I should like to call this basic mode of experiencing existence 'mortality' (see Held 1985). Learning how to die means learning how to cope with mortality.

The power and domination of death over individuals and over whole communities – which was experienced drastically at times of plague, famine and war but which is frequently suppressed today – ranges deeper than anything else which can be claimed to have power. It implies ultimate powerlessness for its victims. To free oneself from the radical power of death means radical freedom. This kind of freedom promises the most perfect possession of life possible between birth and death. The fear of death is its greatest obstacle.

Clearly, then, the art of living must be crucially concerned with unlearning how to be a slave and with learning how to die, as long as its central aim is the best possible possession of life. Skills, techniques, habits and attitudes constitutive of the art have thus to be understood, to be learned and to be exercised in the light of basic modes of experiencing existence, of natality and of mortality. These form the most fundamental tension which permeates the unity of the act of living.

Heraclitus highlights the unity of these opposites, emphasising also that it is far from easy to give an account of it: 'They do not comprehend how, in differing, it agrees with itself – a backward turning connection, like that of a bow and a lyre' (fr. B51DK).

Skills, technologies of the self, ethical and intellectual attitudes to be learned in the art of living, clearly presuppose that individuals as well as communities need to be able to *relate* reasonably to these basic modes of experiencing human existence as a unity in tension. Relating reasonably also presupposes the capacity to take into account, and also to give *an account*, of the act of living in terms of *both* modes and not of one only.

Relating to them and giving an account of them imply a special mode of thinking, feeling and experiencing. I should like to call this 'dually reflective experience'. It is a mode of experiencing which cultivates an awareness of the ambiguous but nonetheless complementary nature of both modes of being in the world. As a habit informing perception and sensibility, thinking, feeling and action, it provides a basic structure to life-knowledge both as knowledge *of* life and as knowledge of *how* to live.

In so far as this is the habituation most adequate for understanding a human life, it is presupposed in any attitude-, skill- or technology-formation of the art of living. Conversely, attitudes or technologies of the art of living will re-enforce dually reflective experience.

Although sensibility and reflective experience are necessary preconditions of the art of living, they are not yet its most fundamental condition. A further habit is required to enable us to accept the tension of the unity of opposing emotional modes of experiencing existence, *to admit in self-reflection* that this tension exists and to *affirm* it deliberately rather than to revolt against it or simply to be resigned to our fate. Nonetheless, learning this habit may frequently be far from easy or pleasurable. I should like to call this kind of 'letting be' by the German word '*Gelassenheit*', since there is no adequate equivalent for it in English. 'Serenity' or 'acceptance' might come close to its meaning. *Gelassenheit* is neither a necessary nor a merely accidental concomitant of living. It has to be acquired as a permanent disposition to relate to living, if the act of living itself is to succeed. Permanent revolt, resignation, denial of its ambiguous nature or indifference to living as a human being can hardly form the basis of an art of living.

Due to *Gelassenheit* human beings are able to become involved autonomously, willingly and consciously with their existence – which otherwise they merely cannot help living because they are thrown into it. It is through the affirmation of life with its fundamental complementary tension that we give life to ourselves. *What makes us human is precisely the capacity to let be the basic tension of living, dying and death, to persevere in it and to give it a specific form.*

Acts of individual or collective suicide, acts of genocide or potential threats of omnicide demonstrate the opposite. They show that individuals or whole societies are frequently not prepared to persevere in this tension, to accept it or to think of its practical consequences. The same can be said of social, economic, health or educational policies in societies which marginalise older people instead of paying close attention to their narratives of experience of living as humans – not to mention the marginalisation of the dying and of death itself. It is true that we have difficulties with the state of being human. It is part of our freedom that we *can* but need not be human.

FEAR OF DYING AND PLEASURE IN LIVING

Naturally, serenity (*Gelassenheit*), sensibility and dually reflective experience do not guarantee *per se* that those who have these dispositions thereby lose the fear of death. They may take a person quite a long way, however, provided that these dispositions are united with technologies of the self as well as with ethical and intellectual habits which also constitute the art of living. They may provide a kind of life-knowledge which makes us inclined to think of dying and death as things which have not to be feared to the extent that we are dominated by our fears.

Not to be dominated by the fear of dying and death does not mean denying the uncertainty of things to come, nor does it mean denying awareness of the inevitable processes of physical and mental decay. Nonetheless, an art of living provides the best possible preparation for facing these conditions. Moreover, the sting of dying and death also diminishes – though this is not to say that it ever disappears entirely – when it can contribute *positively* to the success of living our lives now. A reflective awareness of death and dying can involve a deepening and broadening of life-knowledge, allowing us to be more attentive, perceptive and appreciative of our lives as they are present and those of our friends. Time may be spent more diligently and also more freely. An awareness of dying can increase sensibility, focus activities and even increase pleasure in the present. Time and people may be experienced as more precious and valuable than before.

'The feeling of being alive is pleasurable,' says Aristotle in the *Nicomachean Ethics* (IX, 1170b 1). Almost the entire tradition of practical philosophy in antiquity agrees with him. However, he adds a condition under which he supposes this to be the case. The experience of life as pleasurable presupposes that it is in tune with the 'true nature' of the human being in question. This 'nature' is not to be understood as an ahistorical 'essence' but as *the successful process of self-constitution or personal identity*. This kind of pleasure is an integral part of the good life in time; it is not the 'easy' or 'light' life of the deathless gods of antiquity. Any wish to achieve the latter version of life in time or to make it the implicit basis of advertising, health promotion or social policy is not human, simply because it is illusory to deny mortality. The oracle at Delphi, and Socrates too, advised: 'Know thyself.'

Learning how to live a life successfully as a human being on the basis of sensibility, serenity and dually reflective experience also means to learn how to die. *Ars vitae* and *ars moriendi* are one and the same. We cannot master one art and not master the other. A life based on these arts discloses and exemplifies, in individuals as well as in cultural communities, what it means to live as a human being. Therefore, such a life, even one which does not succeed beyond all expectations but nonetheless shows obvious signs of human flourishing, is a work of practical truth. Moreover, it does not need to suppress or to deny any ruptures, mistakes or errors, since it is capable of integrating them productively.

THE CULTURE OF FRIENDSHIP

Serenity (*Gelassenheit*), sensibility and dually reflective experience can neither be acquired nor supported in social isolation, although they belong very much to an individual's own art of living. It is an empirical fact that communication and living together with 'significant others' on a basis of concern and affection – for as long as this is still physically possible – enhances people's perceptions, emotions and actions. Perception becomes *shared* perception, emotions become *sympathy*, thinking becomes *mutual understanding*, acting becomes *mutual aid*. The result is enhanced life-knowledge, self-knowledge and a deepened relish for living. This result is not nullified by the fact that human nature may involve what Kant termed 'unsocial sociability', demanding a delicate balance between social independence and reliance on others until death. This enhanced life-knowledge is even more urgently required at a time when mental and physical capabilities are decaying in old age.

Communicating and living with relevant others in this way is *friendship*. Friendship is a basic form of human excellence. It is an integral part of the art of living, for 'without friends no one would choose to live, though he had all other goods' (Aristotle, *Nicomachean Ethics* VIII, 1155a 5f.). Friendship must be learned, cultivated and supported from youth. It can only be learned, cultivated and supported in communities or societies in which the promotion of friendship is not simply a private affair but part of the priorities of the common culture. This is true of societies with a common concern in the good life.

If we do not wish older people to feel, to act and to say that their lives are not worth living any longer in spite of the fact that days are added to their lives through social, medical and health care, *then* individuals, communities and the State may have to investigate and to invest into people's capacity to form and maintain friendships even under adverse physical, economical or psycho-social conditions. We must investigate and invest into a *culture of friendship*: and we must attempt this more profoundly and more effectively than can be achieved by the contemporary fashion for technical 'life-skills'.

There is no societal nor individual solution to the problem of ageing which could possibly ignore this need.

ACKNOWLEDGEMENTS

This paper is a revised and expanded version of a paper presented at the Symposium 'Erfüllt leben – in Gelassenheit sterben' at the Free University, Berlin, November 1993 (sponsored by the German Ministry for the Family and Senior Citizens). An initial publication of the proceedings of this Symposium can be found in A. Imhof *et al.*, eds., *Erfüllt leben – in Gelassenheit sterben* (Berlin: Publikationen des Friedrich Meinecke Instituts, 1993).

REFERENCES

Arendt, H., 1960. *Vita Activa, oder Vom Taetigen Leben*. Stuttgart.
Aries, P., 1975. *Essais sur l'histoire de la mort en Occident du moyen age a nos jours*. Paris: Editions du Seuil.
Aristotle, *Ethica Nicomachea*, ed. I. Bywater, 1894. Oxford: Clarendon Press.
Aristotle, *Metaphysics*, ed. W.D. Ross, 1924. Oxford: Clarendon Press.
Boethius, *Consolatio Philosophiae*, in J.P. Migne, ed., *Opera Omnia*, vol. 1 Paris.
Edmondson, R., 1997. *Ireland: Society and Culture*. Hagen: University of Hagen: Fachbereich Erziehungs-, Sozial- und Geisteswissenschaften.
Epictetus, [1910]. *Moral Discourses*, trans. E. Carter. London: J.M. Dent.
Foucault, M., 1981. *The Care of the Self*. History of Sexuality, vol. 3. Harmondsworth: Penguin.
Held, M., 1985. 'Entpoliltisierte Verwirklichung des Gluecks – Epikurs Brief an Menoikeus', in P. Engelhardt, ed., *Glueck and Gegluecktes Leben*. Mainz: Grünewald.
Heraclitus, *Fragmente*, in *Fragmente der Vorsokratiker*, trans. H. Diels, ed. W. Kranz, 1964. Zuerich/Berlin: Weidmann.
Homer, *The Iliad*. Harmondsworth: Penguin.
Imhof, A., 1991. *Im Bildersaal der Geschichte*. München: Beck.
Imhof, A., 1992. *Das unfertige Individuum*. Köln/Weimar/Wien: Boehlau.
Montaigne, M. de, [1991]. *The Complete Essays*, transl. M.A. Screech. Harmondsworth: Penguin.
Neuringer, C., 1976. 'Current Developments in the Study of Suicidal Thinking', in E.S. Shneidman, ed., *Suicidology*. New York: Grune and Stratton: pp. 234–52.
Olshansky, S.J., 1990. 'In Search of Methuselah: Estimating the Upper Limits to Human Longevity', *Science*, 250: pp. 634–9.
Olshansky, S.J., 1993. 'The Aging of the Human Species', *Scientific American*, 268, 4: pp. 46–52.

Schmid, W., 1991. *Auf der Suche nach einer neuen Lebenskunst.* Frankfurt/Main: Suhrkamp.

Seneca, *Epistolae morales ad Lucilium* XXVI: *Letters from a Stoic*, trans. R. Campbell, 1969. Harmondsworth: Penguin.

Wagner, H., ed., 1989. *Ars Moriendi. Erwaegungen zur Kunst des Sterbens.* Freiburg/Basel/Wien: Herder.

Wörner, M.H., 1989. 'Eternity'. *Irish Philosophical Journal*, 6: pp. 3–26.

Wörner, M.H., 1996. 'Gelungenes Leben', in A. Imhof, ed., *Die Zunahme unserer Lebensspanne seit 300 Jahren und ihre Folgen* (Schriftenreihe des Bundesministeriums fuer Familie, Senioren, Frauen und Jugend, Band 110). Stuttgart/Berlin/Köln: Kohlhammer: pp. 275–83.

NOTES

1   Between 1901 and 1910, the average life-expectancy of men in Germany, for instance, was 44.82 years. In 1924–6 it was 55.97, in 1960–2 it was 66.86 and in 1983–5 it was 71.18 years. Life expectancy at birth approaches 75 years in the year 2000; see Imhof 1991 for an elaboration of these trends. It is, of course, the case that the biggest contributor to these changes arises from sweeping reductions in infant mortality.

2   For a discussion of the development of distribution of suicides according to age in Europe see Imhof (1992). More recently, the Central Statistics Office in Dublin in the 1990s reports a similar development in Ireland: among those in the age-group 75-plus, there is a rise in numbers of reported suicides and deaths whose cause cannot be determined but where suicide cannot be excluded.

3   It could scarcely be asserted without empirical research that an immediate causal connection exists between rising life expectancy itself and rising suicide rates among older people; effects on philosophical views may be expected to arise somewhat more indirectly than this. But changes in suicide rates do seem to indicate that problems exist, at least for some, about how to relate to the latter stages of a lifetime.

4   'Lacrimarum vallis' is the name for human life on earth according to the 'Salve Regina' of the Compline Prayer in the Catholic Church. In that tradition, the state of happiness than which none greater can be conceived is 'visio Dei beatifica', which is not, for the most part, expected to be experienced in this life.

FOURTEEN

Tuning into Psychosocial Factors in Adolescent Health Risk Behaviour: Implications for Health Promotion Practice

RANDY M. PAGE

The main threats to adolescents' health are the health risk behaviours and choices they make (Resnick *et al.* 1997). The predominant health risk behaviours that threaten the health status of youth in the United States include the following six categories of risk behaviours: behaviours that contribute to unintentional and intentional injuries; tobacco use; alcohol and other drug use; sexual behaviours that contribute to unintended pregnancy and sexually transmitted diseases (STDs, which include human immunodeficiency virus [HIV] infection); unhealthy dietary behaviours; and physical inactivity. These behaviours contribute to substantial mortality, morbidity and social problems. Further, risk behaviours are frequently interrelated, often are established during youth, and extend into adulthood (Centers for Disease Control, 1996). By age 18, only 16% of youth report having engaged in no risk behaviours, while 62% report two or more such behaviours. Even at age 15, less than half of youth (45%) have avoided all risk behaviours, and 30% have experienced two or more of the following risks: used illegal drugs, had 5 or more drinks of alcohol in a row in the past month, had sexual intercourse, dropped out of school before high school graduation and stayed out all night without permission (Moore and Glei 1994).

The Carnegie Council on Adolescent Development (1995) report, *Great Transitions: Preparing Adolescents for a New Century*, characterises the pressures and risks that America's youth face in the following way:

> Across America today, adolescents are confronting pressures to use alcohol, cigarettes, or other drugs and to have sex at earlier ages. Many are depressed: about a third of adolescents report they have contemplated suicide. Others are growing up lacking the competence to handle interpersonal conflict without resorting to violence. By age seventeen, about a quarter of all adolescents have engaged in behaviours

that are harmful or dangerous to themselves and others: getting pregnant, using drugs, taking part in antisocial activity, and failing in school. Altogether, nearly half of American adolescents are at high or moderate risk of seriously damaging their life chances. The damage may be near term and vivid or it may be delayed, like a time bomb set in youth, (p. 2)

The adolescent and pre-adolescent years provide a special opportunity for promoting health that should not be wasted. Health promotion interventions during adolescence and pre-adolescence give the opportunity not only to prevent the onset of health-damaging behaviours, but also to intervene with health-compromising behaviours that may be less firmly established as part of the lifestyle. Health promotion interventions during this time of the lifespan have the capacity to introduce, reinforce and further establish healthy lifestyle patterns (Millstein *et al.* 1993).

Health risk prevention programmes and interventions are often limited to strategies that do not appear to be effective (Dusenbury *et al.* 1997). Some health risk prevention programmes have been limited to providing only factual information about the harmful consequences of risk behaviours such as tobacco and alcohol use. Other programmes have attempted to induce fear in young persons about the consequences of involvement in health risk behaviours. However, these strategies alone do not prevent engagement in health risk behaviours or promote healthy lifestyle. In fact, they may even stimulate curiosity about these risks and prompt some youth to believe that the health hazards of engaging in risk behaviours are exaggerated (Centers for Disease Control 1994; Leventhal and Cleary 1980)

In contrast, successful programmes and interventions address psychosocial factors related to health risk behaviour among children and adolescents (Best *et al.* 1988; Botvin 1986; Clayton 1991; Dusenbury *et al.* 1997; Flay 1985; Tobler 1992). With this in mind, the purpose of this paper is to relate the findings of several investigations conducted by the author concerning psychosocial factors and adolescent health risk behaviour. In particular, this paper examines research regarding shyness and loneliness, perceptions of body image and attractiveness, social normative expectations and school sports participation. These findings have direct implications for health promotion programmes and interventions targeting youth.

The investigations reviewed in this paper were conducted using survey research methodology. Survey instrumentation was administered to selected samples of child and adolescent populations. The instrumentation included established measures of psychosocial factors (such as shyness, loneliness, hopelessness) and health risk behaviour (cigarette smoking, alcohol use, physical inactivity). The relationship between measured psychosocial factors and health risk behaviour was determined by statistical analysis.

SHYNESS AND LONELINESS

The study of two psychosocial characteristics of adolescents, namely shyness and loneliness, in the context of health risk behaviour has largely been neglected by health promotion strategists and researchers (Page 1988). However, research bears out that these psychosocial characteristics are associated with poor health risk behaviour outcomes. In general, my research has found loneliness and shyness to be associated with illicit drug use (Page 1989, 1990b, 1990c; Page *et al.* 1993a), cigarette smoking (Allen and Page 1994; Page 1990b), alcohol abuse (Page and Cole 1991), disordered eating (Page 1990a, Page 1991b), infrequent physical activity and poor physical fitness (Page 1990a, 1990b; Page, *et al.* 1992; 1994a; Page and Tucker 1994; Page and Hammermeister 1995), frequent television viewing (Page, *et al.* 1996a), and potential suicide risk (Page 1991b).

Shyness, which was operationalised in these studies as the discomfort and inhibition that may occur in the presence of others, was measured by the Cheek and Buss Shyness Scale (Cheek and Buss 1981). Therefore, shy adolescents were those scoring high on this scale. The UCLA Loneliness Scale was used to assess loneliness and lonely adolescents were those scoring high on the scale. Loneliness was operationalised as the degree of dissatisfaction with current social relationships (Russell 1982).

The implications from this body of research suggest that shy and lonely youngsters may benefit from health promotion interventions that emphasise social skills training approaches designed to improve social competence with peers, parents and authority figures (Page *et al.* 1994b). Use of role-playing, modelling and reinforcements are important modalities for learning and retention of social skills. Shy students need to learn how to make and maintain friendships, conversational skills, dating skills, and how to participate in group and social gatherings. Because shy adolescents and pre-adolescents may be susceptible to peer pressure, inclusion of refusal skills training should also be a fundamental component of risk behaviour prevention and health promotion programmes.

Relaxation training and other stress reduction techniques also may help shy and lonely adolescents reduce the discomfort they experience in social encounters. Because shyness is often associated with physiological arousal such as pounding heart, dry mouth, blushing and 'butterflies' in the stomach, such training may help reduce the arousal response and consequent symptoms. Consequently, feelings of discomfort and inhibition may be lessened.

Health promotion professionals should bear in mind that adolescence is a developmental period of high risk for loneliness and that loneliness occurs at a higher frequency among adolescents than among any other age group. Although loneliness may occur at any stage of development, it is usually most intense during adolescence. Loneliness is further intensified when it is a result of rejection by peers.

GENDER DIFFERENCES

From a study of the interactive effects of cigarette smoking and gender on four psychosocial characteristics (shyness, loneliness, sociability and hopelessness) emerged a profile of male adolescent smokers as quite distinct from female adolescent smokers (Allen and Page 1994). Male adolescent smokers scored higher on the measures of loneliness and hopelessness than any of the other smoking status–gender groups. As a group, they also scored lower on shyness and sociability (the tendency to affiliate with other people) than any other group. Conversely, female smokers were the group that scored highest on sociability and lowest on shyness.

The results of this study support the hypothesis that adolescent males use smoking as a mechanism to cope with social insecurity, whereas adolescent females who smoke are more socially competent and self-confident. These results also give support to the idea of structuring smoking prevention interventions differently for adolescent males and females. In other words, current smoking prevention strategies which stress social skills training and self-esteem enhancement may not be optimal for adolescent females. Adolescent female smokers (as well as those at high risk for becoming smokers) do not appear to conform to the traditional model often adhered to by smoking prevention programme planners, in which smokers are viewed as having low self-esteem and as using cigarettes to cope with social situations or to fit in with peers.

On the other hand, social skills training and self-esteem enhancement approaches appear to be especially needed as smoking prevention components for adolescent males and should receive high priority. The results from this study describe adolescent male smokers as unsociable and shy. As such, they may have a propensity to be tense and anxious in social settings and could profit from the application of these approaches.

The inclusion of coping skills training in smoking prevention and cessation programmes targeted at adolescent males also seems to be an important component. A lack of coping skills as evidenced by elevated scores on hopelessness and loneliness is apparent in this group. Emphasising stress management and relaxation training as health promotion strategies may be valuable in helping adolescents to respond to conditions of distress using constructive means rather than maladaptive behaviours such as smoking. Smoking prevention programmes directed towards young males should strive to fortify high-risk youth at an early age, enriching their skills and confidence before they are entangled by failure, frustration and the smoking habit.

PERCEPTIONS OF BODY WEIGHT AND ATTRACTIVENESS

Contemporary society is characterised by social norms that equate thinness with attractiveness and social approval. These norms often place enormous pressure upon individuals, particularly children and adolescents, to be thin because 'thin is in'. The message that thinness equals approval is pervasive and often exploited by the advertising and fashion industries. Within this social environmental context, it is not surprising that there is a high prevalence of body dissatisfaction and weight loss. In fact, concern about physical appearance has been reported to be the most worrisome problem for adolescents (Eme *et al.* 1979). Many studies have found a high degree of body weight dissatisfaction among adolescents, particularly adolescent girls (Page 1991a; Paxton *et al.* 1991). Body weight dissatisfaction has also been found to be associated with indicators of psychosocial distress (Page 1991a). Subjective perceptions of weight appear to be intimately bound to female body image, often leading to aggressive efforts to lose weight in quest of an ideal body image (Wadden *et al.* 1991). As a result, the proportion of adolescent females who diet has increased substantially in past decades. Almost half of all high-school girls report dieting in the previous month and nearly 60% report that they are attempting to lose weight (Centers for Disease Control 1994).

Teen girls may be motivated to use smoking cigarettes as a means to control their appetite and weight (Centers for Disease Control 1994). In view of this fact, I conducted a study to assess weight-related concerns and practices of adolescent cigarette smokers and non-smokers (Page *et al.* 1993b). This study also investigated relationships between smoking status and weight-related concerns and practices. In general, male and female adolescents who smoked cigarettes were less satisfied with their weight and more likely to perceive themselves as fat, be concerned about weight gain, and participate in unsafe or unsound weight-regulating practices (such as self-induced vomiting, going on very restrictive diets, taking diet pills) than their non-smoking peers. Yet, smokers and non-smokers did not differ in terms of body-mass index. This study provides evidence that concern about weight and weight-regulation is salient for both male and female adolescent smokers.

The results of this study add to a literature base which suggests that weight-related concerns such as weight dissatisfaction and self-perceptions of overweight may function as aetiological factors in the initiation of cigarette smoking behaviour. As such, health promoters need to inform children and adolescents that the health consequences of smoking outweigh any anticipated or realised effects of smoking on weight-regulation. Because slenderness is highly prized, adolescents may be willing to overlook the long-term consequences of smoking (such as emphysema, lung cancer, chronic bronchitis or heart disease) in order to achieve or maintain a desirable body weight.

Professionals in the field of health promotion should assist children and adolescents to realise that smoking cessation has major and immediate health benefits for males and females of all ages. The health benefits of smoking cessation far exceed any risks from the small average weight gain or any adverse psychological effects that may follow quitting.

This study showed that concern about weight is a salient issue for both adolescent male and female smokers. Therefore, smoking and body weight issues must be addressed adequately in health promotion efforts directed towards young males as well as young females.

I have also examined whether adolescent body weight dissatisfaction, self-perception of body weight, perceived physical attractiveness, and body mass relate to the use of alcohol and illicit drugs (Page *et al.* 1995). Generally, adolescents who were dissatisfied with their weight and considered themselves as unattractive used illicit substances, drank alcohol, and got drunk more often than those who were satisfied with their weight and considered themselves attractive or average-looking. Underweight adolescents also used illicit drugs and alcohol more frequently than overweight and normal-weight adolescents. Further, it was observed that there was an interacting effect of body weight status and perception of attractiveness for females. Having the perception of being unattractive in combination with being underweight appears to place an adolescent at very high risk of illicit substance use (Page 1993). These results strongly suggest that health promotion strategies which focus upon enhancing adolescent perceptions of body weight and attractiveness may provide an important potential pathway for reducing substance use risk.

Another investigation showed a strong relationship between feelings of unattractiveness and adolescent hopelessness (Page 1992). Hopelessness is a significant component of depression and poor emotional well-being. It has also been shown to be a key psychological factor and indicator of suicidal behaviour and risk. Hopelessness is related to desires by individuals to escape from seemingly insoluble problems or distressing situations and/or environments. Thus, the results of this study suggest also that health promotion strategies which focus upon enhancing adolescent perceptions of attractiveness may also provide a potential pathway for reducing depression, poor emotional well-being and suicidal behaviour risk.

NORMATIVE EXPECTATIONS

Health behaviourists agree that behavioural choices made by young people are influenced by how acceptable a behaviour is believed to be among peers

(Ajzen and Fishbein 1980; Berndt 1979; Green and Kreuter 1991; Jaccard 1975). Duryea and Martin (1981) hypothesise that distortions in perceptions of the prevalence of a risk behaviour may be an important factor in adolescents' decisions to engage in the risk behaviour. They suggested that when young people hold a perception that the prevalence of a risk behaviour among their peers is high, then the tendency to experiment and/or adopt the risk behaviour may be that much stronger. In fact, the perception of the normativeness of a behaviour in a peer group may impact on behaviour more than does the actual prevalence of the behaviour.

I recently conducted a study at my university investigating estimations of the prevalence of binge drinking among students. Students were surveyed about their personal binge drinking behaviour and also asked to give their perception of the prevalence of binge drinking by estimating the percentage of students on campus who binge drink during an average week. Estimations of the prevalence of binge drinking (consuming 5 or more drinks during a single occasion) exceeded the percentage of students who reported binge drinking. It was estimated that 65.5% of male and 54.8% of female students binge drink during an average week. However, 49.5% of male and 28.1% of female students reported binge drinking. Compared to non-binge drinkers, binge drinkers gave significantly higher estimations of the percentage of students who binge drink. Students estimating that more than half of males or females binge drink were at elevated risk of being binge drinkers themselves. The risk of binge drinking was particularly high among students who estimated that more than 80% of students binge drink during an average week (Page *et al.* in press).

Other data collected from these students also show a similar 'distortion effect' for other risk behaviours, including cigarette smoking (Page 1998), marijuana use and having four or more sexual partners during one's lifetime. These findings suggest to health promotion professionals the need to accurately communicate the actual prevalence of risk behaviours on college campuses. This information is necessary to dispel misperceptions among students that risk behaviours are the norm or typical behaviour. In fact, communication campaigns to dispel overestimations of binge drinking are increasingly being used as a strategy to lower the rate of binge drinking on college campuses (Haines and Spear 1997). Dusenbury *et al.* (1997) report from their review of effective drug use prevention programmes that normative education positing that drug use is not the norm has been shown to reduce substance use behaviour.

SOCIAL NORMATIVE ATTITUDES REGARDING THE
WEARING OF BICYCLE HELMETS

I have also investigated social normative attitudes regarding the wearing of bicycle helmets among college students (Page *et al.* 1996b). Social normative attitudes appeared to have influenced college students' decisions about wearing bicycle helmets. Only 22% of students agreed that wearing helmets is characteristic of most of their friends. Among frequent bicycle-helmet wearers, 66.7% agreed that helmet wearing was characteristic of their friends. However, only 22.5% of infrequent wearers and 12.4% of non-wearers stated that it was characteristic of their friends. Other findings regarding social normative attitudes also support this influence on helmet-wearing behaviour. For example, a higher proportion of non-wearers (34.3%) agreed that wearing helmets looks 'dorky' or 'nerdy' than did infrequent (25.3%) and frequent users (8.3%). Only 7.6% of the total sample of students agreed that helmets look 'cool'.

These findings imply that health promotion campaigns intent on increasing helmet-use rates on college campuses should include efforts that strive to improve the social image of helmets. For example, enlisting popular personalities on campuses to serve as role models of bicycle helmet use may be one way to positively influence social norms regarding helmet use.

The social norm regarding bicycle helmet use in this sample of college students is generally non-use. Only 13.8% of students agreed that 'wearing bicycle helmets is true for most people on campus'. This was supported by a helmet observation study in which we found 18.6% of males and 14.8% of females wearing helmets while riding their bikes on campus. Health behaviour change is very difficult when current social norms do not support the wearing of helmets.

SCHOOL SPORTS PARTICIPATION

I utilised the Youth Risk Behaviour Survey (YRBS) to investigate the relationship between participation in school sports and adolescent health risk behaviours (Page *et al.* 1998). The YRBS is a school-based risk behaviour survey of a nationally representative sample of 12,272 high-school students. Male and female students reporting participation on both one or two teams and three or more teams were significantly more likely to have not engaged in cigarette smoking and illegal drug use than those not playing on any sports teams. Although sports participation was not significantly associated with the likelihood of not ever having sexual intercourse, females who played on sports teams were significantly more likely to have not ever had a sexually transmitted disease and to have not been pregnant. Also, among sexually active students, sports participation was significantly inversely associated with having four or more sexual partners (both males and females), the non-use of a condom during last sexual intercourse (both males and females), and the non-use of a method to prevent pregnancy during last sexual intercourse (males only). In males, sports participation significantly decreased the likelihood of smokeless tobacco and steroid use. For both males and females, the likelihood of carrying a weapon in the previous 30 days and attempting suicide was reduced in those who played on sports teams compared to those not participating in school sports.

These findings suggesting that participation in school sports yield protective effects against certain risk behaviours raise important issues for health promotion practitioners that will need to be addressed. What is it about sports participation that reduces the likelihood of engagement in cigarette smoking, illegal drug use, having multiple sex partners, not using condoms, getting a sexually transmitted disease and failure to use pregnancy prevention methods? Does sports participation provide protection by increasing prosocial bonding (peer, family, and/or school connectedness)? Does sports participation provide an avenue for association and bonding among non-smoking and non-drug-using peers? Does being involved in sports provide young people with student and adult role models who exhibit non-risky behaviour? Does playing on sports teams exert a protective effect through diversion by allowing adolescents less discretionary time in which they can get involved in risky behaviours? Are adolescents left too tired or physically exhausted to get into trouble because of the physical exertion required by playing sports? Are adolescents who play sports less likely to engage in risk behaviours because of concern about disciplinary consequences (such as not being allowed to play, being suspended or kicked off a team) that could result? Is it possible that whatever it is about school sports participation that provides a protective effect also operates for other extracurricular school activities such as band, drama and debate activities? Do these extracurricular activities also produce a protective effect against health-risky behaviour?

One possible explanation for the findings of this study may be that participation in school sports increases opportunities for young people to bond in a prosocial way with peers and the school. Social bonding theorists assert that the availability of bonding opportunities in the school environment may enhance an individual's social bonding and reduce risk-taking behaviour (Hawkins *et al.* 1992; McBride *et al.* 1995).

This study also points out that school sports participation may be a risk factor for steroid use and smokeless tobacco among male students. This is not surprising because anabolic steroids are used by adolescent athletes to enhance strength and physical prowess. These attributes can be assets in many sports. Smokeless tobacco use may also be attractive to young American male athletes because use is commonly modelled by professional athletes. In addition, it may also be perceived as a safe alternative to smoking cigarettes and as a way to use tobacco that does not adversely affect athletic performance.

SUMMARY

American youth face many pressures to engage in health-risky behaviours. Health promotion interventions which take into account and address psychosocial factors related to the health risk behaviours of adolescents have increased capacity to be successful. This article reviews several studies identifying salient psychosocial factors; health promotion professionals should take into account research findings such as these when designing and implementing interventions targeted to reduce adolescent health-risky behaviour.

REFERENCES

Ajzen, I., and Fishbein, M., 1980. *Understanding Attitudes and Predicting Social Behaviour*. Englewood Cliffs, NJ: Prentice Hall.

Allen, O., and Page, R.M., 1994. 'Gender Differences in Selected Psychosocial Characteristics of Adolescent Smokers and Nonsmokers' Health Values', *The Journal of Health Behaviour, Education and Promotion*, 18, 2: pp. 34–9.

Berndt, T.J., 1979. 'Developmental Changes in Conformity to Peers and Parents', *Developmental Psychology*, 15: pp. 608–16.

Best, J.A., Thomson, S.J., Santi, S.M., Smith, E., and Brown, K.S., 1988. 'Preventing Cigarette Smoking among School Children', *Annual Review of Public Health*, 9: pp. 161–201.

Botvin, G.J., 1986. 'Substance Abuse Prevention Research: Recent Developments and Future Directions', *Journal of School Health*, 56: pp. 369–74.

Carnegie Council on Adolescent Development, 1995. *Great Transitions: Preparing Adolescents for a New Century*. Washington, DC: Carnegie Council on Adolescent Development.

Centers for Disease Control, 1994. 'Guidelines for School Health Programmes to Prevent Tobacco Use and Addiction', *Morbidity and Mortality Weekly Report*, 43(RR–2).

Centers for Disease Control, 1996. 'Youth Risk Behaviour Surveillance – United States, 1995', *Morbidity and Mortality Weekly Report*, 45(SS–4).

Cheek, J.M., and Buss, A.H., 1981. 'Shyness and Sociability', *Journal of Personality and Social Psychology*, 41: pp. 330–9.

Clayton, S., 1991. 'Gender Differences in Psychosocial Determinants of Adolescent Smoking', *Journal of School Health*, 61: pp. 115–20.

Duryea, E.J., and Martin, G.L., 1981. 'The Distortion Effect in Student Perceptions of Smoking Prevalence', *Journal of School Health*, February: 115–18.

Dusenbury, L., Falco, M., and Lake, A., 1997. 'A Review of the Evaluation of 47 Drug Abuse Prevention Curricula Available Nationally', *Journal of School Health*, 67, 4: pp. 127–32.

Eme, R., Maisak, R., and Goodale, W., 1979. 'Seriousness of Adolescent Problems', *Adolescence*, 14: pp. 93–9.

Flay, B., 1985. 'Psychosocial Approaches to Smoking Prevention: A Review of Findings', *Health Psychology*, 4: pp. 449–88.

Green, L., and Kreuter, M., 1991. *Health Promotion Planning: An Educational and Environmental Approach*. Mountainview, CA: Mayfield Publishing Company.

Haines, M., and Spear, S.F., 1997. 'Changing the Perception of the Norm: A Strategy to Decrease Binge Drinking among College Students', *Journal of the American College Health Association*, 45, November: pp. 134–40.

Hawkins, J.D., Catalano, R.F., and Miller, J.Y., 1992. 'Risk and Protective Factors for Alcohol and Other Drug Problems in Adolescence and Early Adulthood: Implications for Substance Abuse Prevention', *Psychological Bulletin*, 112, 1: pp. 64–105.

Jaccard, J., 1975. 'A Theoretical Analysis of Selected Factors Important to Health Education Strategies', *Health Education Monographs*, 3: pp. 152–67.

Leventhal, H., and Cleary, P.D., 1980. 'The Smoking Problem: A Review of Research and Theory in Behavioural Risk Modification', *Psychological Bulletin*, 88: pp. 370–405.

McBride, C.M., Curry, S.J., Cheadle, A., Anderman, C., Wagner, E.H., Diehr, P., and Psaty, B., 1995. 'School-Level Application of a Social Bonding Model to Adolescent Risk-Taking Behaviour', *Journal of School Health*, 65, 2: pp. 63–8.

Millstein, S.G., Petersen, A.C., and Nightingale, E.O., 1993. *Promoting the Health of Adolescents: New Directions for the Twenty-First Century*. New York: Oxford University Press.

Moore, K.A., and Glei, D.A., 1994. 'Taking the Plunge: An Examination of Positive Youth Development', *Journal of Adolescent Research*, 10, 11: pp. 15–40.

Page, R.M., 1988. 'Adolescent Loneliness: A Priority for School Health Education', *Health Education*, 19, 3: pp. 20–1.

Page, R.M., 1989. 'Shyness as a Risk Factor in Adolescent Substance Use', *Journal of School Health*, 59, 10: pp. 432–35.

Page, R.M., 1990a. 'Adolescent Shyness and Wellness Impairment', *Wellness Perspectives: Research, Theory, and Practice*, 7, 1: pp. 3–12.

Page, R.M., 1990b. 'Loneliness and Adolescent Health Behaviour', *Health Education*, 21, 5: pp. 14–17.

Page, R.M., 1990c. 'Shyness and Sociability: A Dangerous Combination for Illicit Substance Use in Adolescent Males', *Adolescence*, 25, 100: pp. 803–6.

Page, R.M., 1991a. 'Indicators of Psychosocial Distress among Adolescent Females who Perceive Themselves as Fat', *Child Study Journal*, 21, 3: pp. 203–12.

Page, R.M., 1991b. 'Loneliness as a Risk Factor in Adolescent Hopelessness', *Journal of Research in Personality*, 25: pp. 189–95.

Page, R.M., 1992. 'Feelings of Unattractiveness and Adolescent Hopelessness', *The High School Journal*, 75, 3: pp. 150–5.

Page, R.M., 1993. 'Perceived Physical Attractiveness and Frequency of Substance Use among Male and Female Adolescents', *Journal of Alcohol and Drug Education*, 38, 2: pp. 81–91.

Page, R.M., 1996. 'Youth Suicidal Behaviour: Completions, Attempts, and Ideations', *The High School Journal*, 80,1: pp. 60–5.

Page, R.M., 1998. 'College Students' Distorted Perception of the Prevalence of Smoking', *Psychological Reports*, 82: p. 474.

Page, R.M., and Allen, O., 1995. 'Adolescent Perceptions of Body Weight and Weight Satisfaction', *Perceptual and Motor Skills*, 81: pp. 81–2.

Page, R.M., Allen, O., Moore, L., and Hewitt, C., 1993a. 'Co-Occurrence of Substance Use and Loneliness as a Risk Factor for Adolescent hopelessness', *Journal of School Health*, 63, 2: pp. 104–8.

Page, R.M., Allen, O., Moore, L., and Hewitt, C., 1993b. 'Weight-Related Concerns and Practices of Male and Female Adolescent Smokers and Nonsmokers', *Journal of Health Education*, 24, 6: pp. 339–46.

Page, R.M., and Cole, G.E., 1991. 'Loneliness and Alcoholism Risk in Late Adolescence: A Comparative Study of Adults and Adolescents', *Adolescence*, 26, 104: pp. 925–30.

Page, R.M., Follett, T.K., Scanlan, A., Hammermeister, J., and Friesen, R., 1996b. 'Perceived Barrier, Risk Perception, and Social Norm Attitudes about Wearing Helmets among College Students', *American Journal of Health Behaviour*, 20, 1: pp. 33–40.

Page, R.M., Frey, J., Talbert, R., and Falk, C., 1992. 'Children's Feelings of Loneliness and Social Dissatisfaction: Relationship to Physical Activity and Physical Fitness', *Journal of Teaching in Physical Education*, 11, 3: pp. 211–19.

Page, R.M., and Hammermeister, J., 1995. 'Shyness and Loneliness: Relationship to the Exercise Frequency of College Students', *Psychological Reports*, 76: pp. 395–8.

Page, R.M., Hammermeister, J., Scanlan, A., and Allen, O., 1996a. 'Psychosocial and Health-Related Characteristics of Adolescents who Watch Television Frequently', *Child Study Journal*, 26, 4: pp. 319–32.

Page, R.M., Hammermeister, J., Scanlan, A., and Gilbert, L., 1998. 'Is School Sports Participation a Protective Factor against Adolescent Health Risk Behaviours?', *Journal of Health Education*, 29, 3: pp. 186–92.

Page, R.M., Page, T.S., and Garlock, S.A., 1994a. 'Adolescent Loneliness Linked to Low Physical Fitness and Physical Inactivity', *Wellness Perspectives: Research, Theory, and Practice*, 10, 3: pp. 56–61.

Page, R.M., Scanlan, A., and Allen, O., 1995. 'Adolescent Perceptions of Body Weight and Attractiveness: Important Issues in Alcohol and Illicit Drug Use?', *Journal of Child and Adolescent Substance Abuse*, 4, 4: pp. 43–55.

Page, R.M., Scanlan, A., and Gilbert, L., in press. 'Estimations of the Prevalence of Binge Drinking among College Students: Distortion or Reality?', *Journal of Health Education*.

Page, R.M., and Tucker, L.A., 1994. 'Exercise Frequency and Psychosocial Functioning: An Epidemiological Study of 1,297 Adolescents', *Adolescence*, 29, 11: pp. 183–91.

Page, R.M., Scanlan, A., and Deringer, N., 1994b. 'Childhood Loneliness and Isolation: Implications for Childhood Educators', *Child Study Journal*, 24, 2: pp. 107–18.

Paxton, S.J., Wertheim, E.H., Gibbons, K., Szmukler, G.I., Hillier, L., and Petrovich, J.L., 1991. 'Body Image Satisfaction, Dieting Beliefs, and Weight Loss Behaviours in Adolescent Girls and Boys', *Journal of Youth and Adolescence*, 20: pp. 361–79.

Resnick *et al.*, 1997. 'Protecting Adolescents from Harm: Findings from the National Longitudinal Study on Adolescent Health', *Journal of the American Medical Association*, 278, 10: pp. 823–32.

Russell, D., 1982. 'The Measurement of Loneliness', in L.A. Peplau and D. Perlman, eds., Loneliness: A Sourcebook of Current Theory, Research, and Therapy. New York: Wiley-Interscience.

Tobler, N.S., 1992. 'Drug Prevention Programmes Can Work: Research Findings', *Journal of Addictive Diseases*, 11: pp. 1–28.

Wadden, T.A., Brown, G., Foster, G.D., and Linowitz, J.R., 1991. 'Salience of Weight-Related Worries in Adolescent Males and Females', *International Journal of Eating Disorders*, 10: pp. 407–15.

FIFTEEN

Meaning and Measurement in Health Promotion Strategies to Combat Substance Abuse

SAOIRSE NIC GABHAINN

Substance use and misuse as an area within health promotion has been characterised by widespread public interest and considerable diversity in activity. Early on, interventions were frequently planned and executed in an emotionally charged atmosphere where objective data on the extent of the problem were not available and the efficacy of potential interventions was essentially an unknown factor. These contextual conditions no longer prevail. Evidence concerning the extent and role of substance use is now widely available and appropriate evaluation research can be more easily located. The major challenges facing health promoters working in this area concern the interpretation and use of such data and the interpretation, development and implementation of policy and practice. It is with these areas, which constitute problems in themselves, that this paper will concern itself. It will take a comparative approach to Irish data and policy-development on substance use and abuse, in order to highlight some of the temptations and some of the pitfalls involved in evolving coherent sets of responses to health-related predicaments.

DATA AND INTERPRETATION

For a long time, Irish professionals in this area were working in an information void. Lacking the research infrastructure and population base of countries like the United Kingdom and the United States of America, but sharing a language, has been somewhat unfortunate. Models and data collected from quite different contexts have regularly been employed, without the willingness, funding or structures to test their validity or veracity. Indeed the adoption of natural-science models did not help, since they assume an observable regularity in behaviour and its precursors.

Nevertheless, data on the extent of psychoactive drug-use in Ireland have been accumulating over the last ten years. The most recent national data are contained in the 1995 European Schools Project on Alcohol and Other Drugs (Hibell *et al.* 1997) for which Mark Morgan was the Irish investigator. The data presented concern the knowledge, attitudes and behaviours of 16-year-olds across 26 countries. Other recent Irish data include the *Midland Health Board* survey (MHB 1996) of second-level school students aged 16 to 18, the National Youth Council of Ireland, *Get Your Facts Right* (NYCI 1998) survey of 15- to 24-year-olds in the Republic and North of Ireland, the Southern Health Board (Jackson 1997) study on *Smoking, Alcohol and Drug Use in Cork and Kerry*, Colohan's (1996) thesis on health-risk behaviour among young urban dwellers in Galway city, which compared data collected in 1993 and 1996 from 15- to 25-year-olds in a defined local authority housing area, and Kiernan's (1995) thesis on substance use among young people aged 13 to 18 in the Western Health Board region. All of these studies vary according to location, sampling techniques, age groups, methods of data collection and questions asked and therefore should not be directly compared with one another. Neither can any one of them be employed to tell us about substance use in Ireland to the exclusion of the others. Therein lies one of the problems for health promotion. Considerable care and skill needs to be exercised in the comparison of databases stemming from different sources. Table 1 below illustrates this point; these are the lifetime use rates reported by the various surveys (with the exception of the NYCI, which does not report use by individual substance).

Study (Year)	ESPAD (1995)	MHB (1996)	WHB (1995)	SHB (1996)	Galway (1993/1996)
Author/ Researcher	Morgan	nr	Kiernan	Jackson	Nic Gabhainn/ Colohan
Age Group	16	16–18	13–18	15–44	15–25
n	1,849	1,654	2,762	1,500	176/200
Ever use any drug	37%	27%	nr	18%	25%/34%
Cannabis	37%	26%	16%	16%	24%/3%
Ecstasy	9%	7%	2%	3%	nr/10%
Hallucinogens	3%	9%	5%	6%	9%/10%
Opiates	2%	nr	1%	1%	1%/0%
Amphetamines	3%	5%	2%	3%	5%/2%
Cocaine	2%	nr	1%	1%	2%/2%
nr = not reported					

Figure 1. Lifetime use rates for various substances across recent Irish Studies.

Variance in the percentages in each cell are attributable to a variety of factors including the age groups, the level of error in each set of data, the year of data collection and the area of the country involved. A further complication is that the data presented here are for lifetime consumption; that is, respondents were asked if they had *ever* tried or taken any of the substances. A positive response does not necessarily indicate that current use or indeed that current misuse or abuse exists. Planning interventions on the basis of lifetime prevalence could therefore result in poor deployment of resources. Data on recent or current use, frequency of use and style of use are more relevant for this purpose and usually available in the same databases. The current use rates vary according to the wording of the question that respondents are asked; recent use usually refers to the last 12 months, while current use usually refers to the last month or four weeks. The current or recent use rates reported by the studies above are presented in Table 2.

These rates are less likely to make headlines – being, by their very nature, lower or less spectacular. It is therefore of utmost importance when planning and making decisions based on data that the nature and quality of the information should be considered.

Other sources of information regarding substance use include the context of drug use. All of the above studies have reported on supplemental

Study (Year)	ESPAD (1995)	MHB (1996)	WHB (1995)	SHB (1996)	Galway (1993/1996)
Author/ Researcher	Morgan	nr	Kiernan	Jackson	Nic Gabhainn/ Colohan
Age Group	16	16–18	13–18	15–44	15–25
n	1,849	1,654	2,762	1,500	176/200
Time period	last 30 days	nr	Previous month	Last year/ Last month	Last six months
Cannabis	19%	nr	9%	7%/4%	15%/24%
Ecstasy	nr	nr	1%	2%/1%	nr/6%
Hallucinogens	nr	nr	3%	1%/0%	5%/2%
Opiates	nr	nr	0%	0%/0%	1%/0%
Amphetamine	nr	nr	1%	1%/0%	4%/1%
Cocaine	nr	nr	1%	0%/0%	1%/0%
nr = not reported					

Figure 2. Current or recent use rates for various substances across recent Irish studies

questions beyond the narrow issue of actual substance use. For example, NYCI (1998) reported that 41% of the 15- to 24-year-olds received their drug information from the media, 80% thought that they were well informed and 45% believed that some drugs should be legalised. This study also presented interesting data on the frequency of drug-taking; of those who had ever taken drugs, 32% reported that they no longer used them and only 12% use them weekly or more frequently (reflecting 6% of the whole sample). The young people surveyed believed that the main reasons for taking drugs was peer pressure or the influence of friends (46%) and curiosity (40%). Kiernan (1995) reported that drug use was associated with the perceived approval of family and friends as well as with less serious perceived consequences of drug use. The SHB study reported that drug-taking was positively associated with attending bars and discos, with having part-time employment and negatively with attending church (Jackson 1997). The profile of the drug-user in the SHB was a young, male urbanite who also smoked cigarettes and drank alcohol. In this study, there was a high level of awareness of drug-related problems in respondents' communities and 31% reported that some or all drugs should be legalised. The Galway city studies reported on frequency of experienced problems; on average 2% had experienced financial problems, domestic problems, or social problems, while 1% reported experiencing work or health problems related to drug use. The major obstacle in interpreting these data is the lack of uniformity in questions asked and the difficulty in matching the questions to theoretical models for predicting health or drug use behaviour. This means that it is difficult to draw a comprehensive picture of the context of drug use. It also follows that resources which have been employed in data collection, analysis and dissemination cannot further be employed to develop our under-standing of the behaviours in question within the Irish context.

One of the most important points that can be drawn from the data is that alcohol consistently emerges as a more frequently consumed substance and as being related to more potential problems. For example, Kiernan (1995) reported that 67% of her sample had ever had an alcoholic drink and 58% had had a drink in the previous month. In total, 55% of the boys and 38% of the girls reported that they had been drunk, about half of them on more than five occasions. Colohan (1996) reports that 66% of his sample had ever had a drink, 54% in the previous week, and that they had consumed a median of 8 units of alcohol during their last drinking session. In addition 10% reported that they were concerned about the amount of alcohol that they drink and 40% of those who drove cars had driven after drinking in the previous year. The ESPAD (Hibell *et al.* 1997) study reported that 91% of Irish 16-year-olds had ever consumed alcohol, 69% had had a drink in the last 30 days, 67% reported that they had been drunk at least once and 31% that they had been drunk more than 10 times. In addition, 12% reported experiencing individual problems and 23% relationship problems because of their alcohol consumption. The MHB (1996) reported that 88% had ever taken an alcoholic drink, but did not report any more detail regarding current use, drunkenness or consequences of use. Jackson (1997) reported that 87% had ever taken a drink and that 78% were current drinkers. Twenty-three per cent of men and 6% of women reported drinking more than the recommended number of units per week. In addition, 44% of under 18-year-olds claimed to be current drinkers.

It is unfortunate that it tends to be no more than lip service which is paid to the importance of alcohol as a substance of use, misuse and abuse. It is the primary drug of choice in our society and as such occupies an unique position, surrounded by the mystique of adult social life, implicated in a variety of negative outcomes, individual, familial and societal. Despite some success in changing social norms in relation to drinking and driving, there has been a relatively strong reluctance to tackle the variety of other components of alcohol use amongst the adult population. Nevertheless, health promoters increasingly consider alcohol and other drugs (AOD) in the same interventions and work on the premise that misuses of substances have common underlying factors. It should, however, be noted that this premise is widely debated outside health promotion and the practicality of offering secondary and tertiary services to alcohol and drug users within a single service is still controversial.

POLICY AND PRACTICE

Policy in the area of substance misuse is well documented (Harkin *et al.* 1997; Nic Gabhainn and Comer 1998), and the major issues appear to be the balance between demand reduction and the control of supply and, within demand reduction, the balance given to primary and secondary prevention. It is widely acknowledged that substance use is a complex psychosocial problem that requires a multifaceted response. There is no single or simple solution and there is a need to regularly review and modify responses to problems, in the aim to achieve efficient and cost-effective services. Consequently, responses need to be adaptable and tailored to local circumstances. Therein lies some of the difficulty for policy makers attempting to match a unified national or regional perspective with local flexibility.

There are substantial policy differences across countries. For example in the United States of America, any drug use among adolescents is perceived as problematic (Peele 1986). Newcomb (1992) discusses the situation in the US and both illuminates and criticises the rationale behind American policies which emphasise punishment, restriction and 'social warfare'. This is a relatively recent development in US policy and certainly contrasts with the European approach which is rooted in public health considerations. In the United Kingdom, government policy emphasises primary prevention and punitive measures to control supply and has also supported the creation of community drug teams to provide a multidisciplinary, community-led consultancy role (Strang *et al.* 1992). Many agencies, particularly those which are community-based, recognise a need for more flexible approaches when working with young people and adopt a harm minimisation approach (Franey *et al.* 1993), one which Campbell (1994) argues appears to be officially advocated and officially denied simultaneously. Indeed the official position on harm minimisation does not appear to support the wealth of activity being conducted in that area.

Irish national policy is informed by two major documents: the Government Strategy to Prevent Drug Misuse (1991) and the Report of the Ministerial Task Force on Measures to Reduce the Demand for Drugs (1996). In relation to demand reduction, both the education and health sectors are charged with a series of responsibilities. In terms of education, the expansion and dissemination of the substance-abuse prevention programmes (Morgan *et al.* 1996) at both primary and post-primary level is advocated, as is increasing the emphasis on pre- and in-service teacher training. Family support services also receive attention with the endorsement of early intervention programmes for children and out-of-school youth, and support for the home–school liaison service and teacher counsellors. In relation to health, the role of the regional health boards is emphasised, particularly in relation to the collection and dissemination of information, the co-ordination of activities and the provision of outreach and low threshold services. The health boards are also responsible for the facilitation of consultation between interest groups and specifically the establishment of regional drug co-ordinating committees. Thus inter-sectoral and multidisciplinary work appears to be the cornerstone of current policy in Ireland.

Prevention practice in the area of substance use has mirrored the history of models in other areas of health education and health promotion, in that the information-led approaches of the 1960s and early 1970s (Blum 1976) gave way to social competence models (Dusenbury and Botvin 1992; NIDA 1986) which posited that rational-decision-making skills would assist individuals in either rejecting substance use or adopting safer use practices. As a reaction to this, particularly in the US, a range of 'Just Say No' initiatives were launched during the 1980s (Dukes *et al.* 1996; Koch 1994). There are various opposing views as to the usefulness and impact of programmes based on different models of behaviour (Hansen 1992; Tobler 1986) and there are no clear leaders in the field. Refinements of both the decision-making models and social-skills enhancement continue to be both popular and widely supported. Social influence models of prevention are also increasingly advocated (Botvin and Botvin 1992; Dorn & Murji 1992).

These target the social influences to which young people may be exposed in relation to drugs, particularly among peers, the family and the wider community; they appear to be particularly effective when employed in conjunction with other techniques such as multimedia campaigns, community or family based approaches (Botvin and Botvin 1992; Hansen and O'Malley 1996; Tobler 1992; Wodarski and Smyth 1994).

The issue of substance use is in an interesting position within health promotion, being an area of concern where a substantial amount of research and activity occurs outside the mainstream of the discipline. In the UK and the US, the prevention of substance use and misuse has developed into a stand-alone multidisciplinary area essentially independent of health promotion. This has both negative and positive consequences. Addiction prevention specialists and drug workers have developed their own networking forums and successfully argued for their own budgets separate from those for health promotion. Although in many geographical areas there is collaboration and a level of shared responsibility, this is not uniform and the scope for shared approaches within settings has regularly been squandered. It frequently appears that the two groups are not aware of the work of the other or indeed the potential synergy that partnership may bring. A number of the issues that the two groups of professionals face are similar, but the drug prevention staff frequently focus on illicit drug use. They often employ quite sophisticated models of personal change and social influences and less frequently employ the models and processes inherent in modern health promotion. Health promoters in turn can leave the thorny issue of drug prevention to the 'specialists' in this area and fulfil their professional requirements through skills-based interventions for school students or other relevant groups (for instance parents or employees). There are certainly historical reasons why these parallel services have developed and the division is not as acute in Ireland, where both were relatively late starters and thus essentially composed of the same small group of individuals.

CHALLENGES

The challenges for health promotion in the area of substance abuse are twofold. The first concerns the interpretation of knowledge and information. Theoretical models borrowed from single disciplines and research conducted without recourse to any theory development and in the context of post-hoc justification for funding leads to inadequate data from which to determine strategy. Time and institutional support for the necessary planning needs to be forthcoming before such a situation can be effectively altered. We are no longer in a situation where we can dismiss calls for action with measured scepticism regarding the state of our knowledge concerning the extent of any 'problem' or the possible efficacy of any intervention. However, neither are we assured of success by following any one particular model of action.

There remains considerable scope for research designed to match the required flexibility of regional and local responses to perceived problems. That is, rather than large-scale epidemiological studies being required, more focused qualitative work is needed to answer specific questions at local level. Evidence of wholesale cultural colonialism does not negate the desirability of local answers for local questions. In the Irish context, qualitative data are largely missing from peer-review journals, although some institutionally funded work has been published in recent reports (e.g. NWHB 1996; WHB, 1998; Dept of Health 1997). The data reported have been of considerable interest as examples of young peoples' views on the issues concerning them and their perspectives on future developments and possible interventions.

A separate issue within this research strand concerns the evaluation of interventions. While we can borrow prevention programmes and activities that have shown the most promise from the international literature, this does not guarantee that they will operate or be effective in the same way across cultures or subcultures in society. Although individual differences may be interpretable from most published work, comparisons at the broader level including those across sub-groups, family structures or societal structures may be considerably more difficult to disentangle. In perspective, attempts at rendering American or British interventions appropriate to the Irish context have rarely been documented and appear to consist of dropping sections which may have the potential to bring offence to children, parents, the Roman Catholic Church or other such interested parties. It may well be that whole intervention programmes can validly and appropriately be adopted, but we do not yet know. Until all interventions are subject to thorough process and outcome evaluations of sufficient quality, and the subsequent findings disseminated through academic journals or scientific reports, there will be little professional confidence in the potential efficacy of such interventions.

The second major challenge concerns effective inter-sectoral work. Models of professional courtesy and co-operation are not sufficient to enable the development of real multidisciplinary and cross-sectoral projects. Too often ignorance regarding the potential contribution of a body of knowledge, or method of working, prohibits or endangers the potential of such work. While it must be acknowledged that in the area of addiction and substance use it is often explicitly recommended and at times required that groups of different professional, voluntary and community groups should work with one another (Department of Health 1991; Strang *et al.* 1992), too often representatives sit on such committees with little recourse to the rest of their organisation or group and with little real responsibility for the implementation of any subsequent recommendations. Perennial problems concern committees comprised of different interest or knowledge groups, many of whom are taking time out of already overcrowded schedules to attend meetings, or else they send representatives who do not have the power or financial clout to confirm joint decisions. The problem is not that there are no guidelines for the effective running of such cross-sectoral or disciplinary groups (Davis 1996, Durfee *et al.* 1994), rather that such guidelines often appear either to be too idealistic and mistakenly to take for granted common goals within the committee, or else, more frequently, they have not been read or adopted by the convenors or members of such committees. Organisations and staff who become involved in such collaborative work must recognise the comparative opportunity cost of such lost hours and begin to train members and employees in effective group work with other bodies and professionals, which should include ongoing appreciation of the specialist bodies of knowledge and skills of others and the mechanics of cross-disciplinary linguistic interpretation. While this may be possible as well as desirable in large organisations where a variety of differently trained workers are based (such as health boards or government departments), a practical way for smaller groups to illustrate real commitment to inter-sectoral work may be for them to come together to provide such training for members and staff.

The most appropriate caveat which needs to be considered in facing both sets of challenges is one which is widely applicable across the area of substance use, health promotion and all areas of applied work which draw from multidisciplinary bases. It is never sufficient to draw from a limited understanding of a given discipline's knowledge. Expanding research programmes and publication outlets have led to a plethora of findings in every area, each growing and changing regularly. A snapshot of the state of the art in a single discipline is not enough to guide successful applied work. Not only is it necessary to have ongoing contact with theory and practice development, but two fundamental interpretative difficulties with academic knowledge must be understood. The first concerns the 'doughnut effect'. Knowledge bases built on shaky foundations may appear to result in stable and usable data or information, but all assume the validity of earlier findings. Basic errors or assumptions encountered at the beginning of a knowledge base may be later refuted or corrected (the hole in the centre of the doughnut is pushed out), but in practice the knowledge built up on that foundation rarely falls with them, even though it may be fatally flawed. An important example of this was the 'General Adaption Syndrome' (Seyle 1956), which postulated a general physiological response to a stress, encouraging a focus on the identification of potentially stressful events and the introduction of the term into popular vocabulary. More recently 'stress' has been conceptualised as the product of an interaction between an individual and their environment (Lazarus and Folkman 1984), rendering substantial amounts of earlier research uninterpretable. The second fundamental problem concerns unequal knowledge-development within a discipline. The history of scientific knowledge acquisition illustrates that particular subsets of issues may become widely researched, debated and disseminated for social, psychological, historical or cultural reasons rather than because of their intrinsic scientific or applied value. A simple example of this is the publication bias towards positive evaluations or theory-confirming investigations. A thorough and ongoing understanding of these mechanisms is a requirement for all those involved in multidisciplinary work, as is the professional responsibility to disseminate findings to those in source disciplines as well as within health promotion itself.

ISSUES FOR THE FUTURE

While most of the work conducted in relation to substance misuse has focused on the use of illegal substances among young people and school students in particular, there are likely to be an increasing number of areas of concern for health promoters. Considerable rates of prescription drug use has been reported amongst Irish youth. Nic Gabhainn and Kelleher (1995) presented data on the percentages of 15-year-old girls and boys reporting having taken medicine or tablets in the previous month for headaches (59%, 36%), stomach-aches (36%, 11%), sleeping difficulties (7%, 4%) and nervousness (7%, 1%). The ESPAD study (Hibell *et al.* 1997) reported that 6% of boys and 9% of girls reported lifetime use of tranquillisers or sedatives, while Jackson (1997) reported lifetime use of sedatives at 3% for 15- to 19-year-olds but did not distinguish whether these were prescribed for the respondent. While the figures vary, as do the databases and questions asked, this issue warrants further investigation, and possibly the development of targeted interventions which should include both parents and medical practitioners.

A related set of issues that require further development in the context of substance use concerns differences across social groups in the experience of drug taking. While almost all databases suggest higher rates of experimentation and current use for males (with the exception of prescription drug rates) and for urban dwellers, the data on social class differences is not yet strong enough in the Irish context to warrant any generalisations. The unemployed predominate among treatment statistics (Harkin *et al.* 1997), and anecdotal reports and data do exist on drug taking in high-risk areas – that is, areas of social disadvantage (Colohan 1996; Murphy 1996) – which suggest relatively high rates of consumption among youth in these geographic areas. However, comparative data reported by Jackson (1997) did not indicate a higher level of substance use among those in areas of deprivation as compared with the general population. Consequently, social class differences in other areas of the country and within more heterogeneous geographical areas requires exploration. While these individual or family-level variables may assist health promoters in targeting prevention initiatives, community – and society-level variables are also required. Too often the social and contextual issues related to drug use have been operationalised by researchers as attributes of the individual rather than the group, and therefore opportunities have been lost to investigate other parameters, predictors or precursors of these behaviours. This is therefore a call for the inclusion of a variety of perspectives in subsequent research activity in this area.

If it is the case that the current generation of young people are being exposed to and are experiencing substance use to a greater degree than previous generations, one consequence may be a change in social norms towards drug-taking as this cohort grows up and takes their place in adult society. Although previous research suggests that young people tend to 'mature out' of drug-taking (e.g. Swadi 1992), this may have been a function of the social norms of the adult world they were entering. If these norms are altered, it may follow that fewer young adults will cease or decrease their substance-use behaviour and there may, therefore, be further alterations to normative behaviour patterns. Although this is likely to have some negative consequences for health, it does not necessarily follow that young adults maturing in such a culture will experience the cluster of other risk factors commonly associated with adult drug-taking (such as loss of earnings and family ties, or poor housing). Notwithstanding legal problems with drug-taking, these young adults may ultimately provide a set of role models for harm-minimising drug-taking, seen as co-existing with the responsibilities of adult social roles in a similar way to that now promoted for adult alcohol consumers. This issue should be further considered by those concerned with the documentation of the natural history of drug-taking.

While peer interventions are currently popular, and the evidence for their efficacy is somewhat promising (Botvin and Botvin 1992; Kroger 1994), they are likely to be subject to the same innovative effect as their precursors. That is, while they are new and exciting and being developed and implemented by enthusiastic and committed staff, they are more likely to illustrate positive effects. It is therefore vital that the process of such interventions be carefully documented and that the factors which work well be transferred onto the next generation of interventions in a way that facilitates practice-led theoretical development. However, the use of peers in substance-misuse prevention is not necessarily limited to their having a tutor or leadership role. Central components of social network or social support interventions could be borrowed from community psychology and social psychiatric epidemiology to assist in primary and secondary prevention in this area. Training members of naturally occurring networks to provide emotional and affirmational social support to others may result in an ongoing network of social support, capable of buffering members from stressful events or life experiences. Evidence already exists regarding the efficacy of such interventions for injecting drug users (Latkin *et al.* 1994; Wiebel *et al.* 1993) and could be expanded to drug users whose behaviour is less risky or indeed to early experimenters or non-drug users.

In conclusion, the area of substance use provides a useful vehicle for examining some of the more generic current issues in health promotion. As Pentz (1993) argued, the more successful initiatives have been theoretically- and research-based, involve integration with other health and prevention programmes and include multiple modalities. The importance of good quality data, both qualitative and quantitative, cannot be underestimated. But the difficulties inherent in developing policy and implementing practice must also be acknowledged. The challenging nature of working with other professionals and the adoption of concepts and theoretical positions from other disciplines and cultures require of us rigorous and self-critical honesty, maintenance of the highest ethical standards and a commitment to thorough ongoing learning.

REFERENCES

Blum, R.H., 1976. *Drug Education: Results and Recommendations*. Lexington, MA: Heath.

Botvin, G.J., and Botvin, E.M., 1992. 'Adolescent Tobacco, Alcohol, and Drug Abuse: Prevention Strategies, Empirical Findings and Assessment issues', *Journal of Developmental and Behavioural Paediatrics*, 13, 4: pp. 290–301.

Campbell, D., 1994. 'Police Chief Wants Drugs Nationalised', *Guardian*, 6 August.

Colohan, S., 1996. *A Study on the Lifestyle Behaviour and Substance Use and Their Relationship to Occupation*. MSc. Thesis, National University of Ireland, Galway.

Davis, W.F., 1996. *Collaborating with Teachers, Parents, and Others to help Youth at Risk*. Paper presented at the American Psychological Association Annual Convention, Toronto.

Department of Health, 1991. *Government Strategy to Prevent Drug Misuse*. Dublin: Stationery Office.

Department of Health, 1997. *Report of the Health Promotion Consultative Committee on Young People*. Dublin: Stationery Office.

Dorn, M., and Murji, K., 1992. *Drug Prevention: A Review of the English Language Literature*. London: Institute for the Study of Drug Dependence.

Dukes, R.L., Ullman, J.B., and Stein, J.A., 1996. 'Three Year Follow-up of Drug Abuse Resistance Education (DARE)', *Evaluation Review*, 20, 1: pp. 49–66.

Durfee, M.F., Warren, D.G., and Sdao-Jarvie, K., 1994. 'A Model for Answering the Substance Abuse Educational Needs of Health Professionals: The North Carolina Governors Institute on Alcohol and Substance Abuse', *Alcohol*, 11, 6: pp. 483–7.

Dusenbury, L., and Botvin, G.L., 1992. 'Applying the Competency Enhancement Model of Substance Abuse Prevention', in M. Kessler, S.E. Goldston and J.M. Joffe, eds., *The Present and the Past of Prevention: In Honour of George W. Albee.* Newbury Park, CA: Sage.

Franey, C., Power, R., and Wells, B., 1993. 'Treatment and Services for Drug Users in Britain', *Journal of Substance Abuse Treatment*, 10, 6: pp. 561–7.

Hansen, W.B., and O'Malley, P.M., 1996. 'Drug Use', in R. DiClemente, W.B. Hansen and L.E. Ponton, eds., *Handbook of Adolescent Health Risk Behaviour: Issues in Clinical child psychology*. New York: Plenum Press.

Hansen, W.B., 1992. 'School-Based Substance Abuse Prevention: A Review of the State of the Art in Curriculum, 1980–1990', *Health Education Research*, 7, 3: pp. 403–30.

Harkin, A.M., Anderson, P., and Goos, C., 1997. *Smoking, Drinking and Drugtaking in the European Region*. Copenhagen: WHO Regional Office for Europe.

Hibell, B., Andersson, B., Bjarnason, T., Kokkevi, A., Morgan, M., and Narusk, A., 1997. *The 1995 ESPAD Report. Alcohol and Other Drug Use among Students in 26 European Countries*. Stockholm: The Swedish Council for Information on Alcohol and Other Drugs, CAN.

Irish Government, 1996. *Report on the Ministerial Task Force on Measures to Reduce the Demand for Drugs*. Dublin: Stationery Office.

Jackson, T., 1997. *Smoking, Alcohol and Drug use in Cork and Kerry. Cork*: Southern Health Board.

Kiernan, R., 1995. *Substance Use among Adolescents in the Western Health Board Area*. MFPHMI thesis, Faculty of Public Health Medicine, Royal College of Surgeons of Ireland.

Koch, K., 1994. 'DARE: Drug Abuse Resistance Education', in J.A. Lewis, *Addictions: Concepts and Strategies for Treatment*. Maryland: Aspen.

Kroger, B., 1994. *Drug Abuse: A Review of the Effectiveness of Health Education and Health Promotion*. Utrecht: Dutch Centre for Health Education and Health Promotion and IUHPE/EURO.

Latkin, C.A., Mandell, W., Oziemkowska, M., Celentano, D., Vlahov, D., and Ensminger, M., 1994. *Using Social Network Analysis to Study Patterns of Drug Use among Urban Drug Users at Risk for HIV/AIDS*. Paper presented at Sunbelt 14, International Social Network Conference, New Orleans.

Lazarus, R.S., & Folkman, S., 1984. *Stress, Appraisal and Coping*. New York: Springer.

Midland Health Board, 1996. *Report on School Survey of Second Level Students in Midland Health Board Area*. Report 58/96.

Morgan, M., Morrow, R., Sheehan, A.M., and Lillis, M., 1996. 'Prevention of Substance Misuse: Rationale and Effectiveness of the Programme "On my own two feet"', *Oideas*, 41: pp. 5–25.

Murphy, E., 1996. *The Teenage Drugs Explosion: Fact or Myth?* MFPHMI thesis, Faculty of Public Health Medicine, Royal College of Surgeons of Ireland.

National Institute on Drug Abuse, 1986. *Adolescent Peer Pressure: Theory, Correlates and Program Implications for Drug Abuse Prevention*. Rockville, ML: NIDA.

Newcomb, M.D., 1992. 'Substance Abuse and Control in the United States: Ethical and Legal Issues', *Social Science Medicine*, 35, 4: pp. 471–9.

Nic Gabhainn, S., and Comer, S., 1998. *Prevalence, Practice and Proposals: Substance Use in the Western Health Board*. Galway: Western Health Board.

Nic Gabhainn, S., and Kelleher, C., 1995. *Lifeskills for Health Promotion*. Galway: Centre for Health Promotion Studies, National University of Ireland, Galway.

North-Western Health Board, 1996. *Young People and Drug Misuse in the North West*. Manorhamilton: North-Western Health Board.

NYCI, 1998. *Get Your Facts Right*. Dublin: National Youth Council of Ireland.

Peele, S., 1986. 'The "Cure" for Adolescent Drug Abuse: Worse than the Problem?', *Journal of Counselling and Development*, 65: pp. 23–4.

Pentz, M.A., 1993. 'Comparative Effects of Community Based Drug Abuse Prevention', in J.S. Baer, A. Marlatt and R.J. McMahon, *Addictive Behaviours across the Lifespan*. Newbury Park: Sage.

Seyle, H., 1956. *The Stress of Life*. New York: McGraw-Hill.

Strang, J., Smith, M., and Spurrell, S., 1992. 'The Community Drug Team', *British Journal of Addiction*, 87, 2: pp. 169–78.

Swadi, H., 1992. 'A Longitudinal Perspective on Adolescent Substance Abuse', *European Child and Adolescent Psychiatry*, 1, 3: pp. 156–69.

Tobler, S., 1986. 'Meta-analysis of 143 Adolescent Drug Prevention Programs: Quantitative Outcome Results of Program Participants Compared to a Control or a Comparison group', *Journal of Drug Issues*, 16: pp. 537–67.

Tobler, S., 1992. 'Drug Prevention Programme Can Work', *Journal of Addictive Diseases*, 11, 3: pp. 1–28.

Wiebel, W.W., O'Brien, M.U., and Murray, J., 1993. *Social Networks as Targets for Intervention and Intervention Impact*. Paper presented at NIDA Technical Review Meeting on Social Networks, Drug Abuse and HIV Transmission, Bethesda, MD.

Wodarski, J.S., and Smyth, N.J., 1994. 'Adolescent Substance Abuse: A Comprehensive Approach to Prevention Intervention', *Journal of Child and Adolescent Substance*, 3, 3: pp. 33–58.

SIXTEEN

The Riddle of the Sphinx:
Why Do Women Smoke?

CECILY KELLEHER AND
JANE SIXSMITH

INTRODUCTION

There continues to be surprise and disappointment among health professionals of all specialities that rates of smoking are not declining and
indeed may even be increasing among women, particularly the young.
Rather like the ancient riddle of the enigmatic sphinx (who appears in
several guises throughout ancient mythology and whose deadly conundrum
of the three ages of man baffled all but Oedipus), smoking too remains a
deadly puzzle to challenge the credibility of the health promotion movement
and one which reflects the complexity of the issues to be tackled. This
review will examine the issue particularly from an Irish perspective, drawing
in the main on studies which have been conducted in recent years through
the Centre for Health Promotion Studies but which are also grounded in the
more general literature. There are essentially four issues that need to be
addressed on this topic. First, what do we know of the prevalence and
incidence of smoking, both in the population generally and according to
different socio-demographic groups? These data should indicate whether
we are justified in being concerned about women particularly or indeed
whether this apparent gender effect is explained by any other factor.
Secondly, it is appropriate to examine the likely influences on behaviour in
relation to the smoking habit, both in taking it up, persisting with the habit
or being successful in cessation. Thirdly, we need to be critical in appraising
such interventions, most typically in settings like the community, schools,
workplace or primary care. Approaches in these situations have either been
based on personal development programmes or on various forms of
supportive social change. There are a range of indirect issues which have
had a bearing on success in this area, including the feminist concept of the
empowerment of women and its association with personal assertiveness and
self-efficacy. Finally, it may be appropriate, based on this evidence, to

246

suggest new strategies for combating the problem, under the general headings of social change and personal development.

ESTIMATES OF PREVALENCE

We recently undertook a review of the prevalence of smoking for the Irish Department of Health. In Ireland recent national health and lifestyle surveys have now confirmed that the overall prevalence of smoking is about a third of the population, with significant socio-demographic variations (Centre for Health Promotion Studies 1999). However, there are considerable cultural variations in rates across Europe. We know from other countries that the proportion of male smokers has halved since a peak in the post-war period and is now reasonably steady at around a third of the general population; on the other hand women never achieved such high rates in the first place, but their rates have failed to decline significantly except in the higher socio-economic groups. The class factor has been very noticeable for both sexes and in some occupational groups instructive differences are now found, in that very few doctors smoke (O'Connor and Kelleher 1998) but rates in nurses remain higher (Clarke *et al.* 1998; Hope *et al.* 1998; Prendergast 1992).

Smoking is the greatest single cause of death and disease in the world (Joossens and Raw 1996). In Ireland 6,000 deaths per year can be attributed to smoking (Department of Health 1994) and this may be an under-representation of the true impact of smoking on mortality (Peto *et al.* 1996). In order to ensure a reduction in morbidity and mortality, national tobacco control measures are crucial. Reid (1996) argues that the first step in the design of an effective national tobacco control programme is to set measurable targets with dates for their achievement. As with other countries, in Ireland such targets have been set, as is documented in the Irish government's health strategy, *Shaping a Healthier Future* (Department of Health 1994). Prevalence is the most useful indicator for this purpose, supported by indirect measures (Lopez *et al.* 1994). The strategy identifies the need to improve the life expectancy of the population by concentrating on the three main causes of premature mortality in Ireland: cardiovascular disease, cancer and accidents. Cardiovascular and cancer mortality are both influenced by smoking behaviour, in that smokers are at increased risk of developing these conditions (Doll *et al.* 1994). Smoking control is one of the few types of prevention activity that can have a broad impact on improving life expectancy of the Irish population. A reduction in smoking had therefore been specifically identified with the target of reducing the percentage of those who smoke by a minimum of 1% per year so that, by the year 2000, 80% of the population will be non-smokers. This requires a combination of quitting among those currently smoking and a reduction in the numbers of those starting to smoke.

On an individual level valid assessment of smoking patterns is critical, both to increase empirical understanding of smoking behaviour and to improve the effectiveness of interventions (Shiffman 1993). Similarly, in order actively to plan smoking control measures at a population-based level, clear, accurate information is required on the patterns and trends of smoking behaviour in the population as a whole. The active planning of interventions in health promotion greatly facilitates the effectiveness of such programmes (Green and Kreuter 1991).

At an international level differences can be seen in the patterns and trends of smoking behaviour between countries. This, coupled with the identification of individual motives for smoking across cultures, suggests cultural influences on smoking behaviour (Shiffman 1993). Therefore each country must have access to information allowing identification of its national pattern in order to facilitate the development of national tobacco control mechanisms. The target of smoking reduction in Ireland is consistent with the target stipulated by the WHO in the 38 targets for *Health for All by the Year 2000*. This international context is important, as policy responses to tobacco control are increasingly initiated at international level.

It is also important to compare patterns of smoking prevalence across countries and regions, as general patterns of tobacco use may be identifiable and assist in the prediction of future trends. Figure 1 indicates estimated smoking prevalence in the six WHO regions by gender. The difficulty of comparing data at a national level is replicated at an international level, where data are also collected using various methods and measures – compromising any comparisons that can be made. The findings should therefore be viewed with caution, especially for the African region, where little survey data are available. The prevalence rates for the Western Pacific region are particularly high due to the rates of tobacco use in China. In global terms the WHO estimates that about one-third of the global population aged 15 and over smoke. The vast majority of the 1,100 million smokers in the world live in developing countries. The pattern of smoking by gender differs in developing countries as compared to developed ones, with about 1 in 3 regular smokers in developed countries being women as opposed to 1 in 8 in the developing world (WHO *Tobacco Alert* 1996).

In Ireland the policy response of other European countries to tobacco use has potentially the most impact on smoking prevalence rates. The European rates are shown in Figure 2, adapted from the review of Harkin *et al.* (1997). The pattern of smoking behaviour by gender in Ireland is similar to that in Sweden, Norway and the UK with little if any difference between the smoking rates of men compared to women. This trend will be reflected in time by increased ill-health and death in women related to tobacco use.

The rates reported above relate to the prevalence of smoking in adults. The rate at which young people are taking up smoking behaviours also reflects future trends in tobacco use. Surveys have been carried out in the countries of the European region, but difficulties, as with the adult surveys, arise with comparison across countries due to the various survey methods and measures used. This is further complicated in studies of youth by the use of various age ranges. An international WHO collaborative study is the *Health Behaviour in School-Aged Children* (HBSC) study, which has provided data on smoking behaviour in youth for some countries of the European region. Ireland has recently joined this initiative so that data on smoking prevalence rates will in future be available that can be directly compared to that of other participating countries.

In Ireland, national surveys had been undertaken annually by a market research company (Lansdowne Market Research Limited), known as the Joint National Readership Research (JNRR). These national surveys were commissioned by the Health Education Bureau and latterly by the Health Promotion Unit (HPU) until 1994. In 1994 the surveys were suspended, as it was felt that market research methods were inadequate for determining precise enough smoking prevalence rates. Therefore no national data had since been collected on a regular basis for the sole purpose of identifying smoking prevalence rates until the National Lifestyle Surveys were undertaken in 1998. A number of regional and local studies, both published and unpublished, had been carried out, but there is no central collation of this information, which restricts the active planning of programmes. We therefore reviewed studies carried out in Ireland between January 1992 and June 1997, a period of five years. Data in relation to smoking prevalence in Ireland are often gathered at regional level by health boards and are not always formally published, so it was decided that both published and unpublished sources of data would be collected and reviewed.

Literature was accessed using a wide variety of sources, both electronic and manual. The key words of 'smoking', 'tobacco use', 'prevalence' and 'Ireland' were used with the on-line databases of 'Medline' and 'PsychLIT' for a search of subjects and words in titles. A search for authors known to publish in this area was also undertaken using these databases. An internet search was carried out using the search engine Lycos and the key words previously mentioned. A manual search was also carried out in relation to all health-related journals and theses held in the university library and within the Department of Health Promotion in the National University of Ireland, Galway. To gain access to unpublished work, all departments of public health and health promotion in all the health boards, all the academic departments of public health medicine and community health and general practice and selected organisations with an interest in smoking prevalence, the Irish Heart Foundation, the Irish Cancer Society, ASH Ireland and the

Garda Research Unit were contacted by letter. A further search was constructed based on the references of research studies obtained.

A total of 43 studies were identified by this means, four of which are still underway. Few studies were identified whose main purpose was to elicit information on smoking-related issues. The studies that focused on substance use were all with groups of young people. The lifestyle studies related mainly to the identification of risk factors associated with coronary heart disease. The majority of the studies reported smoking prevalence rates as an adjunct to the main study purpose. It is therefore likely that some studies which report smoking prevalence rates in the Irish population or a subsample within it have not been identified. This is compounded by studies which are published in international rather than national journals, a problem recognised by Howell (1996). Therefore a review of the identified studies was carried out, rather than a systematic analysis of prevalence-data gathered.

A diverse range of research designs was used in the studies identified. Similarly, the nature and size of the sample varied by study. The range of research designs is reflected in the various data-collection methods, which were either administered, self-administered or postal questionnaires. All studies relied on self-report of smoking behaviour and did not validate this against any other measure. A myriad of measures were used in the assessment and reporting of smoking behaviour. Labels used for smoking behaviours included: 'regular', 'current', 'occasional', 'social', 'recreational', 'experimental', 'lifetime', 'ever', 'never', 'non-smokers', 'weekly', 'less than weekly', 'heavy', 'light' and 'moderate'. The difficulties raised by this varied use of labels were compounded by the various meanings ascribed to one label. For example, in one study 'current smoking' denoted those who smoked in the previous month; in another, 'current smoking' denoted those who smoked less than daily but at least one or two cigarettes in the previous month. This issue was further complicated by the lack in some studies of definitions of terms used. Comparison of rates reported is thus very difficult. Variations are also to be observed in the other risk factors considered, so that the socio-economic group was measured using a variety of scales. Variables consistently reported were gender and age. While a proportion of the studies identified reported youth smoking behaviour, it was noticeable that these were recorded predominantly among post-primary schoolchildren. Data in relation to smoking behaviour appear rarely to be collected from children under the age of 12 years.

The majority of studies refer to cigarette smoking as opposed to other forms of tobacco use. Shelley *et al.* (1992) identify from the comprehensive smoking data gathered during the Kilkenny Health Project that tobacco products other than cigarettes are used by specific groups, notably older men. These data appear to be rarely collected. When studies did refer to other tobacco products this was noted. The smoking prevalence rates reported by the studies are clearly not comparable, due to the range of measures and methods used to ascertain smoking rates. However, while heterogeneity of measures make estimates difficult, the prevalence rates reported range from 23% to 38% in the studies of young people and from 27% to 39% in the adult studies, with the modal point of 35% in both young people and adults. These figures are more pessimistic than suggested by the population quota studies annually commissioned by the Health Promotion Unit until 1994, but they are in keeping with the recent national survey findings in reflecting considerable variation according to socio-economic group. Prevalence rates declined significantly during the 1970s and 1980s, but this pattern appears to have been halted in the 1990s. The studies reporting smoking prevalence by gender appear to indicate that male and female rates have converged, with little difference now seen between regular smoking rates in men and women. This suggests an increase in women smoking over time. This trend is likely to continue, as the youth studies report similar gender patterns in smoking prevalence. In the adult studies that reported smoking rates by socio-economic group, significant differences were found between blue- and white-collar workers such that there were more regular smokers in the blue-collar groups. In the studies of both young people and adults in disadvantaged circumstances it would appear that a majority are smokers.

While prevalence rates are the most direct indicator of the level of tobacco consumption per person, in the absence of these data (or alternatively to go some way to validate self-reported smoking prevalence data) other indirect indicators may be used. Mortality data in relation to smoking-related death may also be used as a proxy measure of tobacco use. Fiscal measures such as levels of taxation generated by the sale of tobacco products and household expenditure on such products as recorded in the household budget survey may also be used.

It is well established that a number of fatal diseases have been positively associated with smoking, notably lung cancer (Doll *et al.* 1994, Surgeon General Report 1989). However, Wald and Hackshaw (1996) categorised diseases according to the extent to which the difference in incidence between smokers and non-smokers is causally attributable to smoking. Lung cancer risk is largely or entirely caused by smoking and therefore incidence of lung cancer in a population reflects tobacco use. This relationship is obviously complicated by the time delay, which can be several decades between starting to smoke and its full effect (Peto *et al.* 1996). In Ireland mortality figures from the National Cancer Registry (1997) indicate a rapid increase in the rates of lung cancer in both women and men since the 1950s, reflecting an increase in the consumption of tobacco products, especially cigarettes. This trend is likely to continue due to the effect of the time delay between starting to smoke and developing lung cancer.

Taxation on cigarettes has been viewed as a useful source of revenue and has been pursued by successive governments. The levying of such tax and subsequent record-keeping provides an indirect indicator of cigarette use in Ireland (Figure 3). However, these figures must be treated with some caution, due to smuggling of tobacco products. A review in 1994 by the European Bureau for Action on Smoking Prevention (BASP 1994) found the issue of smuggling to be more complex in Europe than merely the illegal trade in tobacco products from countries with low levels of taxation to countries with high levels. The WHO has estimated that 6% of tobacco products are smuggled globally (WHO 1996). This figure relates to all tobacco products, while the figures presented below relate only to cigarettes retained for consumption in Ireland. Thus, the levels of taxation provide only a very general guide to tobacco use. This may be further complicated by patterns of imports versus exports, in that Ireland may have reduced the number of cigarettes imported.

The household budget survey is carried out every seven years in Ireland, with the aim of determining the current pattern of household expenditure for the purpose of maintaining the weighting basis of the Consumer Price Index. A record is made of households' expenditure on a number of items including tobacco products. Household expenditure on tobacco products has increased and may reflect tobacco use, but the proportion of a household's total expenditure on tobacco products has decreased. However, this may reflect retail price of tobacco products rather than a decrease in numbers of those smoking (Figure 4).

We conclude from this section of the review that a relatively large body of data was identified reporting smoking prevalence rates, but the variety of measures used makes comprehensive and detailed comparison of studies impossible. Crude comparison of the data confirms that about one-third of the Irish population smoke, with a discernible class gradient and converging gender differences in smoking prevalence rates. It therefore follows that the target identified in the government's health strategy (Department of Health 1994) of 80% non-smokers by the year 2000 is unreachable. A more realistic target would be 75% non-smokers by the year 2005. This reduction would require a concerted programme for disadvantaged groups. However, the lack of accurate direct information on the smoking behaviour of the Irish population severely restricts any attempts at tobacco control. This will be addressed now by a comprehensive series of national lifestyle surveys of adults and young people now underway in Ireland at our research centre (whose preliminary findings are about to be published).

INFLUENCES ON BEHAVIOUR

What factors influence smoking behaviour? Most attention in the last two decades has been based on the assumptions that peer and social influences are highly important but that, as the rates declined in adults, especially men, shrewd marketing strategists started to focus on women and the young, with interesting dividends. Several agencies have reviewed the impact of both smoking promotion and smoking demotion in films, television, print media, including women's magazines, and role models appearing in such settings. A small study on fashion consciousness among a cross-section of young people and a group with eating disorders undergoing treatment demonstrated that fashion-conscious women were significantly more likely to smoke, though the converse applied to a small group of men (O'Connor *et al.* 1997). A majority of those with eating disorders were smokers but this had little to do with identification with role models. It was concluded that smoking could be seen as an assertive act and is not necessarily causally associated with low self-esteem. There is no doubt that smoking continues to be prevalent in women's magazines and one investigator in Ireland maintains that the government warnings printed on Irish magazines are those least relevant to women, including pregnancy-related risks (Howell 1994). The role of public service broadcasting in countering commercial advertising is well documented and has gone from mass campaigns through to micro-campaigns and then somewhere between the two (Reid 1996). Indeed the countries that sustained national anti-smoking campaigns appeared to do better than those who did not. The problem with mass-media campaigns appears to be twofold: if they are not associated with other intervention approaches then readiness to change cannot be built upon constructively. Further, if the campaigns are unfocused they are unlikely to be internalised. In an extensive review of our government's most recent cycle of mass-media campaigns combined with a triangular impact evaluation we found that smokers were aware of the dangers but did not internalise the risk to themselves (Sixsmith and Kelleher 1997). Other data are consistent with this, in that McCluskey (1989) found smokers were less likely than current or ex-smokers to graduate the risk involved as very serious. Another recently published study (Sutton 1998) showed that smokers were as aware as non-smokers of the degree of risk associated with smoking. Media campaigns therefore should move from knowledge impartment to empowerment and fit in with supportive environment approaches.

In May 1998 we finally saw support at Council of Ministers level in Europe for a range of tobacco-restriction measures including advertising controls. There has been equivocation in many countries about controlling advertising and instituting social controls generally. This is connected with a range of issues including reluctance to tackle the economic implications at European level, a free-market ethos which opposes the limitation of a legal product and, it also should be admitted, a pragmatic assumption in some countries that such controls are unpopular and difficult to enforce. This pessimism may have little basis in reality. In Ireland legislation to curb smoking in public places was introduced in 1991. After a slow start it is becoming more widely adopted and accepted and is being enforced by public-sector organisations on pain of fines and penalties. However, not enough 'carrot' has been applied. There are signs that commercial organisations are simply not aware of basic facts such as the prevalence of smoking among their customers. Two studies demonstrated both that restaurateurs were over-estimating the rates (McArdle et al 1993) and that their customers tended to be non-smokers or smokers who accepted the regulations (Hickey 1996). This kind of information should be disseminated by local authorities to their chambers of commerce and other groupings. A major exception to this are publicans, but even here there may be changes. We have introduced a voluntary code of practice for publicans in Galway, a major tourist city, and plan to evaluate the impact (McCarthy, Galway Health Project, personal communication).

This regulatory approach is also criticised by those who represent the disadvantaged and indeed if regulation were undertaken in isolation such criticism might well be valid. There are two distinct issues concerning women and the smoking habit that are worthy of note. The feminist movement has seen smoking as an assertion of equality and independence almost from the outset and nowadays it is presented as an example of the classlessness of sisterhood. On the other hand the association between poverty, deprivation and lack of social control has also been studied in detail (Graham 1984) and implies again that smoking is a social statement that should not be ignored; indeed anti-smoking approaches that fail to address inequity, either in relation to class generally or between the sexes specifically, will not be appreciated. This kind of argumentation is greeted with a range of responses from the predominantly middle-class health professional establishment, especially medical practitioners. The appearance of colluding with such apparently irrational thinking, particularly when any social benefit is weighed against the vast body of biomedical data linking smoking to ill-health, has proved a problem in developing intervention programmes. Yet any analysis of smoking patterns supports the qualitative data. A study on demographic factors influencing dietary behaviours in the workplace showed that the small proportion of exclusively non-meat-eaters were more likely to be students at university and to be either current or ex-smokers (Fleming *et al.* 1997). Our data on nurses show that hospital nurses are more likely to smoke than public health nurses (Prendergast 1993), but the highest rates are among second-year student nurses, who also reported high levels of stress in the transition to ward work (Hope *et al.* 1998). By contrast, older women travellers, who have obviously deprived social circumstances (O'Donovan *et al.* 1995), were more likely to smoke than employed blue-collar women (Hope and Kelleher 1995) and older more affluent women had quite low rates (Nolan *et al.* 1997). An explicit socio-demographic representation of motivation to smoke and expressed support for tackling the underlying issues might therefore be appropriate as a policy approach at this point.

This is a serious issue for policy-makers and if it continues to be ignored then we shall see both a widening class gradient and the use of smoking as a mild expression of social revolt. The drawback of seeing smoking as a single issue is demonstrated in this way. Unfortunately, to date the major international bodies have been constrained by a compartmentalised approach from tackling this head-on. The European Union for instance funds research and training around individual risk factors in the main and even the statement by the newly-appointed director of the WHO (*Irish Times* 12 May 98) that smoking is a major global public health problem was not given social context in reports. We have never seen the WHO's policy of settings-based interventions reported in the mainstream media.

EFFECTIVENESS OF INTERVENTIONS

This leads to the issue of what interventions are likely to be effective. There are essentially two broad strategies in this vast literature. Firstly, there are personal development approaches aimed at preventing people from taking up the habit or at aiding in cessation. Secondly, there are supportive environment strategies that work by a combination of active and passive strategies in specific settings. Smoking cessation programmes for individuals and groups have been developed around a variety of psychological constructs but particularly those that promote self-esteem and self-efficacy. Efforts for young people have focused on schools and peer-led programmes, and have moved over the years from scare tactics to personal development approaches and from single-issue programmes to more integrated and holistic approaches. In general these are regarded as disappointing, particularly so in the target group of young women. Early smoking-related interventions among schoolchildren worked well, but in recent years (with high non-smoking rates anyway in the target populations) there have been disappointing impact evaluations. As a case in point, Nutbeam *et al.* (1993) reported on the apparent failure to influence smoking uptake rates in UK children using modified programmes from Minnesota and Scandinavia. The problem appears to be related to the timing of the programmes, their depth and content and a failure to appreciate fully the motivation of young people for taking up smoking. We have undertaken a comprehensive evaluation of the schools' Lifeskills programme run by one of our regional health boards in its second-level schools over a 12-year period (Nic Gabhainn and Kelleher 1995). The Lifeskills programme was more effective in countering adverse alcohol-related behaviour than smoking and was more successful for girls than boys. On the other hand the primary-school approaches were effective in raising consciousness about health-related issues and this may be a better option in combating behaviour before more extensive peer influences come into play. We concluded that programmes which promote self-esteem were well suited to alcohol, since the circumstances of experimentation were related to feelings of bravado and insecurity. On the other hand smoking is already established as a habit in children entering second-level education and must therefore be influenced earlier. The pilot Health Promoting Schools initiative in Ireland, which we also evaluated (Nic Gabhainn and Kelleher 1998), was not successful in tackling smoking either, but was not primarily intended to influence behaviour at this early stage and focused more on the creation of a conducive environment. If the holistic approach is correct, and intuitively it seems to deserve a try, then presumably in the longer term cross-sectoral approaches which involve parents and early-learning community groups may have an impact.

In adulthood those who find it hardest to quit are heavy smokers and those who started very young. The large-scale COMMIT study (COMMIT Research Group 1995) demonstrated that this is the hardest group to reach. Several reviews on the effectiveness of workplace, community and primary-care interventions (Ebrahim and Davey Smith 1997; Family Heart Study Group 1994; Oxcheck study 1991) have been recently published or are in train. The effects on smoking are disappointing in magnitude but on a population basis could be appreciable. It is often forgotten that simple advice from a health professional could comfortably achieve our own national target (Coleman and Wilson 1996). The problem is that there is an opportunity cost to time spent in this way which has not always been adequately costed. The second approach, in the workplace particularly, is to enforce passive strategies. We undertook a three-year workplace intervention programme which lent support to the preference for passive strategies, particularly among blue-collar women (Hope and Kelleher 1995).

FUTURE STRATEGIES

How then should we approach social change? At the most radical level we can assume that inequities according to sex and social class will continue to influence smoking patterns and that therefore this must be a persuasive issue in influencing social policies that have an effect on these factors. Less ambitious social-change strategies that could achieve more consensus include stringent taxation (justifiable because it affects the young though questionable because it also victimises the poor), media advertising controls, enforcement of under-age sales and distribution, and regulation of smoking in public places. All of these risk conferring the glamour of the forbidden on the habit, which would translate itself into increasing rates among more affluent young people, particularly girls; and there are signs that this could happen. On the other hand such experimentation could be less harmful in the late teens than earlier, and focused cessation programmes directed at those in their twenties might also prove effective, particularly if primary-school education programmes were to prove effective in longer-term evaluations.

Though so much effort has gone into the development of educational materials this was always assumed to be based on the development of self-esteem, and the issue of gender differences was ignored, apart from attempts to make girls feel that boys would not be attracted to them if they smoked. Clearly this has not worked, because boys who may not be smokers themselves do not in reality sanction girls who are and the enjoyment and short-term gain from smoking is so obviously greater than any perceived long-term risk. A positive approach which is inspired by a feminist perspective might be more appropriate. In other words, more debate at school level about exploitation by vested interest groups might be tied in with the natural sympathy of young people for environmental issues. Given the strong policy imperative under which most health education agencies operate this will take political persuasion to achieve.

Pregnancy is a window of opportunity for giving up smoking but few of those affected sustain non-smoking rates afterwards. This could mean that weight control *post partum* coupled with the stress of having a new child are important factors, and so an approach tied in with exercise and breastfeeding might help – though again the class issue here is a major obstacle. More sensitive and focused health professional support might be appropriate (Becker 1998). There is a strong debate now in the health education literature led by Seedhouse (1997) on the fine line between empathy and identification with their clients on the part of health professionals. Community development approaches in the last decade have emphasised a holistic approach that avoids victim-blaming and 'expertism', but the firm imparting of the harmfulness of smoking must be maintained. On the other hand at a top-down level, despite the rhetoric to the contrary, most media campaigns are not focused on young women and accordingly there is little evidence that they internalise the message to stop smoking. The one role-model relationship that has been under-discussed is that of mother/daughter. If young boys are less of a problem relatively speaking than young girls, then it may be because the messages fathers give sons are different from those mothers give daughters. This suggestion is not as politically incorrect as it may seem. We must acknowledge our own empirical evidence on the gender issue if we are to tackle the problem. One way is to target older women more effectively. This may merit further research, and campaigns aimed at older women need to present more specific data on the benefits in reduction of heart disease and cancers, coupled with sustained practical support, particularly in the area of diet and weight control. Needless to say, wider social support policies that address issues of social exclusion and domestic stress are also likely to empower women in making healthier lifestyle choices.

In conclusion, prevalence data do indicate that there is a problem of smoking among young people, particularly women, but this is also tied in with social class and socio-economic status generally. Why therefore do women smoke? Smoking is a habit taken up for a variety of reasons and is difficult to stop. No single strategy can tackle such a complex problem and therefore a multi-sectoral approach is needed. It would be a step forward to achieve consensus on this point among health professionals. We need to distinguish the cosmetic and ineffective from the effective in each sector. It will take major political will to achieve change on this problem but it may help politicians to know that smoking is a minority habit and that there is support from a variety of interests in tackling the problem.

ACKNOWLEDGEMENTS

This review refers in the main to work associated with the Centre for Health Promotion Studies and we thank our many colleagues and postgraduate students for their input. It also includes data on current smoking prevalence collected for the Health Promotion Unit, Department of Health, Republic of Ireland, who provided grant support for Jane Sixsmith to undertake the work. This paper formed the basis for a presentation on the topic of smoking and young people at a workshop hosted by the British Heart Foundation in London in June 1998.

REFERENCES

Becker, G., 1998. *Promoting and Protecting Breastfeeding: Educational Materials for Health Professionals*. Galway: Centre for Health Promotion Studies and Health Promotion Unit Department of Health.

Bonner, C., 1996. *A Survey of 16–18 Year Old School Pupils in the Midland Health Board Region of Smoking, Alcohol and Substance Abuse*. Unpublished.

Brewer's Dictionary of Phrase and Fable, 1981. Revised edition, ed. I.H. Evans. London: Cassell.

Central Statistics Office, 1997. *Household Budget Survey 1994–1995: Preliminary Results*. Dublin: Stationery Office.

Centre for Health Promotion Studies, 1999. *The National Health and Lifestyle Surveys: SLÁN/HBSC.* Dublin: Health Promotion Unit, Department of Health and Children; Galway: Centre for Health Promotion Studies, NUI.

Clarke, A., Daly, L., and Comerford, D., 1998. 'Smoking Rates among Acute Hospital Patients', *Proceedings of 6th Health Promoting Hospitals Conference*, Darmstadt.

Colahan, S., 1996. *A Study of Lifestyle Behaviour and Substance Use and Their Relationship to Occupation.* MSc thesis, Department of Health Promotion, National University of Ireland, Galway. Unpublished.

Coleman, T., and Wilson, A., 1996. 'Anti-smoking Advice in General Practice Consultations: General Practitioners' Attitudes, Reported Practice and Perceived Problems', *British Journal of General Practice*, 46: pp. 87–91.

COMMIT Research Group, 1995. 'Community Intervention Trial for Smoking Cessation (COMMIT): II. Changes in Adult Cigarette Smoking Prevalence', *American Journal of Public Health*, 85, 2: pp. 193–200.

Connolly, C., 1996. *Young People's Attitudes to Breast Feeding.* MA thesis, Department of Health Promotion, National University of Ireland, Galway. Unpublished.

Daly, S.F., Kiely, J., Clarke, T.A., and Mathews, T.G., 1992. 'Alcohol and Cigarette Use in a Pregnant Irish Population', *Irish Medical Journal*, 85, 4.

Department of Community Health and General Practice, University of Dublin, 1996. *A Report from the Tallaght Community Health Group.* Unpublished.

Department of Health, 1996. *Smoking and Drinking Among Young People in Ireland.* Dublin: Department of Health.

Department of Health, 1994. *Shaping a Healthier Future: A Strategy for Effective Healthcare in the 1990s.* Dublin: Department of Health.

Doll, R., Peto, R., Wheatley, K., Gray, R., and Sutherland, I., 1994. 'Mortality in Relation to Smoking: 40 Years' Observations on Male British Doctors', *British Medical Journal*, 309: pp. 901–11.

Doorley, P., 1994. 'Editorial: Prospect for Achieving the National Target on Smoking Prevalence by the Year 2000', *Irish Medical Journal*, 87, 6: p. 158.

Ebrahim, S., and Davey Smith G., 1997. 'Systematic Review of Randomised Control Trials of Multiple Risk Factor Interventions for Preventing Coronary Heart Disease', *British Medical Journal*, 314, 7095: pp. 1666–74.

European Bureau for Action on Smoking Prevention, 1994. *Tobacco and Health in the EU: An Overview.* Brussels: Commission of the EU.

Family Heart Study Group, 1994. 'Randomised Controlled Trial Evaluating Cardiovascular Screening and Intervention in General Practice: Principal Results of British Family Heart Study', *British Medical Journal*, 308: pp. 313–20.

Fleming, S., Kelleher, C., and O'Connor, M., 1997. 'Eating Patterns and Factors Influencing Likely Change in the Workplace in Ireland', *Health Promotion International*, 12, 3: pp. 187–96.

Graham, H., 1984. *Women, Health and The Family*. Herts, UK: Harvester Wheatsheaf/Health Education Council.

Green, L.W., and Kreuter, M.W., 1991. *Health Promotion Planning: An Educational and Environmental Approach*. California: Mayfield Publishing.

Harkin, A.M., Anderson, P., and Goos, C., 1997. *Smoking, Drinking and Drug Taking in the European Region*. Copenhagen: WHO Regional Office for Europe.

Heywood, S., 1996. *Survey of Tipperary Post Primary Students' Views and Experiences of Illegal Drugs, 1995–1996*. Unpublished. Garda Síochána College, Garda Research Unit.

Hickey, P., 1996. *Smoking Control in Restaurants: A Questionnaire Study of Patrons Knowledge and Attitudes Regarding the Tobacco Regulations 1995*. MA thesis, Department of Health Promotion, National University of Ireland, Galway. Unpublished.

Hope, A., Kelleher, C., and O'Connor, M., 1998. 'Lifestyle Practices and the Health Promoting Environment of Hospital Nurses', *Journal of Advanced Nursing*, 28, 2: pp. 438–47.

Hope, A., and Kelleher, C., 1995. *Health at Work* Galway: Centre for Health Promotion Studies.

Howell, F., 1996. 'Smoking in Irish Journals: A Content Analysis 1960–1994', *Irish Medical Journal*, 89, 1: pp. 18–19.

Howell, F., 1994. 'Tobacco Advertising and Coverage of Smoking and Health in Women's Magazines', *Irish Medical Journal*, 87: pp. 140–1.

IMS for the *Irish Independent* (17.8. 1996). 12–17 year olds 513 interviews (from ASH Ireland).

Joossens, L., and Raw, M., 1996. 'The Health Impact of the Tobacco Regime', in M. Whitehead and P. Nordgren, eds., *Health Impact of the EU Common Agricultural Policy: A Policy Report of the Swedish National Institute of Public Health*.

Kiernan, R., 1995. *Substance Abuse of Adolescents in the WHB Region*. Thesis to Faculty of Public Health Medicine, Galway. Unpublished.

Lopez, A.D., Collishaw, N.E., and Piha, T., 1994. 'A Descriptive Model of the Cigarette Epidemic in Developed Countries', *Tobacco Control*, 3: pp. 242–7.

Mannix, M., O'Reilly, O., Shelley, E., and Collins, C., 1992. *The Need to Refocus Health Promotion Strategy for Young People*. South Eastern Health Board. Unpublished.

McArdle, M., Kelleher, C., and Ward, J., 1993. 'Consumer Choice and Ireland's Tobaco Regulations: Do Restaurateurs meet their Clients' Needs?', *Health Promotion International*, 8, 4: pp. 275–80.

McCluskey, D., 1989. *Health: People's Beliefs and Practices*. Dublin: Government Stationery Office.

Midland Health Board Lansdowne Market Research. 'Re Family Planning in the Region 503 Women 18–45 Year Old Women 39.8% Current Smokers.' Unpublished.

Moroney, L.J., 1993. *Smoking, Alcohol and Other Drug Use: Among Post Primary School Pupils in County Roscommon and the Elphin Diocese Area of County Galway. Preliminary Findings*. Roscommon Regional Youth Services.

Morgan, M., 1990. *Cigarette Smoking among Adolescent Boys in 1990: A Study of Prevalence and Influences*. Dublin: ESRI.

Morgan, M., Doorley, P., Hynes, M., and Joy, S., 1994. 'An Evaluation of a Smoking Prevention Programme with Children from Disadvantaged Communities', *Irish Medical Journal*, 87, 2: pp. 56–7.

Morgan, M., and Grube, J.W., 1994. 'Lifestyle Changes: A Social Psychological Perspective with Reference to Cigarette Smoking among Adolescents', *The Irish Journal of Psychology*, 15, 1: pp. 179–90.

Morgan, M., and Grube J.W., 1989. 'Adolescent Cigarette Smoking: Developmental Analysis of Influences', *British Journal of Developmental Psychology*, 7: pp. 179–89.

National Cancer Registry Board, 1997. *Cancer in Ireland, 1994, Incidence and Mortality: Report of the National Cancer Registry*. Cork: National Cancer Registry Board.

Nic Gabhainn, S., and Kelleher, C., 1995. *Lifeskills for Health Promotion*. Galway: The Centre for Health Promotion Studies.

Nic Gabhainn, S., and Kelleher, C., 1998. *The Irish Network of Health Promoting Schools 1993–1996: Preliminary Evaluation Report*. Galway: The Centre for Health Promotion Studies.

Nolan, G., Friel, S., and Kelleher, C., 1997 'Comparative Diet and Lifestyle Study between Irish and West Virginian Women'. Poster presentation, Nutrition Society, Irish Section. Dublin: Trinity College.

Nutbeam, D., Macaskill, P., Smith, C., Simpson, J.M., and Catford, J., 1993. 'Evaluation of Two School Smoking Education Programmes under Normal Classroom Conditions', *British Medical Journal*, 306, 6870: pp. 102–7.

O'Connor, E.A., Friel, S., and Kelleher, C.C., 1997. 'Fashion Consciousness as a Social Influence on Lifestyle Behaviour in Young Irish Adults', *Health Promotion International*, 12, 2: pp. 135–9.

O'Connor, M., and Kelleher, C., 1998 'Do Doctors Benefit from Their Profession?', *Irish Medical Journal*.

O' Donovan, O., McKenna, V., and Kelleher, C., 1995. *Health Service Provision for the Travelling Community in Ireland*. Galway: Centre for Health Promotion Studies.

OXCHECK Study Group, 1991. 'Prevalence of Risk Factors for Heart Disease in OXCHECK Trial: Implications for Screening in Primary Care. Imperial Cancer Research Fund OXCHECK Study Group', *British Medical Journal*, 4, 302, 6784: pp. 1057–60.

Peto, R., Lopez, A.D., Boreham, J., Thun, M., Heath, C., and Doll, R., 1996. 'Mortality from Smoking Worldwide', in. R. Doll and J. Crofton, eds., 'Tobacco and Health', *British Medical Bulletin*, 52, 1: pp. 12–21.

Prendergast, M., 1992. *A Study of Attitudes, Lifestyles and Training in the Context of Health Promotion and Health and Safety Among Nurses*. MSc thesis, Department of Health Promotion, National University of Ireland, Galway. Unpublished.

Reid, D., 1996. 'Tobacco Control: Overview', in. R. Doll and J. Crofton, eds., 'Tobacco and Health', *British Medical Bulletin*, 52, 1: pp. 108–20.

Seedhouse, D., 1997. *Health Promotion: Philosophy, Prejudice and Practice*. Chichester: Wiley and Sons.

Shelley, E., Collins, C., and Daly, L., 1992. *Trends in Smoking Prevalence: The Kilkenny Health Project Population Surveys 1985–1991*. Dublin Department of Public Health Medicine and Epidemiology, UCD. Unpublished.

Shelley, E. *et al.*, 1997. 'The Happy Heart National Survey 1992 of Health Behaviours Associated with CHD', *The Irish College of Physicians and Surgeons*, 26, 2: pp. 96–102.

Shiffman, S., 1993. 'Assessing Smoking Patterns and Motives', *Journal of Consulting and Clinical Psychology*, 61, 5: pp. 732–42.

Sixsmith, J., and Kelleher, C., 1997. *Evaluation of the Health Promotion Unit's Mass Media Anti Smoking Campaign: Final Results*. Unpublished Report. Dublin: Department of Health.

Steptoe, A., and Wardle, J., 1992. 'Cognative Predictors of Health Behaviour in Contrasting Regions of Europe', *British Journal of Clinical Psychology*, 31: pp. 485–502.

Surgeon General Report, 1989. *Reducing the Health Consequences of Smoking: 25 Years of Progress. US Department of Health and Human Services*. Publication No. CDC 89–8411.

Sutton, S., 1998. 'How Ordinary People in Great Britain Perceive the Health Risks of Smoking', *Journal of Epidemiology and Community Health*, 52, 5: pp. 338–9.

Wald, N.J., and Hackshaw, A.K., 1996. 'Cigarette Smoking: An Epidemiological Overview', in R. Doll and J. Crofton, eds., 'Tobacco and Health', *British Medical Bulletin*, 52, 1: pp. 3–11.

World Health Organisation, 1996. *Tobacco Alert. The Tobacco Epidemic: A Global Public Health Emergency*. Geneva: WHO.

World Health Organisation, 1997. 'Tobacco Epidemic: Much More than a Health Issue', WHO Fact Sheet, May, No. 155.

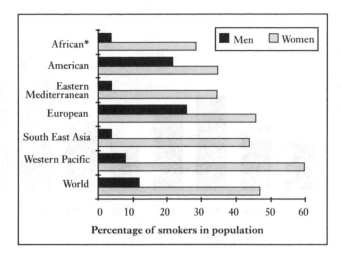

Figure 1. Percentage of smokers in WHO regions 1996.
* Use figures with caution as estimates only. (WHO 1996)

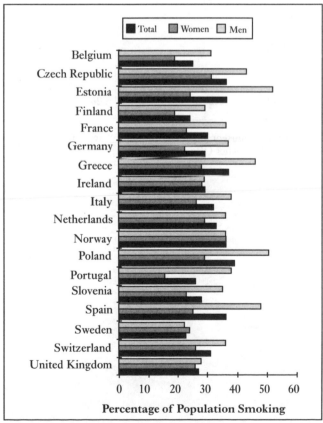

Figure 2. The European perspective. Smoking prevalence in adults by gender and country in WHO European region with data from 1993/4. Adapted from Harkin et al. 1997.

No. of cigarettes

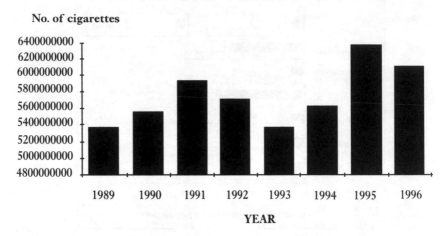

Figure 3. Cigarettes retained for home consumption in Ireland 1989–1996.
Source: The Revenue Commission Statistical Report 1997

	1987		1994/5	
Tobacco products	£	% Total expenditure	£	% Total expenditure
	7.30	3.27	8.26	2.65

Figure 4. Comparison of household expenditure on tobacco products between 1987 and 1994/5. Source: Central Statistics Office 1997).

APPENDIX

Study, Methods and Smoking Prevalence by Gender and Socio-economic Group in the Youth Studies

Study, Year & Author	Method	Smoking Prevalence	Gender Male Female		Socio-economic Group	Other
E. O'Connor, S. Friel & C. Kelleher (1997) *Fashion Consciousness as a Social Influence on Lifestyle Behaviour in Young Irish Adults*	*Sample*: 150 men & women aged 15–30 years Quota presenting sample *Method*: Cross-sectional street questionnaire survey *Area*: Irish cities	Current 32%	30%	33%		Fashion conscious women more likely to smoke 42% than others 23%(p=0.05)
Department of Health & ESRI (1996) *Smoking & Drinking Among Young People in Ireland*	*Sample*: 1) 4,000 Post primary school students Random, stratified schools; 2) 157 early school leavers Snowball sample *Method*: Self-administered questionnaire survey *Area*: National	*At age 17*: 1) Lifetime 55% Regular16% Current 29% 2) Lifetime76% Regular 57% Current 67%	57% 24% 38% 73% 57% 61%	54% 22% 36% 86% 60% 76%	No clear association found between smoking & socio-economic group Tentatively suggest prevalence slightly decreased	Compared with data from similar Dublin studies* (1986, 1991)
C. Bonner (1996) *Report of School Survey of 2nd Level Student s in MHB Region*	*Sample*: 1,654 post primary school students Random selection of schools *Method*: Self-administered questionnaire survey *Area*: Midland Health Board Region	Ex-smoker 10% Current 34% Non-smoker 56%	Study specifies that no gender difference was identified.			
S. Colohan (1996) *A Study of Lifestyle Behaviour & Substance Use & their Relationship to Occupation*	*Sample*: 200 aged between 15–25, resident in one area. Random *Method*: Door to door administered questionnaire *Area*: Urban area	Lifetime 55% Current 47%				Comparison with similar 1993 data found decrease in current & regular smokers from 46.5% to 53.8%
C. Connolly (1996) *Young People's Attitudes to Breast Feeding*	*Sample:* 178 post primary school students in one town *Method*: Self-administered questionnaire *Area*: One town in West of Ireland	Current 30%	38% Significant difference	16% gender (p<.0005)		
U. Diamond (1996) *Irish Network of Health Promoting Schools: Post primary schools*	*Sample*: 218 post primary school students. Stratified schools in network *Method*: Self-administered questionnaire *Area*: National	Lifetime 72% Current 38%	Study specifies no significant gender difference found			Comparison with recipients of MWHB lifeskills & the control. differences found in lifetime smoked with 72% versus 51% of lifeskills recipients & 54% of controls
C. Dring (1996) *Evaluation of a Mass Media Anti Smoking Campaign Among Adolescents*	Sample: 134 post-primary school students. Stratified school s by region *Method*: Self-administered questionnaire *Area*: National	Regular 33% Occasional 12% Non-smoker 55%	31%	39%	Groups collapsed to blue collar and white collar. No significant difference found	

* Morgan & Grube 1986/1991

Study, Year & Author	Method	Smoking Prevalence	Gender Male Female	Socio-economic Group	Other
B. Dineen & U. Fallon (1996) *GP/Schools Intervention Programme*	Sample: 313 8–15 year olds attending GP practice *Method*: Administered questionnaire parents in attendance *Area*: Galway county	Lifetime 6.7% Regular (1) Occasional (2)			
S. Haywood (1996) *Survey of Tipperary Post Primary School Pupils' Views & Experiences of Illegal Drugs*	*Sample*: 617 post primary school students. Random & representative sample of 23 schools in County Tipperary *Method*: Self-administered questionnaire *Area*: Tipperary	Lifetime 66%	Study specifies no significant gender difference found		
Irish Independent Newspapers (1996) *IMS Survey*	*Sample*: 513, population quota *Method*: Administered questionnaire survey *Area*: National	Regular 12% Occasional 10% Non-smoker 78%	No significant difference by gender found in figures reported		
S. Nic Gabhainn & C. Kelleher (1995) *Lifeskills Evaluation*	*Sample*: 2,407 post primary school students *Method*: Administered questionnaire *Area*: North Western Health Board & North Eastern Health Board	Current Lifeskills pupils 23%			Comparison made between Lifeskills & comparison students. No difference observed
R. Kiernan (1995) *Substance Use Among Adolescents in the WHB Area*	*Sample*: 2,787 post primary school students & early school leavers. Random sample of schools in Western Health Board area *Method*: Self-administered questionnaire survey *Area*: Western Health Board	Lifetime 67% Regular 27% Occasional 12% Non-smoker 60%	No significant difference found by socio-economic group based on either mother or fathers occupation		Significant difference found in smoking prevalence in relation to students income. The higher the income the more likely to smoke
L. Moroney (1993) *Smoking, Alcohol & Other Drug Use in Roscommon and part of Galway County*	*Sample*: 2,632. All students in post primary schools in one area *Method*: Self-administered questionnaire *Area*: County Roscommon & Elphin Diocese area of County Galway	Lifetime 58% Regular Occasional Non-smoker	69% 75% 16% 9% 14% 16% 70% 75%		
M. Mannix *et al.* (1992) *The Need to Refocus Health Promotion for Young People*	*Sample*: 527 post primary school pupils. Random sample of pupils stratified by age *Method*: Self-administered questionnaire *Area*: County Kilkenny	Lifetime 69% Weekly Less than weekly Non-smoker	26% 16% 8% 11% 67% 73%		Comparison made with similar data collected in students 1987. Slight decrease in experimenting with tobacco 1987 71%, 1992 69%

→

Study, Year & Author	Method	Smoking Prevalence	Gender Male Female		Socio-economic Group	Other
E. Shelley *et al.* (1997) *The Happy Heart National Survey 1992 of Health Behaviours Associated with Coronary Heart Disease*	*Sample*: 1,798 random location technique with quota controls for age & sex from electoral register *Method*: Administered questionnaire survey *Area*: National	Current smokers	38%	29%		'In men & women the prevalence of smoking was substantially higher in the manual as compared to the non-manual classes' p. 99
Department of Education and the Health Promotion Unit (1996) *A National Survey of Involvement in Sport and Physical Activity*	*Sample*: 3,300, population quota *Method*: Administered questionnaire *Area*: National	Current: cigarettes 32% cigars 1%				
B. Dineen & U. Fallon (1996) *GP/Schools Intervention Programme*	*Sample*: 196 parents of children in GP intervention programme *Method*: Administered questionnaire *Area*: County Galway	Regular smokers 13% Occasional 16% Ex-smoker 22% Never smoker 47%				
P. Hickey (1996) *Smoking Control in Restaurants Patrons Knowledge and Attitudes to the Tobacco Regulations 1995*	*Sample*: 190 quota of restaurant patrons from 6 randomly chosen restaurants *Method*: Self-administered questionnaire *Area*: Galway city	Current 27% Never smoker 59% Ex-smoker 14%				
A. Hope (1996) *Agri Workers: Health & Safety*	*Sample*: 1,399 population quota *Method*: Administered questionnaire *Area*: National	Current 35%	34% Gender not significant	36% difference statistically	Groups collapsed to ABC1 & C2DE Statistically significant difference found	
The Midland Health Board & Lansdowne Market Research (1996) *Family Planning Needs Assessment*	*Sample*: 503 women population quota *Method*: Administered questionnaire *Area*: Midland Health Board Region	Current 40%				
J. Sixsmith & C. Kelleher (1996) *Evaluation of the Mass Media Anti-Smoking Campaign*	*Sample*: 1,400 population quota *Method*: Administered questionnaire *Area*: National	Regular 30% Occasional 5% Ex-smoker 19% Never smoker 46%	31%	29%	difference not significant	Groups collapsed to ABC1 & C2DE Statistically significant difference found
M. Wiley & B. Merriman (1996) *Women & Health Care in Ireland*	*Sample*: 3,940 drawn from the electoral register using RANSAM system *Method*: Administered questionnaire *Area*: National	Regular 29% Occasional 6% Ex-smoker 16% Never smoker 49%			'Smoking behaviour is significantly related to social class'	

Study, Year & Author	Method	Smoking Prevalence	Gender Male	Female	Socio-economic Group	Other
A Report from Tallaght Community Health Group (1996)*	*Sample*: 396 households. Identified from the electoral register from 12 DEDS in Tallaght. ESRI RANSAM *Method*: Administered questionnaire *Area*: Tallaght	*In household No one smokes 35% One smokes 36% More than one smokes 29%				
S. Nic Gabhainn & C. Kelleher (1995) *Lifeskills Evaluation*	*Sample*: Young adults – lifeskill graduates. Presenting sample *Method*: Self-administered questionnaire *Area*: NWHB Region	Current 48%				
A. Hope & C. Kelleher (1995) *Health at Work*	*Sample*: pre-test 2,528 & post test 1,834 *Method*: Pre and post intervention measures by self-administered questionnaire *Area*: West of Ireland	Current smokers	25.4%	21.4%	Groups collapsed to social class 1–3 & 4–6, 7 = unknown Significant difference found	
O. O'Donovan, V. McKenna & C. Kelleher (1995) *Health Service Provision for the Travelling Community*	*Sample*: 200 stratified by accommodation type in Galway & Dublin *Method*: Administered questionnaire *Area*: Galway & Dublin	Current 62%				
E. Shelley *et al.* (1995) *The Kilkenny Health Project*	*Sample*: 1) Kilkenny 802 2) Offaly 631 Independent, geographical, clustered, stratified random sample from the electoral register *Method*: Administered questionnaire survey *Area*: Counties Offaly & Kilkenny	1) Current cigarettes 25% Current pipe/cigar 3% Current mixed 1% Total current smokes 29% Total Ex-smokers 32% Never smoked 39% 2) Current cigarettes 25% Current pipe/cigar 4% Current mixed 1% Total current smokes 30% Total ex-smoker 26% Never smoker 43%	25% 4% 3% 31% 40% 28% 25% 8% 2% 36% 34% 30%	25% 1% 0 30% 23% 51% 24% 0 0 24% 19% 57%		Comparison made with similar data from Kilkenny 1985 & Offaly 1986
S. Nic Gabhainn (1994) *Attitudes to Cardiovascular Disease*	*Sample*: 57 random selection from local authority employment organisation West of Ireland *Method*: Background questionnaire to focus groups *Area*: West of Ireland	Current				
M. McMahon (1993) *A Survey of the Occupational Health Risks & Concerns of Prison Personnel*	*Sample*: 460, Quota sample *Method*: Postal survey *Area*: National	Current 26% Ex-smoker 31% Non-smoker 43%			No statistically significant difference found by gender	No statistically significant difference found by smoking prevalence & age, stress, activity level

Study, Year & Author	Method	Smoking Prevalence	Gender Male	Female	Socio-economic Group	Other
A. Steptoe & J. Wardle (1992) *Cognative Predictors of Health Behaviour in Contrasting Regions of Europe*	*Sample*: 7,153 of which 786 Irish. Dublin students aged 17–30 *Method*: Self-administered questionnaire survey *Area*: Dublin	*ambiguity over reported prevalence rates as tables labelled women indicate higher prevalence rates than men. Text states significant difference found between sexes, men smoking more.				
M. McArdle (1991) *Social Marketing & the Anti-Smoking Campaign*	*Sample*: 100 adults who eat out. Quota of age ranges *Method*: Administered questionnaire *Area*: Galway	Current 35% Ex-smoker 20% Non-smoker 45%	20% 12% 18%	15% 8% 27%		
S. Henry, S. McErlain & G. Bleakney (no date) *Public Attitudes to Smoking Related Issues*	*Sample*: 1,075 quota sample *Method*: Administered questionnaire *Area*: Eastern Health Board	Current 39% Ex smoker 23% Never smoked 38%				
Joint National Readership Research 1990/91, 1991/92, 1992/93, 1993/94, for the HPU	*Sample*: Range for years 1990–1994 2,580–2,646 Multistage probability sample *Method*: Administered questionnaire *Area*: National	1990/1 Current 28% 1991/2 Current 30% 1992/3 Current 28% 1993/4 Current 29%	30% 30% 31% 29%	27% 30% 26% 28%	Groups collapsed to ABC1 & C2DE statistically significant differences found in each year.	

Index